Outpatient Surgery
Clinical Decision Making and Board Review

Edited by

ALAN DARDIK MD PhD FACS

Associate Professor, Department of Surgery
Interdepartmental Program in Vascular Biology and Therapeutics
Yale University, New Haven, CT, USA
Chief, Peripheral Vascular Surgery
VA Connecticut Healthcare Systems, West Haven, CT, USA

and

MICHAEL GAUNT MA MD FRCS

Consultant Vascular Surgeon, Cambridge University Hospitals NHS
Foundation Trust, Cambridge, UK
Associate Lecturer, Cambridge University, UK

T0132713

Radcliffe Publishing
London • New York

Radcliffe Publishing Ltd
33–41 Dallington Street
London
EC1V 0BB
United Kingdom

www.radcliffepublishing.com

_____

British Library Cataloguing in Publication Data

A catalogue record for this book is available from the British Library.

ISBN-13: 978 184619 595 2

Typeset by Kate Broome, Auckland, New Zealand
Printed and bound by Cadmus Communications, USA

Contents

Preface

Welcome to the third edition of *General Surgery Outpatient Decisions*. This edition of the book has been updated and expanded to appeal to North American surgeons. Although we have simplified the title to *Outpatient Surgery*, we have not changed the focus of the book; we still focus on answering questions that are relevant to your everyday practice and in preparation for your professional examinations.

In this edition, we have recruited some of the most prestigious American academic surgeons to rework and review a chapter in their specialty. This allowed us to update the book to both modern American practice style as well as to include the most up-to-date information since the last edition of the book. In addition, a general surgery resident reviewed each chapter, ensuring that each chapter is understandable from a trainee's point of view and degree of experience. We have also added several review questions for each chapter; we believe that this type of rapid review will both increase understanding as well as retention of the material. These new approaches have led to an entirely new edition, which we believe you will enjoy.

Alan Dardik and Michael Gaunt
January 2012

About the Editors

Alan Dardik graduated from Yale University summa cum laude and with distinction in the major of Computer Science in 1986. He then received both the MD and PhD degrees from the University of Pennsylvania in 1993; his graduate work, describing a role for TGF-alpha in preimplantation embryo development, was supported by a Doctoral Fellowship from the Howard Hughes Medical Institute and was awarded the Balduin Lucke Memorial Prize. Dr. Dardik then completed his general and vascular surgical training at the Johns Hopkins Hospital, including a postdoctoral fellowship training supported by an NIH Postdoctoral Research Award. In 2001 Dr. Dardik joined the faculty at Yale University, where he continues to teach, take care of patients, and carry out research. He has received several teaching awards including the C. Elton Cahow award for outstanding faculty teaching. Dr. Dardik is the Chief of Vascular Surgery at the VA Connecticut. He also runs a busy basic science research laboratory funded by the NIH in which he studies the effects of vascular interventions such as vein graft adaptation to the arterial circulation. He has published over 140 peer-reviewed research papers, is active in several surgical societies, and lectures widely. Dr. Dardik is currently the course director of the Vascular Research Initiatives Conference sponsored by the Society for Vascular Surgery.

Michael Gaunt qualified in medicine with distinction at Leicester University in 1988 and undertook his surgical training in hospitals around the British Midlands. He was elected Fellow of the Royal College of Surgeons of England in 1992 and undertook a period of research leading to the award of a doctorate of medicine with distinction. During his training he received a number of research awards, including the Moynihan Medal of the Association of Surgeons of Great Britain and Ireland, the Founders Prize of the Vascular Society of Great Britain and Ireland, and the European Vascular Surgery Prize. Mr Gaunt was elected Hunterian Professor of Surgery of the Royal College of Surgeons of England in 1996. In 1999 he was appointed consultant vascular surgeon at Addenbrooke's Hospital and associate lecturer at Cambridge University. Mr Gaunt has published over 120 peer-reviewed research papers and is actively involved in both undergraduate and postgraduate medical education.

List of Contributors

Malcolm V. Brock, MD
Associate Professor of Surgery and Oncology
Johns Hopkins University
Baltimore, MD

Anees B. Chagpar, MD, MSc, MA, MPH, FACS, FRCS(C)
Director, The Breast Center – Smilow Cancer Hospital at Yale-New Haven
Associate Professor, Department of Surgery
Yale University School of Medicine
New Haven, CT

Michael J. Collins, MD
Resident, General Surgery
Department of Surgery
Yale University School of Medicine
New Haven, CT

John A. Curci, MD, FACS
Assistant Professor of Surgery, Washington University in St. Louis
Associate Program Director, Vascular Surgery
Staff Surgeon, John Cochran VAMC
Section of Vascular Surgery
St. Louis, MO

David T. Efron, MD, FACS
Associate Professor of Surgery, Anesthesia and Critical Care Medicine
Chief, Division of Acute Care Surgery: Trauma, Critical Care,
Emergency and General Surgery Director of Adult Trauma,
Department of Surgery
The Johns Hopkins Hospital
Baltimore, MD

Jason S. Gold, MD
Assistant Professor of Surgery
Harvard Medical School (Brigham and Women's Hospital)
Chief of Surgical Oncology
VA Boston Healthcare System
West Roxbury, MA

Steven B. Goldin, MD
Associate Professor of Surgery
Vice Chairman of Surgical Education
University of South Florida
Tampa General Hospital
Tampa, FL

Lynn S. Model, MD
Resident, General Surgery
Department of Surgery
Yale University School of Medicine
New Haven, CT

Clinton D. Protack, MD
Resident, General Surgery
Department of Surgery
Yale University School of Medicine
New Haven, CT

George A. Sarosi Jr., MD, FACS
Associate Professor of Surgery
Robert H. Hux Professor of Surgery
Program Director, General Surgery
University of Florida College of Medicine
Staff Surgeon, NF/SG VA Medical Center
Gainesville, FL

Julie Ann Sosa, MD MA FACS
Associate Professor of Surgery and Medicine (Medical Oncology)
Division of Endocrine Surgery and Surgical Oncology
Department of Surgery
Yale University School of Medicine
New Haven, CT

Seth A. Spector, MD, FACS
Associate Professor of Surgery
University of Miami Miller School of Medicine
Department of Surgery, Division Surgical Oncology
Chief of Surgery – Miami VA Healthcare System
Miami, FL

Philip Wai, MD
Assistant Professor of Surgery
Division of Intra-Abdominal Transplantation
Department of Surgery
Maywood, IL

Kenneth R. Ziegler, MD
Resident, General Surgery
Department of Surgery
Yale University School of Medicine
New Haven, CT

List of Abbreviations

14C	radio-carbon
123I	radio-iodine
131I	radio-iodine
131MIBG	meta-iodobenzylguanidine
5-ASA	5-aminosalicylate
5FU	5-fluorouracil
5-HIAA	5-hydroxyindoleacetic acid
5-HT	5-hydroxytryptamine
99mTc	technetium-99m
AAA	abdominal aortic aneurysm
ABI	ankle–brachial index
ACE	angiotensin-converting enzyme
ACTH	adrenocorticotropic hormone
ADH	atypical ductal hyperplasia
AFP	alpha-fetoprotein
AIDS	acquired immunodeficiency syndrome
AJCC	American Joint Commission on Cancer
ALH	atypical lobular hyperplasia
ALP	alkaline phosphatase
ALT	alanine transaminase
ANA	antinuclear antibodies
ANCA	antineutrophil cytoplasmic antibody
ANCA	antineutrophil cytoplasmic autoantibodies
APA	aldosterone-producing adenoma
APR	abdominoperineal resection
APT	abnormal prothrombin antigen
ARDS	acute respiratory distress syndrome
ASCA	anti-*Saccharomyces cerevisiae* antibodies
AST	aspartate aminotransferase
AV	arteriovenous
AXR	abdominal X-ray
BBC	benign breast change
BC	breast cancer
beta-hCG	beta human chorionic gonadotropin
BFHH	familial hypocalciuric hypercalcemia
BI-RADS	Breast Imaging Reporting and Data System
BMI	body mass index
BT	Breslow thickness
BUN	blood urea nitrogen
C&S	culture and sensitivity test
CA 19-9	carbohydrate antigen 19-9
CAD	cystic adventitial disease
CBC	complete blood count
CBD	common bile duct
CBT	carotid body tumor
CDH	congenital diaphragmatic hernia

CE	capsule endoscopy
CEA	carcinoembryonic antigen *or* carotid endarterectomy
CEAP	Clinical-Etiology-Anatomy-Pathophysiology
CHD	common hepatic duct
CHOP	cyclophosphamide, doxorubicin, vincristine and prednisone
CIN	contrast-induced nephropathy
CLO	campylobacter-like organisms
CML	chronic myeloid leukemia
CNS	central nervous system
CRH	corticotrophin-releasing hormone
CRP	C-reactive protein
CT	computed tomography
CTA/MRA	computed tomography angiography/magnetic resonance angiogram
CTD	connective tissue disease/disorders
CWD	continuous wave Doppler
CXR	chest X-ray
CXR-PA	chest X-ray, posterior anterior view
DCIS	ductal carcinoma in situ
DCP	Des-gamma carboxyprothrombin
DES	diffuse esophageal spasm
DMSA	dimercaptosuccinic acid
DSA	digital subtraction angiography
DVT	deep-venous thrombosis
EATL	enteropathy-associated T-cell lymphoma
ECG	electrocardiogram
EGD	esophago-gastro-duodenoscopy
ELISA	enzyme-linked immunosorbent assay
ENT	ear, nose, and throat
ERCP	endoscopic retrograde cholangiopancreatography
ER/PR	estrogen/progesterone receptors
ESR	erythrocyte sedimentation rate
EUA	examination under anesthetic
EUS	entoscopic ultrasound
EVAR	endovascular aneurysm repair
EVLA	endovenous laser ablation
FA	fibroadenoma
FACS	follow-up after colorectal surgery
FAP	familial adenomatous polyposis
FHH	familial hypercalcemic hypocalciuria
FIT	fecal immunochemical test
FMD	fibromuscular dysplasia
FNAC	fine-needle aspiration cytology
FNH	focal nodular hyperplasia
FOBT	fecal occult blood test
GEJ	gastro-esophageal junction
GERD	gastro-esophageal reflux disease
GHRH	growth-hormone-releasing hormone
GI	gastrointestinal
GIST	gastrointestinal stromal tumor
GnRH	gonadotropin-releasing hormone

GTT	gamma-glutamyl-transpeptidase
H2RA	H2-receptor antagonist
HALO	Hemorrhoidal Artery Ligation Operation
Hb	hemoglobin
HBsAg	hepatitis B surface antigen
HCC	hepatocellular carcinoma
hCG	human chorionic gonadotropin
HDL	high-density lipoprotein
HIB	*Hemophilus influenzae* type b
HIDA	hepatobiliary iminodiacetic acid
HNPCC	hereditary non-polyposis colorectal cancer
HPV	human papillomavirus
HRT	hormone replacement therapy
IBD	inflammatory bowel disease
IgA	immunoglobulin A
IgG	immunoglobulin G
IgM	immunoglobulin M
IMA	inferior mesenteric artery
INR	international normalized ratio
IPSID	immunoproliferative small intestine disease
iPTH	intact parathyroid hormone
LCIS	lobular carcinoma in situ
LDL	low-density lipoprotein
LES	lower esophageal sphincter
LFT	liver function test
LUQ	left upper quadrant
MALT	mucosa-associated lymphoid tissue
MAOI	monoamine oxidase inhibitor
MCV	mean corpuscular volume
MDM	multidisciplinary meeting
MDT	multidisciplinary team
MEN	multiple endocrine neoplasia
MI	myocardial infarction
MIBG	meta-iodobenzylguanidine
MIBI	methoxyisobutylisonitrile
MRCP	magnetic resonance cholangiopancreatography
MRI	magnetic resonance imaging
MRSA	methicillin-resistant *S. aureus*
MSH	melanocyte-stimulating hormone
MTBE	methyl tert-butyl ether
MTC	medullary thyroid cancer (medullary carcinoma of thyroid)
NAC	nipple areolar complex
NCCN	National Cancer Center Network
NCI	National Cancer Institute
NICE	National Institute for Health and Clinical Excellence
NP59	6-beta-iodomethyl-19-norcholesterol
NSAID	non-steroidal anti-inflammatory drug
OCP	oral contraceptive pill
OPSI	overwhelming postsplenectomy infection

PAIR	percutaneous fine-needle puncture, aspiration, injection of hypertonic saline and reaspiration
PAN	polyarteritis nodosa
PAS	p-aminosalicylic acid
PCP	primary care physician
PDT	photodynamic therapy
PEC	percutaneous endoscopic colostomy
PET	positron emission tomography
PGE1	prostaglandin E1
PID	pelvic inflammatory disease
PPI	proton-pump inhibitor
PPPD	pylorus-preserving pancreatoduodenectomy
PTC	percutaneous transhepatic cholangiography
PTFE	polytetrafluoroethylene
PTH	parathyroid hormone (parathormone)
PV/ESR	plasma viscosity/erythrocyte sedimentation rate
PVD	peripheral vascular disease
RA	rheumatoid arthritis
RAS	renal artery stenosis
RET	proto-oncogene reticuloendothelium
RFA	radiofrequency ablation
RUQ	right upper quadrant
SBE	small bowel enema
SBFT	small bowel follow through
SCC	squamous cell carcinoma
SeHCAT test	75-selenium homotaurocholic acid retention test
SEPS	subfascial endoscopic perforator surgery
SFA	superficial femoral artery
SFJ	saphenofemoral junction
SGOT	serum glutamic oxaloacetic transaminase
SGPT	serum glutamic pyruvic transaminase
SICU	Surgical Intensive Care Unit
SLE	systemic lupus erythematosus
SMA	superior mesenteric artery
SOD	sphincter of Oddi dysfunction
SPECT	single photon emission computed tomography
SS	systemic sclerosis
SSRI	selective serotonin reuptake inhibitor
SSS	subclavian steal syndrome
TAA	thoraco-abdominal aneurysms
TACE	transarterial chemoembolization
TART	transanal resection of tumor
TB	tuberculosis
TBI	toe–brachial index
TEM	transanal endoscopic microsurgery
TENS	transcutaneous electric nerve stimulation
TIA	transient ischemic attack
TIPS	transjugular intrahepatic portosystemic shunt
TOS	thoracic outlet syndrome
TPN	total parenteral nutrition

TRAb	thyrotrophin-receptor antibodies
TSH	thyroid-stimulating hormone
UC	ulcerative colitis
UCSF	University of California, San Francisco
UES	upper esophageal sphincter
US	ultrasound
UTI	urinary tract infection
VIPoma	vasoactive intestinal peptide tumor
VBI	vertebrobasilar ischemia
VMA	vanillylmandelic acid
WBC	white blood-cell count
WCC	white cell count
ZE	Zollinger–Ellison syndrome
ZN	Ziehl–Neelsen

Acknowledgments

We would like to thank our expert contributors to this book for their hard work and dedication to the cause. We thank the authors of the chapters in the first two editions of the book, Tjun Tang, Stewart Walsh, Fiona MacNeill, Bill Flemming, Edward Cheong, Richard Hardwick, Al Windsor, Neville Jamieson, Satyajit Bhattacharya, Adrian O'Sullivan, Henry Tilney, Paris Tekkis, Umar Sadat, David Cooper, Miles Banwell, and Michael Irwin, for building the chapters upon which this edition is based.

We must thank Drs Jordan Pober and John Bradley, co-founders of the joint Yale–Cambridge University Biomedical Research Program, as well as Dr. Bill Sessa, who has continued to facilitate this program as the current director of Yale's Program in Vascular Biology and Therapeutics. This joint program between the two universities has been fostering collaboration for 10 years. We believe that one of its highlights has been the friendship between the two editors, which has led directly to this edition.

We thank our wives and children for never letting us forget, through the long nights and weekends editing this book, that our jobs as husbands and fathers never ends and supersedes our editorial responsibilities. We thank the editorial staff of our publisher for agreeing with them and, despite this, producing this edition in record-breaking time.

General Outpatient Issues
Michael Gaunt and Alan Dardik

ONE

The Outpatient Consultation Process
The Purpose of the Surgical Outpatient Consultation
It is worth emphasizing the simple but fundamental point that each surgical consultation has a specific purpose which the surgeon must address. If the attending surgeon cannot identify a purpose for another consultation then the patient should be discharged back to the referring physician. Discharging a patient does not mean casting them off without care. Patients should be discharged with a plan and instructions for re-referral if appropriate.

The Structure of the Consultation
Each consultation should have a structure which becomes routine. In this way, important stages and information are not overlooked. Each doctor develops their own routine, but, for example, a simple structure might consist of:
1. Read the referral letter.
2. Read the previous clinic letters and old notes.
3. Be clear about the purpose of the consultation before entering the room.
4. Introduce yourself and who you work for.
5. Put the patient at ease; ascertain who has accompanied the patient.
6. Explain what you are going to do, e.g. take a history then perform an examination.
7. Take the history.
8. Perform the relevant examination.
9. Take a moment and decide what to do.
10. Discuss any further diagnostic tests or treatments with the patient.
11. Answer any questions.
12. Synthesize and deliver concluding remarks and instructions.
13. Write notes or draw any necessary diagrams, etc.
14. Dictate the clinic letter or note.

The Referral Letter
The consultation begins before the patient is seen by reading the referral letter in the case of new patients or the last clinic letter in the case of follow-ups. For new patients, the referral letter usually contains the reason why the patient has been sent to the office or clinic plus other useful information such as a list of coexisting medical conditions and a list of current medications. The referral letter sets the scene and provides useful information, but this should not be allowed to unduly influence the consultation. Once patient contact is made, the diagnostic process starts again from scratch with the history and examination.

The Previous Clinic Letter and Notes
The previous notes are in the clinic for a purpose – they are there for you to read. In general, it is better to have as much information as possible before starting a consultation. Reading the notes puts the current presenting illness in context and prevents any repetition of diagnostic tests. An apparently successful consultation can be undermined by the patient informing you that they have already had the tests you were proposing and they were all normal. You are embarrassed and the patient leaves with the impression that you didn't know what you were doing.

Reading a very large set of notes during a busy clinic is not feasible. This is where a detailed previous clinic letter is invaluable in summarizing what has gone before.

The Purpose of the Consultation
New Patients
For new patients, the objective of the consultation is either to reach a diagnosis or to exclude any serious pathology related to that specialty. If it is suspected that the patient's symptoms may be caused by a potentially serious or malignant condition, then diagnostic tests will need to be performed and reviewed promptly.

Follow-up Patients
Seeing follow-up patients in a busy clinic is often a task often delegated to junior staff that may lack a clear understanding of the consultation objectives. In surgery, follow-up patients can be divided into a) new undiagnosed conditions returning with the results of tests, b) chronic conditions which are being monitored, and c) post-operative patients.

New Conditions Under Investigation
These patients are returning to clinic to receive the results of diagnostic tests performed so far. Either the patient will have been seen previously by yourself or by a colleague. Read the previous clinic letter and review the notes to remind yourself of the case. It is useful to ensure that the results of all tests are available before you meet the patient. This may involve calling the relevant department for the results of the test out of ear-shot of the patient. Decide whether the results are diagnostic or whether further tests are necessary. If the results are diagnostic and the result is bad news, e.g. cancer, plan how you will break the news to the patient. If the results are equivocal, it may be necessary to repeat the history and examination to detect new features which may have developed and aid in the diagnosis. Think about possible further tests and the timescale for obtaining these results. It may be that the results are not diagnostic but serious causes have been excluded and the need to obtain a diagnosis is less urgent. If the results are diagnostic and good news, decide whether further follow-up will be required or whether the patient can be discharged with advice alone.

If the results of the tests require medical or surgical therapy, then decisions to treat should always be reviewed with the responsible attending. Medical therapy can be prescribed, depending on the urgency, and it is often performed in conjunction with the referring physician. Surgical therapy often requires coordination of several steps, including reviewing the options for different procedures, discussing them with the patient and family, obtaining informed consent, and preparing the patient for the procedure. Final preparations for the procedure can include filling out hospital paperwork, obtaining pre-operative laboratory and blood bank studies, and consultation with additional specialists, such as anesthesia or cardiology specialists, in preparation for the procedure.

Chronic Conditions
The purpose of the consultation in these patients is to detect whether the patient's condition is stable, improving or deteriorating, and to detect any complications of the underlying condition or treatment. Ideally, the previous clinic letter should contain the reason for the follow-up, what to look for, and an objective description of the clinical condition at that time to allow comparison with the present. It may be time for routine investigations to be performed, e.g. yearly mammogram, or fecal occult blood screening. If the patient's condition has been stable for some time, it may be appropriate to decrease the frequency of outpatient consultations or discharge the patient with clear instructions

to the patient's primary care physician (PCP) and the patient when to re-refer. Do not automatically bring the patient back at the same time interval as the last visit.

Another useful option is the "open appointment." With an open appointment the patient is not given another clinic date but is instructed to call and make a new appointment if their condition recurs. This system works best for reliable patients, familiar with their clinical condition, who have been stable for a long period but who may relapse and require prompt treatment. Depending on the condition and the patient's reliability, you may want to restrict open appointments to a time limit, e.g. a year, after which you schedule a follow-up appointment with them or they should return to their PCP for follow-up. Never underestimate the importance of the PCP as gatekeeper to the proper functioning of the healthcare system.

Post-operative Patients

The purpose of these consultations is to decide whether the operation has been successful in achieving its objectives, e.g. relieving the patient's symptoms or completely removing a tumor. Prior to seeing the patient, read the clinic and operative notes and determine the operation performed and whether there were any intra-operative or post-operative complications which require long-term follow-up, e.g. damage to the common bile duct. If tissue was removed at the time of operation and sent to pathology, make sure you read the pathology report even if the procedure was performed for a non-malignant cause. Occasionally, routine pathology can reveal occult cancer which was never suspected but which may necessitate further management. If the operation was to remove cancer, determine whether this was completely removed or whether the tumor extended to the radial or longitudinal resection margins, indicating residual disease that requires further surgery or adjuvant therapy. The histological grade of the tumor and any evidence of lymph node spread or vascular invasion may indicate that adjuvant radiotherapy/chemotherapy is required. Decide the basics of a treatment plan before breaking any bad news to the patient. These days, the patient may have been discussed at a multidisciplinary team meeting (MDT) and decisions made regarding treatment and follow-up – make sure you have the results of these decisions. The patient may want to modify the plan according to their own preferences, but uncertainty on the part of the doctor at this difficult time is to be avoided.

Meeting the Patient

The doctor should enter the consultation room thoroughly prepared. Ascertain which person in the room is the patient, and introduce yourself. Many patients will be expecting to see the consulting attending physician immediately because that is the name on their appointment card. Who you are and your position in the hierarchy needs to be explained. Determine the relationship of other people in the room to the patient. Do not automatically assume that they are relatives. In this way you will avoid an embarrassing exposure of a patient in front of a neighbor or volunteer driver.

It may be appropriate to put the patient at ease with some friendly comments before launching in to the formal consultation, e.g. apologize for the long wait.

It is often useful to explain the structure of the consultation to the patient: "What I'd like to do is to ask you some questions, then examine you and then we'll discuss what we are going to do."

History and Examination

Obtain the relevant history and perform the relevant examination. Examination of outpatients can be difficult. The patient may be relatively immobile or encased in numerous layers of clothing which take a long time to remove. It is frustrating to wait, but more frustrating to miss an obvious and vital clinical sign due to inadequate examination. Often it is helpful to ask the clinic ancillary staff to help the patient undress or remove items of clothing, such as shoes or pants, which are routinely examined, after the staff member places the patient in the exam room.

Have a Think: The Management Plan

Many doctors seem embarrassed to be seen thinking, but it is actually what we are paid to do. Once the history and examination are complete and the patient is getting dressed, this provides time to record and reflect on the findings and formulate a management plan. For simple and routine problems this will be brief, but for more complicated problems this may be the time to obtain more senior advice or consult a helpful text.

Medicine is a partnership between patient and doctor. The more the patient understands about what is trying to be achieved, the more likely they are to comply with the investigations or treatment. Therefore, take time to make sure your patient understands their condition and your management plan. Additionally, although you may have a specific management plan in mind, you must be prepared to modify this depending on the patient's preferences. Always allow time for the patient to ask any questions and answer them as fully as you can.

Concluding Remarks

The consultation has to be brought to an end. Ideally this occurs when all questions are answered and everyone understands what is involved. However, there may be occasions when a more formal signal that the consultation is drawing to a close is needed. Usually, standing up and closing the notes folder is taken as the relevant cue. Final remarks may consist of "You'll receive an appointment for an ultrasound through the mail in a few weeks' time and we'll see you again in the clinic a week after the test to discuss the results."

Hand-written Entry in the Notes

A hand-written or electronic note is necessary as a contemporaneous record of the consultation and the management plan. Diagrams can be included to illustrate clinical findings which are difficult to incorporate in a typed letter. Also, a detailed initial note is invaluable some days later if the dictation recording system of the clinic becomes corrupted and you need to dictate the letters again.

Dictate the Clinic Letter

Matters concerning the composition of clinic letters and other forms of communication are covered in the next section.

Communication

Good communication is at the heart of good medicine, and this is particularly the case in outpatient medicine. A doctor needs to communicate effectively with the patient and the patient's relatives at the time of the consultation. The importance of this has been recognized in most medical schools, and communication with patients, in particular breaking bad news, now forms part of most curriculae. However, a more neglected area is communication with other healthcare professionals; the most common means of communication in the clinic is the outpatient letter.

Communication with the Patient

This mainly consists of verbal communication during the consultation itself. The importance of introductions and determining the relationship to the patient of any accompanying person has already been emphasized. If the patient is accompanied by a member of staff from a nursing or residential home, they may be a useful source of information and may be able to relay instructions back to the nursing home. Relatives may be another useful source of information, but alternatively may try to dominate the consultation with their own interpretation of events. Generally if the patient is capable of answering questions then they should be allowed to do so without interference and relatives should be encouraged to keep quiet. However, the relative may be an important caregiver for the patient, so it is worth avoiding alienation. An explanation that you wish the patient to answer their own questions at this point in the consultation but you would be interested in the relative's observations at the end may control the situation.

Breaking Bad News
This usually means a diagnosis of cancer or other serious disease. Prior to the consultation, decide how certain the information is or whether further investigation is needed. If there is no reasonable doubt, then a plan of how to break the news is needed.

There are numerous helpful texts on the subject of how to break bad news which cover the subject in more detail than is available here. But several basic principles which are applicable to the outpatient setting will be described. If possible a patient should not be given bad news in isolation and ideally a relative or close friend should be there when the news is given. Hospitals vary in their provision for these circumstances, but a trained counselor or nurse in attendance is also useful to provide comfort and further explanation if required.

Another principle is that bad news should be tempered with good news. One of the first questions a patient tends to ask after receiving an adverse diagnosis is, "Is there anything that can be done?" It is reassuring to be told that reasonably effective treatment is available and that the hope of cure exists. The best interpretation should be put on the situation without instilling false hope. Uncertainty on the part of the doctor at this stage will make a bad situation worse. Therefore, the management plan needs to be decided before the consultation begins. This may involve talking with the senior surgeon and deciding on the best course of action before meeting the patient.

Answer as many questions as you can and then withdraw, giving the patient some time to come to terms with what has been said and receive the comfort and reassurances of relatives and nurses. During this time further questions may occur, and you should return to see the patient to verify that new questions have been answered. The clinic nurse should also determine how the patient is getting home. Probably, no patient should be allowed to drive immediately after receiving this kind of news. They are unlikely to be concentrating fully on their driving. It may be more sensible to order a taxi or for the patient to arrange for a relative to pick them up.

The Outpatient Letter
This letter is unusual because one letter is written to several different potential readers who require different information and may interpret the same information differently.

The first person you are writing the letter to is yourself. This letter is your record of what happened during the consultation, which you can refer to if a subsequent question arises. The letter is best dictated immediately after a consultation when all the details are fresh in your memory. There may be the temptation not to record certain facts in the belief that you will remember them. This may be true for a week or two, but six months and possibly a thousand patients later this will not be the case. If you think that something might be relevant, note it down. We strongly recommend that any portion of the physical exam be recorded as part of the letter, as these objective findings are easily forgotten but often critical at later points in the patient's care.

The next person is the PCP, who receives a mountain of mail every week and does not have the time to wade through a lot of flowery prose. They basically want to know the diagnosis and the management plan including further tests, treatments and the timing of the next outpatient appointment. The PCP also wants this information as soon as possible after the consultation, not two months down the line. Some doctors prefer letters which consist of a list of headings, such as Diagnosis, Diagnostic Tests, Treatments, and Follow-up, etc., therefore removing the need to compose a letter at all.

The next person to read the letter is the next outpatient doctor, who has never seen the patient before. This doctor requires a summary of the original complaint or symptoms, what has happened in terms of tests or interventions, and an outline of the current management plan. The alternative to a letter summarizing this information is the task of wading through the whole set of notes trying to read other people's handwriting and trying to find pathology or radiology reports – which is a considerable waste of time that could have been spent with the patient.

Finally, remember this letter may be read by a hospital manager investigating a complaint or, ultimately, a prosecution lawyer. Humorous or apparently witty statements which seemed funny at the time may appear at best insensitive and at worst patronizing and disparaging when read in the light of subsequent adverse events.

The majority of letters are dictated and typed some time after the clinic by a medical transcriptionist.

Dictating the Letter

There are many different versions of dictating machines around, including tapes, digital audio recorders, and telephone dictation systems, so before dictating a whole clinic's worth of letters make sure you know how the system operates. If there is a tape, check that the tape and the machine are compatible and what you are saying is recording and can be played back in an intelligible form. Nothing is worse after a long clinic to find that none of your carefully composed letters have been recorded and you have to do it all again.

Decide whether you are going to state the punctuation as you dictate (comma), or leave it to the secretary to put in the punctuation based on your sentence construction and voice intonation (period). If possible, discuss this with the secretary who is going to be typing the letters to find out what the secretary prefers. Some secretaries are expert at making sense of the worst dictation, and they can also advise you as to the preferred style of the senior doctor you work for.

Start by stating the date and the title of the clinic, e.g. "Dr. Big's endocrine clinic," and who you and the patient are, e.g. "Dr. Small dictating. The first patient is . . ." This enables the recording to be identified even if it is separated from the patient notes.

At the start of each letter, state the patient's full name and hospital identification number or date of birth. Next, state who the letter is to, e.g. "Letter to the PCP, Dr. Good, with a copy to the stoma care nurse, Ms Ostomy, RN."

The style of the letter may largely be determined by the "house style" of the group in which you are working. This may be a structured letter under set headings, with or without a section of text. For text, it is a good idea to allocate a new paragraph to the introduction, history, examination, investigations, and treatment, etc.

Letter to the Primary Care Physician (PCP)

The PCP wants to know the following points. What is the diagnosis, or which tests are being performed to reach a diagnosis? When do you expect to make a diagnosis? What should be done about the symptoms in the meantime? What have you told the patient? If the diagnosis has been made, what is the treatment plan and what is the prognosis?

As stated earlier, the average PCP receives a mountain of mail every week and, therefore, short and concise communications are appreciated.

The style of letters varies from hospital to hospital, and the style which you adopt will largely be determined by the preferred format adopted by the department in which you are working. Increasing in popularity is the formulated letter consisting of a series of headings such as Diagnosis, Diagnostic Tests Awaited, Results, Medications, etc. This is a very efficient letter, but some consider it too impersonal and not explanatory enough. At the other end of the scale is the flowery prose consisting of long sentences and paragraphs which many PCPs skip to read the bottom line. A combination of the two exists which starts with a structured summary under relevant headings and then a section of text explaining how the diagnosis was reached and why a specific series of tests have been requested. Whatever the style, all good letters contain the following information:

1. A summary of why the patient was referred.
2. A summary of the history.
3. A summary of examination findings.
4. A list of differential diagnoses.
5. A list of diagnostic tests.
6. The treatment plan.
7. The time course for further tests or treatments.
8. What the patient and relatives were told.
9. Arrangements for follow-up, open appointment, or if the patient has been discharged, the conditions under which the patient should be re-referred.

Follow-up Patients
For follow-up patients, letters should include the following information:
1. A summary of the course of the illness and any interventions so far, which sets the consultation in context.
2. A reason why the patient is being followed.
3. Current history and examination findings.
4. Results of recent tests.
5. An explanation of the symptoms and signs to look out for.
6. How long the follow-up is likely to continue.
7. When the patient is likely to be discharged.

Note/Letter to the Next Surgical Clinic Doctor
It is important to write the clinic note or letter bearing in mind that the next doctor to see the patient may not be yourself. In the case of new patients returning for the results of tests, the needs of the next clinic doctor are the same as the PCP, and a note or letter containing the information outlined in the previous section is adequate.

Follow-up notes which consist of "I have reviewed Mrs Smith and her condition is unchanged and we will see her again in 3 months' time" are completely unhelpful.

Each note should start with a summary which sets the consultation in context, e.g. "I reviewed the history of this 43-year-old woman who in April 1996 underwent a right simple mastectomy with a level 1 axillary node dissection. Her pathology report revealed this to be a 1 cm tumor, which was a moderately differentiated (grade II) ductal carcinoma with 3 out of 8 axillary lymph nodes involved. Following surgery she was treated with a full course of adjuvant chemotherapy from which she made a good recovery and on her last two outpatient visits she has been well with no signs of recurrence . . . etc." The next doctor now knows exactly what the original problem was without having to search for the operation note, the oncology notes or the several pathology reports. Once this trend is established, it is a simple matter for the next doctor to use the same paragraph, modified appropriately, to start the next letter.

Referrals to Other Clinicians

There may be occasions when referral of a patient to another specialty is indicated, either because the original complaint is not your specialty or the original complaint is your specialty but there is a coexisting condition which merits treatment in its own right. Many PCPs have their preferred referral pathways, and therefore non-urgent cases should be referred back to the PCP with reasons why an additional referral is indicated. However, on other occasions a referral may be urgent or closely related to surgical treatment, e.g. a cardiology assessment prior to a surgical procedure in a patient with an existing heart condition. In these instances it is probably advisable to refer the patient yourself but send a copy of the referral letter to the PCP.

Prior to referring to another specialty, it is wise to discuss the case with your attending physician who can confirm a referral is indicated and advise you as to the correct referral pathway. In this case, the referral letter should start by indicating that your attending has been involved in the decision to refer. Then outline the reason why the patient was referred to your specialty and what your main findings have been. Next explain why a referral to another specialty is indicated and how this impacts your treatment plan, if this applies. Finally, express a potential timetable for when you would like the patient to be seen and how this fits in with your own timetable for follow-up and treatment.

Ordering Diagnostic Tests

Diagnostic tests tend to be classified as either urgent or routine. Difficulty arises for tests that are not urgent but if the result was postive the surgeon would want to know immediately. For example, during the investigation of rectal bleeding the decision may be made to investigate the condition further with a colonoscopy. The test is performed to exclude a colon carcinoma but there may be a four-week waiting time to schedule for routine colonoscopies. If the result is negative, there are few consequences; but if a colon cancer is detected, a month has been wasted during which potentially life-saving treatment could have been administered. When deciding on whether a case is urgent or not, one must always consider the consequences of a positive result.

Routine Tests

Routine tests are usually arranged by completing the relevant request form or using the hospital's computerized ordering system. An experienced clinic nurse can usually advise you as to the correct process. If not, one can always call the relevant department and ask their advice. One assumes there is no pressing need to know the results as long as they are available for the next consultation. However, for certain tests, there may be long waiting times – once again, contact the relevant department for more advice.

Urgent Tests

Obtaining urgent tests is an art form. Just writing "urgent" on the request form is no guarantee that the request will be treated as urgent. Clearly stating the timescale of when the result is needed by helps departments plan and prioritize their work appropriately. However, many departments have set procedures for dealing with urgent requests, and unless these procedures are followed precisely the request fails. This information is often known to the people who have worked in the hospital for many years but is a mystery to newly rotating doctors. A telephone call to the relevant department to obtain advice regarding these procedures or a specific appointment time is useful. Always record the name of the person you spoke to in case of future difficulties. In a legal sense, if you do not record the name of the person and the date and time of the conversation, then that conversation never took place. Telephone calls can use up a lot of time in the clinic and it may not be possible to contact the relevant person. It may be possible to delegate these calls to the clinic secretary and only get involved if difficulties arise.

In very difficult cases, admitting the patient to the hospital and performing the tests as an inpatient is one option, but, it may be inappropriate in many cases and is often wasteful of hospital resources.

Finally, a phone call or visit to the senior physician in charge of the testing department in question, explaining the clinical features and asking them to ensure the investigation is performed within a certain time, tends to ensure the right result – even if you get a less than friendly response.

Performing Procedures in Clinic

Performing procedures in clinic may be an integral part of the investigation or treatment of the patient's condition. Procedures commonly performed in the outpatient setting include abscess drainage, fine needle aspiration, Tru-cut biopsy, rigid sigmoidoscopy, proctoscopy, injection of hemorrhoids and rectal biopsy. Other procedures may be performed depending on the specialty; details of these procedures are described in the relevant chapters.

Obviously, one should never perform an invasive procedure unless one has been trained to do so. In addition, the issue of consent has been increasing in importance in recent years. Although in past years it was unusual for patients to sign a consent form prior to these procedures, more recently most procedures require written informed consent. In addition, these procedures, if performed in a hospital clinic setting, require performance of the hospital standard of procedures, including pre-operative paperwork, creation of a sterile field, performance of a time-out procedure, statement of the operative checklist, and post-operative discharge planning.

The Discharge Plan

Permanently discharging patients from clinic can be a contentious issue. On the one hand, if all patients were followed up indefinitely the clinics would soon become overburdened and cease to function. On the other hand, if discharge is handled insensitively there can be criticism that the patient has been abandoned or that an unfair onus of further management has been placed on the PCP.

The decision to discharge a patient from the clinic is easy when the patient originally presented with a relatively simple condition which was treated and the symptoms resolved. However, for other patients the decision to discharge can be more difficult. Earlier in the text we emphasized that if a reason for follow-up cannot be identified, the patient should be discharged. This seems like common sense and for an experienced clinician this is a relatively simple decision, but junior surgeons may fear that the reason why they cannot identify a reason for follow-up is because their knowledge is deficient, i.e. a good reason does exist but they fear they are ignorant of it. In this situation there is a strong temptation to "play safe" and follow the course of the previous clinic doctor and review the patient in the clinic at the same interval as before. Inappropriate outpatient visits are wasteful of healthcare resources and cause an inconvenience for the patients and their caretakers. Therefore, every effort should be made to reserve outpatient consultations for those patients who really need them.

Another problem with multiple inappropriate clinic visits is that some patients become accustomed to attending the hospital and may actually look forward to their appointments. These patients may have adopted the sick role and frequent hospital visits legitimize their "illness." This may have certain sociological and economic benefits, e.g. being excused from work, receipt of disability benefits, etc., which they may feel will be threatened if they are discharged. These can be difficult patients to manage, and to avoid conflict it may be necessary to delay discharge until the attending has stepped in and finalized this decision with them.

For some chronic conditions or after major surgery, follow-up intervals become very long, e.g. yearly. In these situations the doctor should question whether further clinic follow-up is appropriate. After all, it is unlikely that the occurrence of new symptoms will coincide with the next appointment date. More likely, within that time if new symptoms arise the patient will seek the advice of their PCP, who in turn will ask for the appointment to be brought forward and the original appointment will become irrelevant. If the patient had been discharged with instructions to consult their PCP if new symptoms arose the same procedure would have been followed and the patient seen in the same time but without the inconvenience of the original clinic appointment.

An alternative arrangement is the time-limited open appointment, where the patient has open access to the clinic to make their own appointment if the symptoms recur within a certain time after discharge, e.g. one year.

Discharging a patient should not be considered as casting them off into the unknown void. Patients should be discharged with a plan which includes instructions as to when they should seek medical opinion. These instructions should be included in the clinic letter in the form of what the patient was told and additional instructions to the PCP.

Breast
Lynn S. Model and Anees B. Chagpar

In the US, the female breast has a cultural, psychologic and sociologic significance far beyond its function as a milk-producing organ. Indeed, breast health issues have become increasingly politicized as a consequence of powerful advocacy and lobbying and high media exposure. According to National Cancer Institute (NCI) reports, the incidence and mortality of breast cancer (BC) have decreased since 1990. The decrease in incidence has been mainly in the population greater than 50 years old, and has largely been attributed to the reduction in hormone replacement therapy (HRT) use. The decrease in mortality is attributed to earlier detection and better treatments, such that many patients now survive their cancer in extended remission. The five-year survival rate for localized cancers is 98%, and overall five-year survival regardless of stage is 89%. Breast cancer management requires a multidisciplinary team effort, comprised of dedicated surgeons, plastic surgeons, radiologists, pathologists, medical oncologists, radiation oncologists, geneticists, nurses, social workers, physical therapists, and allied staff. Often delivered in the setting of a highly specialized multidisciplinary breast center, such coordinated care has been shown to improve patient outcomes and enhance the quality of care and overall patient experience. The delivery of high-quality care is rarely dependent on the skills of one clinician, but rather is the result of good organization as part of a functional, patient-focused team.

Practical Tips for the Trainee
◇ Understand the American Joint Commission on Cancer (AJCC) staging system.
◇ A number of professional organizations have standardized treatment guidelines and algorithms – be familiar with these, especially the National Cancer Center Network (NCCN) treatment guideline.
◇ Multidisciplinary teams (MDTs) have a strong educational value and are a powerful learning resource for new team members. You will be able to learn how to function within an MDT, and observe the complexity of team dynamics and leadership styles. Collaborative working represents the future model of healthcare. Working within an MDT means you will never be making decisions in isolation.
  ∝ Participate in multidisciplinary conferences as often as possible when the opportunity arises.
◇ Your team will have its own protocols for breast assessment and diagnosis, and a standard treatment plan; ask if these protocols are written down and available, as they are a useful guide.
◇ At your first breast clinic, ask if you can sit in and watch someone more experienced or senior do the first few assessments.
◇ If possible, early in your rotation follow a patient through the whole process from diagnosis to surgery. This provides the opportunity to:
  ∝ understand the process from the patient perspective
  ∝ interact with the rest of the MDT and introduce yourself to the whole team.

Breast Assessment
Breast referrals are made for a wide variety of breast/chest wall and axillary problems, pain being the most common symptom and breast lump being the most common sign. The

TABLE 2.1 Age-related risk rates of breast cancer in the general population (these rates are likely to be slightly higher in a symptomatic breast clinic population)

Age Range (years)	Risk Rate
30 to 39	1 in 233
40 to 49	1 in 69
50 to 59	1 in 42
60 to 69	1 in 23
Lifetime risk	1 in 8

majority of patients (90%) will have normal breasts: the breast is a dynamic organ under constant hormonal influence, especially between puberty and menopause. Therefore, the majority of breast changes are indeed functional or physiologic alterations secondary to the normal hormonal shifts associated with this extended time period. These include physiologic transformations associated with pregnancy and lactation, and the progressive involution of the breast which begins around the age of 35 years and accelerates after menopause.

Pain, a palpable mass, or nipple discharge often draws a patient's attention to their breast. Common benign causes of breast mass vary in incidence with patient age. For patients under 25 years old, benign fibroadenoma is the most common cause of breast mass. For those between 35 and 50 years old, fibrocystic changes are very common (1 in 3 women) and may cause mass-like lumps in the breast. Mastitis and breast abscess may cause mass-like abnormalities in the breast, and are mostly found in lactating women. Phyllodes tumors commonly affect women in their 40s and 50s, and papillary adenoma of the nipple is also common in women in their 40s. Above the age of 50 years, the incidence of cancer in a mass increases, and in those aged 60 years or more it is the most likely diagnosis. Table 2.1 lists the age-related risk rates for the general population.

The safest course of action is to assume that each lump might be a cancer whatever the age, until proven otherwise.

Breast Assessment Process
Assessment of the breast is a three-part process consisting of clinical assessment, mammography/ultrasound/magnetic resonance imaging, and cytology/biopsy. This system allows rapid and accurate diagnosis or exclusion of a cancer diagnosis, allowing most patients to be discharged back to their PCP after one comprehensive clinic visit.

The appropriate use of all three modalities reduces but *does not eliminate* the chance of missing a cancer, as no combination of tests is 100% sensitive or specific. Not all cancers present with classic clinical or radiologic features. Of note, lobular cancer is the most commonly "missed"; its clinical and radiologic presentation can be subtle and cytology may have a bland appearance.

The following sections describe the use of this assessment strategy in the breast clinic.

Clinical Assessment
Breast History
As with all clinic visits, the first step is to introduce yourself and explain your status to the patient; it is important that the patient understands that you will see them first and then discuss their management with the senior doctor/attending, who may also then wish to see them.

You and the patient should ideally be seated during the history taking. The patient's breasts should not be exposed at this stage of the consultation; they should be covered either by the patient's own clothes or by a specially designed breast evaluation gown.

While taking the history, you have the opportunity to assimilate other sensitive issues, for example your patient's concerns and fears: What drove them to report their symptoms and come to see you? What do they want from this clinic visit? This is not always obvious.

Try to establish a rapport, as the patient may already be nervous and embarrassed about the intimacy of the forthcoming breast examination. Make eye contact, smile and try to appear friendly and relaxed as well as confident and calm.

Rarely, a female patient will refuse to see a male doctor. Usually the nursing staff will have anticipated and managed this situation. This can seem personal, but bear in mind it isn't; be sensitive, not offended.

The Stressful Consultation

Occasionally a consultation will be tense and stressful, usually because the patient is frightened of the possibility of an unfavorable diagnosis. A patient may scrutinize your facial expressions, and over-interpret (usually negatively) your words or actions. Additionally, they may be cold and withdrawn, or angry and aggressive. Patients may be tearful, or may ask repeatedly whether everything is OK. Such emotional situations can cause you to feel intimidated and pressured to make statements you are not certain about. Try not to give blind reassurances, or distance yourself from the encounter. Attempt to understand their vulnerabilities, but be honest. If the breast feels normal, say so; if you are not sure, say so; and if you are concerned, express your concerns. Explain that the examination is only one part of the assessment process and you may not be able to confidently tell what the problem is until (for example) imaging has given you additional information.

The History – Specifics

Age is the most important factor in assessing the likelihood of a new breast change being cancerous. However, you should always have a high index of suspicion as even young women can get BC, and when they do, it tends to be aggressive.

History of presenting problem: Determine the time course of each symptom and any variation within the menstrual cycle, as this is often a clue to the diagnosis. Is the mass getting bigger or smaller? Does it vary in size with periods? Is there associated pain or tenderness?

Pain may be cyclical or non-cyclical. Note when the pain first started, its duration, site and severity, relieving and exacerbating factors, associated symptoms, timing of recurrences, and timing in relationship to menses.

✧ *Cyclical breast pain* is related to ovarian function; breasts are swollen and tender and/ or lumpy 3–10 days (or longer) prior to menstruation; pain is usually relieved by menstruation.

✧ *Non-cyclical breast pain* is pain caused by specific conditions of the breast not related to ovarian function, e.g. trauma and fat necrosis, infected cyst, mastitis (periductal or lactating), abscess, fistula.

✧ *Non-breast pain* may be angina, cholelithiasis, cervical spondylosis, hiatal hernia, nerve entrapment, Tietze's syndrome, esophageal lesions, lung conditions, etc.

Lump: have the patient describe it to you – "pea," "marble," "grape," etc., are useful comparisons. How was the lump noticed? How long has it been present?

Nipple discharge may be spontaneous or may occur upon stimulation (after a bath, for example). Ask about color (bloody, clear, yellow, white, green). Is it associated with pain?

Any previous breast imaging: check date and location of last mammogram.

General: Check general health and comorbidities.

Breast cancer risk factors:
- ✧ Family history: Maternal and paternal, first- and second-degree.
- ✧ Past history of radiation to the chest wall (i.e. radiotherapy for Hodgkin's lymphoma).
- ✧ Any previous breast problems – nature, investigation, and outcome.

Other risk factors:
- ✧ Endogenous estrogen exposure: Menarche, menopause, age at first pregnancy, number of pregnancies, breastfeeding history.
- ✧ Exogenous estrogen exposure: oral contraceptive pill (OCP), HRT.

The Breast Examination

Always have a chaperone present, regardless of your gender. The room and your hands should be warm. Explain at each stage what you are going to do and why (this serves as verbal consent for the exam). There are many breast examination techniques. A common technique is to imagine the breast as a clock and work your way around the clock face from 12 to 12, examining the breast from the outer margin toward the nipple (*see* Figure 2.1).

Start with **inspection**:
- ✧ Ask the patient to expose their whole torso, displacing long hair and jewelry, and to sit facing you.
- ✧ Ask them to point to the area they are concerned about: the patient's use of hand and fingers will give you a clue to whether it is a focal or a generalized problem.

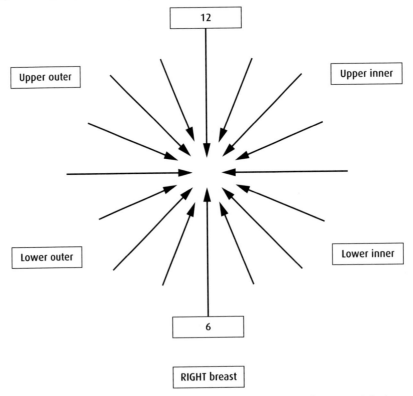

FIGURE 2.1   Breast quadrants. Most breast glandular tissue lies in the outer quadrants, especially the upper outer quadrant.

✧ **Look** for asymmetry, visible lumps, skin dimpling or peau d'orange. Inspect the nipple–areolar complex (NAC). Look for signs of locally advanced cancer: ulceration, fixation to chest wall (ribs, muscles), erythema of the skin, satellite nodules, invasion of the skin, etc.

✧ **Look** for skin dimpling or distortion as the patient slowly raises both hands above the head.

✧ **Look** for retraction as the patient squeezes in with their hands on their hips, tightening their pectoral muscles.

Next, **palpate**:

✧ Palpate the cervical, supraclavicular, infraclavicular and axillary lymph nodes. Supporting the patient's arm in your non-examining hand may allow for better evaluation of the axilla.

✧ Palpate the breasts in two positions: with the patient seated upright, and then lying supine. Examining patients in two positions allows you to feel masses that you may miss if you examine them in only one.

✧ Examination of the breast requires palpation of the entire breast: from the clavicle to the sixth rib, and from the sternum to the anterior axillary line. There are a variety of ways to do this; one of these is described below.

  ∝ Have the patient lie supine but not flat, with a pillow under the head, arms elevated with elbows flat on the bed, and hands tucked under the head.

  ∝ If the patient is symptomatic, examine the asymptomatic breast first to gain some idea of the normal texture of the breast.

  ∝ Palpate all breast tissue with the flat of the fingers, following the pattern you feel most comfortable with. Focus on the area of patient concern, remembering the axillary tail and the NAC.

  ∝ If you find a lump, note its site, size, consistency, surface, whether there is skin/muscle tethering.

  ∝ If the problem is nipple discharge, ask the patient to massage the breast/nipple to demonstrate the discharge: assess color, and number of ducts involved (uniduct or multiduct).

  ∝ Repeat the process for the opposite side.

What is a Lump?

Do not agonize over "whether there is a lump or not." If the patient feels that her breasts have changed and/or she thinks there is a lump, you need to prove she doesn't have cancer. A lump is any tissue or area that feels more prominent or asymmetric compared with the patient's normal breast tissue. Clinical examination, although helpful, is unreliable and subjective. Each woman has a different "normal" feel to her breasts, so it is important to compare the two breasts; asymmetry is a useful guide for the need to proceed to imaging and other investigations.

   Lumps can be obviously discrete and circumscribed, i.e. with fibroadenoma, cyst, lipoma or cancer; or feel like an area of asymmetric lumpiness, e.g. benign breast changes, fibroadenoma, cyst, lipoma or cancer. The texture of the patient's tissue and skin and the proportion of fat to glandular tissue will also affect your ability to feel a lump. A young breast with low fat content and a tight skin envelope may have little laxity and feel generally firm (dense), making it difficult to feel even a superficial discrete lump. An older breast with a greater fat to glandular tissue ratio and a more mobile skin envelope is softer, often making lumps more obvious to palpation.

✧ *Benign breast changes* – generalized islands of nodularity; occasionally focal or asymmetric.

✧ *Fibroadenoma* – firm, round, very mobile, may be multiple. Cannot usually be compressed.
✧ *Breast cysts* – firm, round, mobile, may be multiple; as the fluid can be compressed, may have a "rubbery" feel; sometimes tender.
✧ *Breast cancer* – classic signs are hardness, irregularity, dimpling, tethering, ulceration, etc. Smaller, earlier cancers frequently do not demonstrate these signs. Virtually any type of breast change *can* indicate a cancer.

The Nipple
Nipple Discharge
Pre-menopausal discharge is common and usually stops with menopause; therefore, all post-menopausal discharge must be regarded as suspicious. In younger women, bloody discharge can be a sign of ductal carcinoma in situ (DCIS) or invasive cancer, although the most common cause of bloody nipple discharge remains intraductal papilloma.
  Physiologic discharges:
✧ Multi-duct, multicolored (yellow to dark green-brown) discharge is relatively common and normal. It is often secondary to nipple massage or a hot bath/shower. It is occasionally spontaneous, although more often is expressed. This is generally bilateral. It is usually seen pre-menopausally.
✧ Ectatic ducts produce a sticky yellow fluid or white toothpaste-like material on massage.
✧ Milk-like fluid can be expressed by most pre-menopausal women who have lactated. True galactorrhea (pituitary adenoma – associated with increased prolactin levels) is rare and the discharge is spontaneous and copious.

Pathologic discharges: Usually, these are blood-stained, single duct, spontaneous, unilateral and persistent. They may be pre- or post-menopausal. Causes are:
✧ Intraductal papilloma.
✧ Cancer (especially a presenting feature of DCIS).

Nipple Inversion/Retraction
✧ *Inversion* is usually slit-like and may be congenital; it is often due to fibrosis and shortening of the periductal tissue and major ducts. If acquired, the nipple can often be everted with gentle manipulation, and the areola is soft and healthy.
✧ *Retraction* may be due to a retro/periareolar cancerous process or mass pulling the NAC inwards. Often the nipple is visible but distorted and the surrounding areolar tissue hard, inflexible and drawn in in a saucer-like manner.

Inversion and retraction look different, but may be confused. Regardless, any new finding of nipple inversion or retraction should be approached with a high degree of suspicion.

Eczema and Paget's disease
Eczema and Paget's can look identical, especially in the early stages of Paget's.
✧ *Eczema* of the breast often affects the areola and surrounding skin; it can be bilateral and associated with a generalized eczematous skin change and breastfeeding. It presents with flaking, weeping, or itchy skin.
✧ *Paget's* usually begins with similar symptoms centrally, destroying the nipple architecture and spreading outwards onto the areola. There may be an associated underlying mass. These signs are not pathognomonic, and a scaling/excoriated NAC should undergo a punch biopsy.

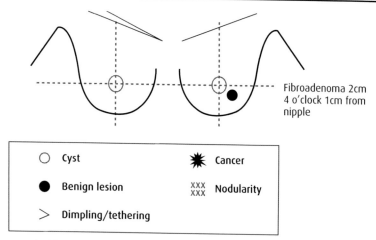

Fibroadenoma 2cm
4 o'clock 1cm from
nipple

○	Cyst	✳	Cancer
●	Benign lesion	XXX XXX	Nodularity
>	Dimpling/tethering		

FIGURE 2.2 A method for recording the examination

Recording the Examination
✧ Record examination findings and your clinical impressions (*see* Figure 2.2).
✧ Always mark the site of patient concern.
✧ Imagine the breast as a clock face, and describe the site of the lesion accordingly.
✧ Record the distance from the nipple.
✧ Give the size of the irregularity.

Imaging
Most women who attend a diagnostic clinic will be offered imaging regardless of their presenting symptom or sign: clinical examination is poor at discriminating between cancer and normal changes, particularly in the pre-menopausal woman with dense nodular breasts.

General indications for imaging (in normal-risk patients) are as follows.
✧ All women over 40 years:
  ∝ Mammography – to screen both breasts.
  ∝ Targeted ultrasound – focused on the symptomatic area, or to direct biopsy.
✧ Women <35 years with focal lumps, nodularity, pain or tenderness:
  ∝ Targeted ultrasound – focused on the symptomatic area, or to direct biopsy.
✧ Young women with a high-risk genetic profile:
  ∝ MRI (currently under investigation).

Mammography
Mammography uses soft-tissue X-rays to image the breast, which is compressed between two plates while the image is taken. Mammography is the gold-standard breast imaging and screening tool due to its high sensitivity and specificity. Usually two views (oblique and cranio-caudal) are obtained, using 1 mGy of radiation. The breast is more radio-dense below the age of 35, making mammography less sensitive.

Mammography is particularly good at detecting early non-palpable lesions, and micro-calcifications. Radiologists indicate their suspicions regarding the imaging based on the BI-RADS classification (Table 2.2).

TABLE 2.2 BI-RADS classification: Breast Imaging Reporting and Data System

BI-RADS category	Assessment	Clinical management recommendation(s)
0	Assessment incomplete	Need to review prior studies and/or complete additional imaging
1	Negative	Continue routine screening
2	Benign finding	Continue routine screening
3	Probably benign finding	Short-term follow-up mammogram at 6 months
4	Suspicious abnormality	Perform biopsy, preferably needle biopsy
5	Highly suspicious of malignancy; appropriate action should be taken	Biopsy and treatment, as necessary
6	Known biopsy-proven malignancy, treatment pending	Assure that treatment is completed

Ultrasound

Acoustic water-based gel, which is a good medium for the transmission of ultrasound waves, is applied to the breast and an ultrasound probe manipulated over the breast by the ultrasonographer. This technique involves no radiation exposure, and is often helpful in patients under the age of 35 or those with dense breast tissue. It may also be used specifically to look at retroareolar tissue, which is not well seen using mammography. Ultrasound allows solid and cystic lesions to be distinguished but is operator dependent, and not as sensitive as mammography. Ultrasound is a poor screening tool, and thus scanning an asymptomatic breast is not recommended.

Other Breast Imaging Modalities (Secondary Imaging)

If a patient has changes that are suspicious or diagnostic for cancer on ultrasound, the ultrasonographer should scan the axilla. If a node appears to be suspicious for cancer (local criteria), fine-needle aspiration cytology (FNAC) is performed. Pre-operative identification of axillary nodal disease will allow a more appropriate management of the axilla, e.g. full axillary lymph node dissection rather than sentinel lymph node biopsy.

There are many other types of breast imaging techniques available whose roles are unclear or are still in the research or developmental arena. These include positron emission tomography (PET) and scintimammography. Magnetic resonance imaging has high sensitivity and is especially useful in imaging the difficult breast (very young and dense, and post surgery and radiotherapy) or assessing multifocality, but its expense, the low specificity, and the difficulty of MRI-guided biopsy restrict use to very specific indications.

Tissue Diagnosis

Techniques for tissue diagnosis include:
◇ Fine-needle aspiration.
◇ Punch biopsy.
◇ Percutaneous wide-bore needle (core) biopsy.
◇ Excisional biopsy.

In general, you should only proceed to obtaining tissue by these techniques if there is a focal or discrete *solid* change evident either on imaging or clinical examination or, as is more usual, both modalities. Random aspiration of a lumpy area is to be avoided. Most clinics prefer to perform FNA or core biopsy after the clinical exam and imaging, as any invasive procedure can cause tissue inflammation or bleeding and can reduce the accuracy of later clinical and radiologic findings.

Increasingly, core biopsy is the preferred technique for obtaining tissue, as it gives histology with architecture rather than just cytology. Histology is the gold-standard diagnostic modality. Core biopsy will give a definitive diagnosis of benign lesion (i.e. will confirm that the lesion is a fibroadenoma and can be safely followed by clinical/self exam alone), and will give more specific information about the particularities of a cancer, thus allowing better pre-operative planning.

Cysts are only aspirated if they are symptomatic and/or patients request aspiration; asymptomatic cysts do not require aspiration. After aspiration, cyst fluid can generally be discarded if there is no blood-staining or residual mass – which can indicate a papilloma, intracystic carcinoma or necrotic cancer with cystic degeneration. Occasionally, on aspiration you will perforate an unseen vessel and blood will enter the cyst fluid in your syringe. If you are in doubt, request cytology.

Tissue/cyst drainage can be performed either under guidance by palpation (usually by the surgeon) or under image guidance (by radiologist, sonographer, or surgeon). Image guidance (ultrasound or stereotactic mammography) is the preferred method, especially for smaller lesions, as it reduces the risk of missing the lesion and limits false-negative results due to poor sampling. If your clinic performs these procedures exclusively in the radiology department, you should still attempt to take part in them as this is a key step in BC diagnosis.

Fine-Needle Aspiration

This is to perform and gives almost immediate results, although information is limited to "cancer" or "benign." It can be difficult to get an adequate number of epithelial cells. Results are very dependent on the experience of the clinician doing the FNA (sensitivity 52–95%, depending on operator) and on that of the cytologist interpreting the result. It is not useful for assessing microcalcifications.

Fine-needle aspiration requires a 10 mL syringe and a 21–23 gauge needle. The method is as follows:

✧ Explain the procedure and obtain written consent.
✧ Position the patient as for examination of the breast.
✧ Clean the skin with an alcohol swab; a small amount of lidocaine can be injected subcutaneously if desired.
✧ Fix the lesion with one hand while using the other to insert the needle, applying suction to the syringe and passing it 5–6 times through the lesion.
✧ Release suction and withdraw the needle. Deposit the sample either onto glass slides or into cytologic preservative fluid.
✧ As soon as the needle is withdrawn, apply pressure with a cotton-wool ball to the area of aspiration for 3–4 minutes, to minimize bruising. Apply a bandaid or other covering to prevent staining of the patient's garments.

Punch Biopsy

This is useful for the breast skin or for very superficial lesions in the skin (e.g. skin tumor deposits), especially in the area of the NAC (e.g. if you want to exclude Paget's disease); it is also helpful in the diagnosis of inflammatory breast cancer (dermal lymphatic invasion).
✧ Explain the technique and obtain written consent.
✧ Position the patient as for breast examination. Clean the NAC skin and infiltrate skin with local anesthetic.

✧ Punch biopsy cutting blades are provided on a handle in a range of sizes from 2–6 mm. Using a screwing motion, push the round cutting blade through the skin and underlying tissue. Lift the tissue above the skin using forceps or a needle, and cut the tissue free with scissors. Place tissue in formalin. Sutures may not be required. Apply a suitable dressing.

Percutaneous Wide-Bore Needle (Core) Biopsy

This tissue diagnosis technique provides histologic diagnosis. If cancer is found, it provides information about morphology, grade, estrogen/progesterone receptors (ER/PR) and HER2/neu status. It takes slightly more time to perform than FNA, is slightly more traumatic (more bruising), and results take 24–48 hours to obtain.

✧ Explain the technique and obtain written consent.
✧ Position the patient as for breast examination.
✧ Clean the skin and infiltrate with local anesthetic. Make a small incision with a number 11 blade in the skin over the lesion.
✧ Hold the lesion between thumb and forefinger, and insert the special biopsy needle (gun) up to the lesion. Fire the gun, remove the needle in the closed position and open it to deposit the core of tissue into formalin. Several cores are often taken.
✧ Core biopsies can be done under palpation guidance as described here, or using ultrasound or stereotactic guidance.
✧ In addition, vacuum-assisted core biopsy devices are available, and can often provide larger samples. With some of these, removal of the device is not required after each sample, such that multiple cores can be taken without having to remove and re-insert the device each time.
✧ As soon as the needle is removed, apply pressure with a cotton-wool ball to the biopsy site to minimize bleeding and bruising. A suitable small dressing is applied.

Excisional Biopsy

This is used for surgical excision of a lesion or microcalcifications with or without a localizing guidewire. It is performed when simple image-guided or manually guided biopsy is not possible.

Microductectomy or *Hadfield's procedure* (major duct excision) may be useful to diagnose the underlying cause of a bloody nipple discharge, as a large amount of tissue is provided for histology. If the lump is found to be benign, this provides both diagnosis and treatment. It requires a formal operation which leaves a scar. If the mass proves to be malignant, a second operation may be needed for staging and wider excision. Only a small number of lesions – namely very small mammography-detected cancers or small foci of microcalcifications – require a formal surgical excision to make a diagnosis.

Other Diagnostic Breast Investigations

Staging: If the patient is diagnosed with breast cancer, they may require staging. Routine pre-operative staging is not recommended and is reserved for those with advanced disease or with specific symptoms and signs that may indicate metastatic disease.

Staging tests include bone scan and computed tomography (CT) scan of chest, abdomen and pelvis, along with routine blood tests.

The Multidisciplinary Meeting

Multidisciplinary meetings (MDMs) or tumor boards provide an opportunity for the team to discuss the diagnostic results of newly diagnosed cancers, review their imaging and pathology results, and discuss the multidisciplinary treatment plan. Often, this will involve complex problem solving and decision making among team members. Try to understand this process; if it is not clear, then ask questions.

After the Patient Assessment – What to do Next
Advice and Education
After thorough assessment and diagnosis of a patient's condition, you need to formulate a management strategy. For benign breast conditions or changes, management consists of advice and education regarding normal age-related breast changes, guidance on breast awareness, and the use of breast-cancer screening techniques, as appropriate. Your job includes making sure patients know that they are always welcome back if they have further problems, and explaining when it is advisable to visit their PCP first. If you inadvertently cause a patient to feel embarrassed that they have wasted your time because they have normal breasts, they are more likely to fail to report future changes in their breasts for fear of looking foolish.

Most patients do not fully understand the complex nature of the female breast and the hormonal influences that cause breast changes. Understandably, patients often believe that breast pain is a sign of disease. A well-informed patient will have greater confidence in managing their own breast signs and symptoms in the future, and this will help to reduce the number of unnecessary clinic visits for benign breast conditions. Note that the breast clinic will frequently have abundant literature available. Use leaflets judiciously: handing out information sheets is no substitute for a careful face-to-face explanation.

Breast Awareness
This is more than just breast self-examination – it is about patients knowing their breasts so that if there is a change they will notice it and report it to their doctor. Patients can then repeat their exam at a different stage of their menstrual cycle (in a pre-menopausal woman) or be referred straight to a breast clinic (in a post-menopausal woman).

The Anxious Patient
Occasionally you will meet a patient who finds it difficult to accept that the "lumpiness" of their breasts is normal for them. They may thus require more time and careful repeat examinations and explanations of the results. A patient may have a cancer phobia or other underlying psychologic/psychosocial problems. These patients need to be identified early and seen by the senior clinician, rather than having numerous unnecessary tests or treatments.

The Dissatisfied Patient
Sometimes a patient will not be satisfied that the assessment has been carried out properly. These patients require careful handling; always involve the senior clinician and do not be dismissive. Listen to their concerns with courtesy and sympathy – you might be wrong and their concerns justified: remember, no test is infallible.

Breaking Bad News
You may need to explain the diagnosis of cancer to a patient. Although this is difficult for you, it is even more difficult for the patient. It is normal for a patient with a new diagnosis of breast cancer to be distressed, and it is your job to allow them time to express their feelings and fears. Sitting in on these discussions with more experienced clinicians is a good way to start developing your own technique for handling these difficult situations.

Management of Specific Breast Conditions

Breast Cancer

The specific details of the medical and surgical management of breast cancer is beyond the scope of this book. The AJCC breast cancer staging system is, however, given below.

AJCC Breast Cancer Staging System

Primary Tumor (T) Categories

TX	Primary tumor cannot be assessed.
T0	No evidence of primary tumor.
Tis	Carcinoma in situ (ductal carcinoma in situ, lobular carcinoma in situ, or Paget's disease of the nipple with no associated tumor mass).
T1	Tumor is 2 cm (¾ of an inch) or less across.
T2	Tumor is more than 2 cm but not more than 5 cm (2 inches) across.
T3	Tumor is more than 5 cm across.
T4	Tumor of any size growing into the chest wall or skin. This includes inflammatory breast cancer.

Nodal (N) Categories

NX	Nearby lymph nodes cannot be assessed (for example, removed previously).
N0	Cancer has not spread to nearby lymph nodes.
N1	Cancer has spread to 1–3 axillary (underarm) lymph node(s), and/or tiny amounts of cancer are found in internal mammary lymph nodes (those near the breast bone) on sentinel lymph node biopsy.
N2	Cancer has spread to 4–9 lymph nodes under the arm, or cancer has enlarged the internal mammary lymph nodes (either N2a or N2b, but not both).
N3	Any of the following:
N3a	*Either*: Cancer has spread to 10 or more axillary lymph nodes, with at least one area of cancer spread greater than 2 mm *Or*: Cancer has spread to the lymph nodes under the clavicle (collar bone), with at least one area of cancer spread greater than 2 mm.
N3b	*Either*: Cancer is found in at least one axillary lymph node (with at least one area of cancer spread greater than 2 mm) and has enlarged the internal mammary lymph nodes *Or*: Cancer involves 4 or more axillary lymph nodes (with at least one area of cancer spread greater than 2 mm), and tiny amounts of cancer are found in internal mammary lymph nodes on sentinel lymph node biopsy.
N3c	Cancer has spread to the lymph nodes above the clavicle with at least one area of cancer spread greater than 2 mm.

Metastasis (M)

MX	Presence of distant spread (metastasis) cannot be assessed.
M0	No distant spread is found on X-rays (or other imaging procedures) or by physical exam.
M1	Spread to distant organs is present. The most common sites are bone, lung, brain, and liver.

Staging

Stage 0	*Tis, N0, M0*: This is ductal carcinoma in situ (DCIS); lobular carcinoma in situ (LCIS) is sometimes also classified as stage 0 breast cancer. Paget's

disease of the nipple (without an underlying tumor mass) is also stage 0. In all cases the cancer has not spread to lymph nodes or distant sites.

Stage IA   *T1, N0, M0*: The tumor is 2 cm (about ¾ of an inch) or less across (T1) and has not spread to lymph nodes (N0) or distant sites (M0).

Stage IB   *T0 or T1, N1mi, M0*: The tumor is 2 cm or less across (or is not found) (T0 or T1) with micrometastases in 1–3 axillary lymph nodes (the cancer in the lymph nodes is greater than 0.2 mm across and/or more than 200 cells but is not larger than 2 mm) (N1mi).

Stage IIA   One of the following applies:
T0 or T1, N1 (but not N1mi), M0: The tumor is 2 cm or less across (or is not found) (T1 or T0) and *either*:
It has spread to 1–3 axillary lymph nodes, with the cancer in the lymph nodes larger than 2 mm across (N1a), *or*:
Tiny amounts of cancer are found in internal mammary lymph nodes on sentinel lymph node biopsy (N1b), *or*:
It has spread to 1-3 lymph nodes under the arm and to internal mammary lymph nodes (found on sentinel lymph node biopsy) (N1c).
Or: T2, N0, M0: The tumor is larger than 2 cm across and less than 5 cm (T2) but hasn't spread to the lymph nodes (N0).

Stage IIB   One of the following applies:
T2, N1, M0: larger than 2 cm and less than 5 cm across (T2). It has spread to 1–3 axillary lymph nodes and/or tiny amounts of cancer are found in internal mammary lymph nodes on sentinel lymph node biopsy (N1).
Or: T3, N0, M0: larger than 5 cm across but does not grow into the chest wall or skin and has not spread to lymph nodes (T3, N0).

Stage IIIA One of the following applies:
T0 to T2, N2, M0: less than 5 cm across (or cannot be found) (T0 to T2). It has spread to 4–9 axillary lymph nodes, or it has enlarged the internal mammary lymph nodes (N2).
Or: T3, N1 or N2, M0: larger than 5 cm across but does not grow into the chest wall or skin (T3). It has spread to 1–9 axillary nodes, or to internal mammary nodes (N1 or N2).

Stage IIIB *T4, N0 to N2, M0*: The tumor has grown into the chest wall or skin (T4), and one of the following applies:
It has not spread to the lymph nodes (N0).
It has spread to 1–3 axillary lymph nodes and/or tiny amounts of cancer are found in internal mammary lymph nodes on sentinel lymph node biopsy (N1).
It has spread to 4–9 axillary lymph nodes, or it has enlarged the internal mammary lymph nodes (N2).
Inflammatory breast cancer is classified as T4 and is stage IIIB unless it has spread to distant lymph nodes or organs, in which case it would be stage IV.

Stage IIIC *Any T, N3, M0*: The tumor is any size (or can't be found), and one of the following applies:
Cancer has spread to 10 or more axillary lymph nodes (N3).
Cancer has spread to the lymph nodes under the clavicle (collar bone) (N3).
Cancer has spread to the lymph nodes above the clavicle (N3).

Cancer involves axillary lymph nodes and has enlarged the internal mammary lymph nodes (N3).

Cancer has spread to 4 or more axillary lymph nodes, and tiny amounts of cancer are found in internal mammary lymph nodes on sentinel lymph node biopsy (N3).

Stage IV   *Any T, any N, M1:* The cancer can be any size (any T) and may or may not have spread to nearby lymph nodes (any N). It has spread to distant organs or to lymph nodes far from the breast (M1). The most common sites of spread are the bone, liver, brain, or lung.

Normal or Benign Lumps

✧ *Fibroadenoma*: If you have histologic proof of a fibroadenoma (FA), no further tests are required. The majority of FAs involute and have no increased cancerous potential. Some women prefer to have the lump removed for cosmetic reasons; however, this is at the expense of a scar, possible chronic pain, and the inherent risks of surgery. Other reasons for surgical removal are increasing size and discomfort, or pain. Due to the benign nature of this condition, patients can always be discharged from clinic and re-referred if symptoms do not improve.

✧ *Cysts*: After tests (ultrasound) confirm a simple cyst, no further treatment is required. A large dominant cyst that causes pain or infection may require aspiration. Aspiration is performed with a fine needle, and may be repeated. Cytology of aspirated fluid is not requested unless the fluid is blood-stained (possible intracystic carcinoma or papilloma) or the lump does not disappear after aspiration (possible necrotic cancer with cystic degeneration).

✧ *Benign breast change (BBC)*: BBC is normal. Once you have confirmed BBC, no further action is required.

✧ *Other benign lump (e.g. lipoma)* – If histologic assessment is benign, no further action is required.

Pain

The vast majority of breast pain complaints stem from benign conditions. Common causes include *cyclic mastalgia*, which is breast pain that is worse before menstruation and lessens when period flow begins; it is common in women <40 years old and is believed to be related to hormonal changes. *Non-cyclic pain (non-cyclic mastalgia)* is more common in women >40 years old and is more likely to be related to a fibroadenoma or cyst. These patients are usually best managed by diagnostic work-up and exclusion of cancer, followed by education and self-management of symptoms.

Masses that cause pain may be excised, but surgery is never an option for cyclic breast pain. Complementary therapies such as acupuncture, reflexology, and evening primrose oil have anecdotally been shown to help some women, but evidence for these therapies is scant. Certain medications that alter hormone cycles can be of help in cyclic breast pain if patient self-management fails. These include the OCP, danazol, bromocriptine, ramoxifen, and growth-hormone-releasing hormone (GHRH) analogues. These drugs have significant side effects and should never be recommended without consultation with the senior clinician and a careful and detailed risk–benefit discussion.

Other causes of breast pain to be aware of and include in your differential diagnosis are mastitis/breast sepsis, nursing, estrogen therapy, costochondritis, injury to chest wall, shingles, medications (digoxin, methyldopa, chlorpromazine, oxymetholone, aldactone), and breast cancer.

Nipple Inversion (of Benign/Congenital Origin)

Congenital nipple inversion is very common, usually caused by short lactiferous ducts. It can also occur with profound weight loss, breastfeeding, and breast trauma. Once cancer is ruled out as a cause, gentle manipulation may encourage the nipple to evert to allow breastfeeding. With severe inversion and duct fibrosis, breastfeeding may not be possible.

Cosmetic surgery is an option to correct nipple inversion, but this procedure usually requires division of the major lactiferous ducts, eliminating the possibility of breastfeeding.

Breast Sepsis

✧ *Mastitis*: Most common form of breast sepsis. Presents with pain, tenderness, erythema, swelling, and flu-like symptoms. The most likely causative organism is *Staphylococcus aureus*, with *S. epidermidis* and streptococci falling closely behind. Mastitis is most commonly associated with breastfeeding, where it is termed puerperal mastitis; it is more common in women with diabetes and other chronic illnesses.
✧ *Non-lactating infection*: Periductal mastitis, mammary duct fistula, infected cysts.
  ∝ Infected sebaceous cysts are common in the sternal and inframammary regions of the breast.
  ∝ Variations of hidradenitis suppurativa can be seen in the breast, especially around the nipple and axilla.
  ∝ Other rare causes of sepsis or breast inflammation need to be considered if the sepsis does not clear with appropriate antibiotic treatment. There may be diagnosis of exclusion (e.g. granulomatous mastitis).
✧ *Inflammatory breast carcinoma*: May present with the history and appearance of an acute breast infection/mastitis.
✧ *Periductal mastitis*: Affects young or middle-aged women who have a history of smoking, which damages the periareolar ducts. Infection of the damaged ducts causes inflammation with or without a mass (organisms responsible include enterococci, anaerobic streptococci, *Bacteroides* sp. and *S. aureus*).
✧ *Mammary duct fistula*: A communication between the skin and a major duct, usually in the periareolar region. This often follows a history of periductal mastitis with periareolar inflammatory mass which drains spontaneously. It is occasionally seen after a biopsy of an area of inflammation or incision and drainage of a non-puerperal abscess.

Treatment

If infection is suspected (erythema, warmth, pain, swelling, fever), it is justified to start antibiotic treatment based on clinical judgment and modify according to the results of later tests. If the patient appears septic, they may require admission for intravenous (IV) antibiotics (broad-spectrum or methicillin-resistant *S. aureus* (MRSA) coverage).
✧ *Abscess* – regardless of etiology, the majority may be treated in the clinic or emergency room with ultrasound-guided aspiration under local anesthetic. Overlying thinned or necrotic skin needs to be removed to allow free drainage of the cavity. Antibiotics should be administered. If the patient is currently breastfeeding, encourage manual expression of milk and/or feeding. Repeat aspirations every 24–48 hours as required. Surgery is indicated for refractory, large, or multiloculate abscesses.
✧ *Periductal mastitis* – antibiotic treatment with a penicillinase-resistant beta-lactam antibiotic is usually sufficient. If inflammation persists or anaerobes are cultured, the addition of metronidazole is helpful. If ultrasound demonstrates abscess, repeat aspiration is a better treatment option than incision and drainage, as the latter results in a mammary fistula in up to one-third of patients. Smoking cessation also reduces recurrence.

✧ *Mammary duct fistula* – treatment consists of antibiotics and surgical excision of affected ducts.

Follow-up

Follow-up is determined by the specific diagnosis and course of the condition. Periductal mastitis requires special attention, as it is difficult to treat and may have a relapsing course. Treatment for recurrent disease is surgical excision of the diseased duct system under antibiotic coverage. The cosmetic outcome can be very poor. Periductal mastitis usually resolves after menopause.

Male Breast Problems
Gynecomastia and Breast Cancer

More men are attending breast clinics because of:
✧ Increased awareness of male breast cancer – 1970 new cases (2010) per year, resulting in 390 deaths per year in the US.
✧ Distress at the appearance of gynecomastia.

Gynecomastia is a diffuse enlargement of the breast ductal/stromal tissue behind the male nipple, which often results in tenderness in the early stages of the process. This tissue becomes enlarged due to alterations in the male estrogen : testosterone ratio. Obesity accompanied by the deposition of fatty tissue in the pectoral region is commonly mistaken for gynecomastia.

The two most common causes of true gynecomastia are puberty and senescence. It is often asymmetric and may be either painful or painless. Other causes involve alterations in the estrogen : testosterone ratio, as mentioned above, resulting from use of antiandrogen drugs (cimetidine, digoxin, spironolactone), cirrhosis, malnutrition, primary or secondary hypogonadism, hyperthyroidism, renal disease, lung cancer, and testicular tumors.

History and Examination

Male breast patients require a complete general medical history, including a detailed drug, alcohol and smoking history. A full physical examination, including the genitalia, is mandatory. Male BC can mimic gynecomastia but usually presents with similar features to locally advanced female BC, i.e. an asymmetric lump with skin dimpling, nipple distortion, etc. The diagnosis of male BC is often more straightforward than in women, as there is no surrounding glandular tissue to cause diagnostic uncertainty, and men often do not present until a palpable lump is present due to the lack of mammographic screening.

Diagnostic Tests

Male BC is rare, especially in those aged less than 50 years with a negative family history. However, it does occur, and all patients should be approached with a high index of suspicion. If the physical exam and history trend toward the diagnosis, appropriate tests should be performed. Mammography is possible in the male breast. If tissue is required, core biopsy is the preferred technique as cytology can be misleading in the male breast.

Treatment

Male BC is staged and treated in a similar fashion to female BC.

Physiological gynecomastia requires no specific treatment other than explanation and reassurance. Cosmetic surgery for gynecomastia is an option, but patient expectations should be appropriately managed.

Breast Follow-up Clinics

The purpose of the three-stage breast-mass work-up is to exclude cancer and confirm a normal/benign breast, so as to allow prompt discharge from the breast clinic. Women with normal breasts do not require regular check-ups at the breast clinic. Before scheduling a follow-up visit, ask yourself why you want to bring this patient back. If you are not confident about the reliability of the results of the initial diagnostic tests, then go with your instincts: repeat tests or the performing of further tests to rule out cancer need to be expedited. If in doubt, discuss with a senior clinician.

As with everything, there are exceptions to the rules. A few examples are given below.

✧ Occasionally a patient with a cancer phobia may respond to a structured follow-up schedule over a few years, until her underlying fears have been addressed through counseling or other appropriate interventions.
✧ Women with high risk of BC, due either to a strong family history or a known genetic predisposition (BRCA 1/2, or other genetic syndromes), should be included in an aggressive high-risk screening program – the process will vary from clinic to clinic.
✧ Women with known cysts who get recurrent lumps may find that continued access to a breast clinic for limited exams can be useful.

The Post-operative "Results" Clinic

The format of a post-operative clinic visit may vary, but usually the surgeon and the breast care nurse are in attendance. Same-day follow-up with the breast oncologist can be a helpful addition if further treatment will be necessary.

Histology results are available, on average, between 7 and 14 days after surgery. Post-operative follow-up should be held, if possible, after the weekly MDM, when all of the necessary information has been discussed and a management plan is in place.

Patients can become distraught while awaiting results, especially if there is uncertainty about the diagnosis. Breast care nurses bear the brunt of this distress. Patients with benign lesions can be contacted by letter or phone to save them a journey or to relieve anxiety before the clinic appointment. However, there must be reliable mechanisms in place to ensure that this happens.

At the clinic:
✧ Examine the patient for possible complications of surgery before discussing the results.
✧ Once you have completed the examination, ask the patient to dress.
✧ Ensure the patient is comfortable and sitting next to their partner or a family member.
✧ Explain the results.
✧ It can be very helpful to have the breast care nurse present, especially if the information is complicated or the results indicate poor prognosis.
✧ *Never* give results while the patient is undressed or in the process of dressing.
✧ During the consultation, assess the patient's physical and emotional recovery.

Pain

Breast and axillary surgery is not painful; any pain is generally mild and controlled with simple analgesia. However, when present, neurogenic pain can be difficult to manage, so early involvement of a pain specialist is essential to prevent a chronic pain syndrome from developing.

✧ If pain has been difficult to control since surgery, consider nerve damage.
✧ If pain was mild but is getting worse, consider infection.
✧ Poor mobility can increase pain due to disuse atrophy and stiffness; if this occurs, consider intensive physical therapy.

Wound
✧ Infection occurs in 5–10% of breast surgery wounds. It is normally minor and self-limiting. Take swabs or aspirate fluid for culture, and prescribe antibiotics.
✧ Abscess formation is rare but needs prompt drainage in the clinic.
✧ Delayed hematoma may occur: the wound will be bulging and oozing blood. The clot should be evacuated; this can often be done in the clinic.

Seroma Formation
This is common after any breast and axillary surgery (>50%). It requires aspiration only if very large and uncomfortable (stretching the wound to dehiscence) or appears infected. Most seromas will reabsorb over a few weeks. If aspiration is required, use an aseptic technique. Insert the needle or trocar through the insensate scar for minimum patient discomfort.

Lymphedema
Early, very mild post-operative edema of the arm or breast is common after axillary node dissection, and improves as other routes for lymph flow are established.
    Cording (lymphatic thrombosis) is common and can be traced from the axilla, down the inner aspect of the arm, across the elbow to the wrist. It is self-limiting.

Nerve Damage
Intractable pain or hyperesthesia in the affected nerve distribution is often the clue to nerve damage. Physical therapy may help to lessen any disability.
✧ *Intercostal brachial nerve*: sensation altered for the inner aspect of the arm, axilla and posterior axillary fold.
✧ *Long thoracic nerve (serratus anterior muscle)*: may see winging of the scapula.
✧ *Thoracodorsal nerve (latissiumus dorsi muscle)*: wasted posterior axillary fold, difficulty with arm/shoulder abduction.

Shoulder Mobility
It is normal to have slightly restricted movement in the first few weeks after axillary surgery due to pain and scarring of the incision, but the importance of physical therapy exercises should be reinforced to prevent the development of a frozen shoulder as scar tissue starts to mature and contract. Early identification of potential shoulder problems and referral for intensive therapy is crucial to preventing long-term disability.

The Breast Oncology Clinic
Patients who have completed their cancer therapy are generally followed on a regular basis in the breast oncology clinic. In general, clinical follow-up is suggested every six months for the first three years and then yearly for five years. Patients should continue to have mammograms on a yearly basis.
    The value of routine clinical examination in detecting recurrent or new cancers is debatable, as most recurrences are detected through mammography or by the patient. It is clear that patients value follow-up consultations however, as they provide reassurance and the opportunity to discuss concerns and worries.

History – A Few Prompts
✧ How is the patient? How is their general health? How is life?
✧ Are they menstruating?
✧ Are they taking their prescribed anti-cancer treatment? Do they have any side effects?
✧ Have they noticed any new symptoms or breast changes?

Examination

Examination mainly focuses on checking for loco-regional recurrence, i.e. the breasts and nodal basin; but take general note of the patient's state of health – advanced metastatic disease is usually obvious.

✧ *Skin and chest wall* – local recurrence may present as scattered skin lesions in the vicinity of the previous surgery or on the chest wall.

✧ *Breasts* – local recurrence after breast-conserving surgery may be difficult to detect because of the fibrous changes that occur following surgery and radiotherapy. Contralateral cancers occur in 5% of patients.

✧ *Nodal basin* – axilla, infra- and supra-clavicular fossa, intramammary chain (sternal intercostal spaces).

✧ Other sites for clinical examination, such as the abdomen or chest, will be determined by the history.

Investigations

✧ If the patient is asymptomatic and well, routine follow-up investigations such as bone scan, chest X-ray (CXR) or tumor markers are *not* recommended.

✧ Suspected local recurrence needs to be proven; ideally with targeted imaging and histology. Systemic recurrence is mainly diagnosed on imaging studies, as histology can be difficult to obtain.

✧ On confirmation of recurrence, there is a need to restage the disease.

Treatment

Results are discussed at the MDM and the treatment plan is instituted: the details are beyond the scope of this handbook. When a patient relapses, it is a demoralizing experience and the patient's fears about dying will resurface. Most patients regard the diagnosis of recurrence as a greater psychological blow than the original diagnosis. It is important to be honest about the implications of relapse, especially if the patient has very advanced disease with poor prognosis. Considerable psychologic support will be needed, and time should be allocated during the clinic session to deal adequately with all these aspects.

✧ A local relapse may predict early systemic relapse, or it may indicate that the original local control attempt was inadequate and further treatment may still be curative.

✧ A systemic relapse indicates that the disease is not curable, and thus further treatment is designed to control and contain the disease. Despite this, second-line treatments can lead to remissions that are measured in terms of years, especially if the disease is bony rather than visceral. Newer monoclonal antibody and tyrosine–kinase inhibitor targeted therapies are offering extended remission.

Finally

✧ Never forget that your duty is to care for the patient to the best of your ability.

✧ Do not make decisions beyond your level of training or competence; if you are not sure, check and check again. A patient may pay a very high price for your uncertainty.

✧ Never be afraid to ask for help or advice; do not work in isolation, as you are a member of the MDT, and they are there to both train and support you.

Enjoy your time with the breast team. It will be a demanding, but rich and stimulating, professional and personal experience.

Primary Care Physician Guidelines
"Urgent" Referrals
<5% of breast cancers occur in women aged <40 years. Urgent referrals should be made for women:
- ✧ <35 years whose symptoms/signs are *highly* suggestive of breast cancer.
- ✧ >35 years and pre-menopause with any discrete lump that persists over a menstrual cycle.
- ✧ >35 years and post-menopause with any discrete lump.

1. Signs of Breast Cancer
- ✧ Lump with skin dimpling or ulceration.
- ✧ Nipple retraction (new), distortion, or ulceration (unilateral).
- ✧ Other: Change in skin contour, peau d'orange, dimpling, or fungating mass.

2. Lumps
- ✧ Discrete lump: any lump in a post-menopausal woman should warrant a high index of suspicion.
- ✧ Asymmetric, discrete, nodular lumps: especially those that are persistent and do not change with menstrual cycle.
- ✧ Post-menopausal abscess/infection: refer for urgent treatment and investigation.

3. Nipple Discharge
Multi-ductal or multicolored discharge is usually simple duct ectasia. Refer if:
- ✧ There is any post-menopausal discharge.
- ✧ Discharge is blood-stained (note that 85% of bloody nipple discharge is benign, e.g. intraductal papilloma).
- ✧ Discharge is persistent: single-duct discharge, especially if bloody.
- ✧ Discharge is excessive: sufficient to stain clothes (i.e. socially embarrassing).
- ✧ Discharge is unilateral.
- ✧ Discharge is spontaneous.

4. Pain
<5% of breast cancers present with pain and no lump. Refer if pain is:
- ✧ Associated with a lump (usually benign breast changes or cyst).
- ✧ Intractable (first try reassurance, a well-supporting bra, and dietary and lifestyle changes).
- ✧ Unilateral, and persistent (>3 months) in post-menopausal women.

Women who can be Managed by Primary Care Physician
- ✧ Recurrent cysts: PCP cyst aspiration should only be performed in women with proven cystic changes (following previous assessment at breast center). Always request cytology.
- ✧ The majority of women under 30 years of age, especially with cyclical, tender, lumpy breasts or symmetrical nodularity, with no focal or discrete abnormalities.
- ✧ The majority of breast pain.
- ✧ Most nipple discharge, especially if multi-duct/multicolored (as above).
- ✧ Negative family history: asymptomatic women with average risk.
- ✧ Simple lactational sepsis that responds to antibiotics.

Breast Screening Eligibility
Breast screening only suitable for *asymptomatic* women:

✧ Mammography recommended annually starting at age 40 years (American Cancer Society).

✧ Clinical breast examination annually starting at 20 years old. Note that breast self-examination monthly starting at age 20 has no *proven* survival benefit.

"High risk" patients in whom annual MRI would be recommended:

✧ Have a known BRCA1 or BRCA2 gene mutation.

✧ Have a first-degree relative (parent, brother, sister, or child) with a BRCA1 or BRCA2 gene mutation, and have not had genetic testing themselves.

✧ Have a lifetime risk of breast cancer of 20–25% or greater, according to risk assessment tools that are based mainly on family history (eg. BRACAPRO) (National Cancer Institute).

✧ Had radiation therapy to the chest when they were between the ages of 10 and 30 years.

✧ Have Li–Fraumeni syndrome, Cowden syndrome, or hereditary diffuse gastric cancer syndrome, or have one of these syndromes in first-degree relatives.

"Moderately increased" risk patients who should get yearly mammograms starting at age 30 (flexible):

✧ Have a lifetime risk of breast cancer of 15–20%, according to risk assessment tools that are based mainly on family history (National Cancer Institute).

✧ Have a personal history of breast cancer, ductal carcinoma in situ (DCIS), lobular carcinoma in situ (LCIS), atypical ductal hyperplasia (ADH), or atypical lobular hyperplasia (ALH); consider tamoxifen or raloxifene for risk reduction and referral to a high-risk clinic.

✧ Have extremely dense breasts or unevenly dense breasts when viewed by mammography (consider MRI).

Questions and Answers

Q1   Evaluation of gynecomastia should include:
    A   An assessment of medications.
    B   Questioning the patient about marijuana use.
    C   Examining the patient's testicles.
    D   A and B.
    E   All of the above.

A1   E: Medications and other substances, like marijuana, can cause gynecomastia. In addition, testicular examination is important as gynecomastia may be a symptom of testicular cancer.

Q2   Treatment of mastitis includes all of the following except:
    A   Antibiotics.
    B   Surgical incision and drainage.
    C   Mastectomy.
    D   Smoking cessation.
    E   Management of diabetes.

A2   C: Mastitis is treated with antibiotics, with incision and drainage for those that progress into abscess. Smoking and diabetes are factors that exacerbate mastitis, and control of these is important. However, mastitis is a benign condition, and mastectomy is not indicated.

Q3 All of the following may be used in the management of breast pain except:
  A   Anti-inflammatories.
  B   Evening primrose oil.
  C   Danazol.
  D   Venlafaxine.
  E   Bromocriptine.

A3 D: All of the above, with the exception of Venlafaxine, are known to help breast pain. Venlafaxine is a selective serotonin reuptake inhibitor (SSRI) type antidepressant, which has been used effectively in the management of hot flashes.

Q4 Bloody nipple discharge is most likely caused by:
  A   Invasive carcinoma.
  B   Intraductal carcinoma.
  C   Intraductal papilloma.
  D   Pituitary adenoma.
  E   Paget's disease.

A4 C: The most common cause of bloody nipple discharge is intraductal papilloma. Intraductal carcinoma (also known as ductal carcinoma in situ, DCIS) and invasive cancers account for 10–15% of bloody nipple discharge cases. Pituitary adenomas may cause nipple discharge, but this tends to be milky in color, and Paget's disease is more often characterized by an excoriation of the nipple rather than bloody nipple discharge, although both can occur.

Q5 Since the 1990s, which of the following statements describes trends related to breast cancer?
  A   Both the incidence and the mortality associated with breast cancer has declined.
  B   Incidence has increased, while mortality has declined.
  C   Incidence has decreased, while mortality has increased.
  D   Both the incidence and the mortality have increased.
  E   There are no consistent trends noted.

A5 A: The incidence of breast cancer has declined since 2000, largely thought to be related to the decline in the use of hormone replacement therapy. Mortality has also declined, in part due to screening and early detection, but also in part due to improved therapies.

Endocrine

Lynn S. Model and Julie Ann Sosa

The referral pattern of endocrine problems and neck masses is variable; endocrine problems may be seen initially by an internist, family practice physician, or endocrinologist who refers suitable cases for surgery; or may present directly to general surgical or specialist endocrine surgical clinics. At large academic medical centers, patients may have access to multidisciplinary endocrine clinics incorporating both medical physicians and surgeons. Neck masses also can be referred to otolaryngologists/head and neck surgeons, who may re-refer patients to an endocrine surgeon or handle the disease themselves. Given these diverse patterns of referral, the surgical trainee needs a working knowledge of endocrine conditions so that the patient is managed appropriately, regardless of whether there has been prior endocrinologic work-up.

Assessment of Endocrine Disorders

If a patient is referred with a mass near or in an endocrine gland, there are certain principles that should be followed:

✧ Make the endocrinologic diagnosis (which is often biochemical, based on laboratory tests).
✧ Specifically localize the tumor; biopsy if appropriate.
✧ Decide if the patient needs an operation.
✧ Decide what operation is appropriate.
✧ Ensure the patient is medically and physiologically safe for the proposed surgery, if necessary.

The manner in which these principles are applied depends to a large degree on the particular gland being assessed, and will be discussed later in the chapter in the gland-specific sections. Keep in mind that, at the first physician–patient interaction, a careful full history and physical examination is required for all patients, followed by targeted diagnostic and biochemical tests to elicit the correct endocrine diagnosis.

Endocrine History

The majority of endocrine problems are found in the thyroid and parathyroid glands, but adrenal and endocrine pancreas diseases can also occur. There is no single endocrine history; rather, symptoms vary widely according to the affected endocrine system. The objectives of each consultation are similar: to determine whether the mass in question is associated with an endocrine abnormality and/or with any other abnormalities, and whether the mass is benign or malignant.

Pituitary disorders will not be discussed in this chapter, and pancreatic endocrine lesions and the Zollinger–Ellison syndrome are described in the pancreatic chapter. The carcinoid syndrome is described in the chapter on small intestine disorders.

Endocrine Physical Examination

The physical examination is directed toward the specific endocrine system affected. An endocrine gland lesion may be associated with a mass, but may also have an associated endocrine syndrome that produces specific physical characteristics or effects, e.g. Cushing's syndrome. Endocrine masses are generally only palpable in the neck, as the pancreas and adrenal glands are found in an intra-abdominal or retroperitoneal location that is not generally amenable to palpation.

Tests for Endocrine Disorders

As with the history and the physical examination, diagnostic tests are targeted toward the endocrine gland in question. Laboratory tests can examine hormone levels in serum and/or urine, and help to assess tumor function. Imaging is used to localize a tumor and possibly determine the likelihood of malignancy, depending on tumor size, its relationship to neighboring structures, and lymph node involvement.

Tissue biopsy, usually in the form of fine-needle aspiration (FNA), may aid in diagnosis of malignant masses and direct the appropriate surgical approach. This is particularly important in the diagnosis of thyroid lesions.

Some of the specific diagnostic tests used in endocrine disease diagnosis will be described below.

Biochemical Tests

Serum Tests

Biochemical assays are available to determine the levels of most hormones in the serum as a measure of disease.

✧ Thyroid, parathyroid, adrenal, and gastrointestinal hormones all can be measured directly to determine their relative production rates.

Tumor markers are particularly useful in follow-up after total thyroidectomy, as they can act as an early warning of recurrence. They include:

✧ Thyroglobulin in differentiated thyroid cancer, including papillary, follicular, and Hürthle cell cancers.

✧ Calcitonin and carcinoembryonic antigen (CEA) in the case of medullary carcinoma of the thyroid.

Urinary Tests

✧ Particularly useful in patients with primary hyperparathyroidism: 24-hour urinary calcium excretion should be normal or elevated.

✧ Low excretion of calcium (<2 mmol/day) may indicate the rare condition of benign familial hypocalciuric hypercalcemia (BFHH), which can mimic hyperparathyroidism but which does not result in the clinical sequelae and complications of that disease.

✧ Functional adrenal tumors can be detected by excess adrenal hormone breakdown products in the urine, and/or urine electrolyte changes.

✧ Elevated 24-hour urinary catecholamines are indicative of pheochromocytoma; these include epinephrine, norepinephrine, metanephrines, normetanephrines, vanillyl-mandelic acid (VMA), and dopamine.

✧ Estimation of 24-hour urinary cortisol excretion is used in the assessment of Cushing's syndrome. This should be combined with a serum adrenocorticotropic hormone (ACTH) level to exclude Cushing's disease; alternatively, a low-dose dexamethasone suppression test can be employed.

✧ Conn's syndrome is associated with a low serum potassium and elevated excretion of potassium in the urine.

Provocative Tests

Often, standard laboratory measurement of serum hormone levels does not accurately identify the disease or the ectopic production of a hormone. Provocative tests involve administrating an agent which normally stimulates the production/release of the hormone in question. Subsequent to agent administration, serum levels are monitored to determine whether levels of the hormone rise in response to the stimulus.

For example, most ectopic sources of ACTH are not responsive to corticotrophin-releasing hormone (CRH), while most pituitary lesions are responsive to CRH. Administration of CRH produces a rise in serum ACTH if there is a pituitary source, but no rise if there is an ectopic source.

A provocative test also can be combined with selective venous sampling to localize the specific site of the lesion producing the hormone. For example, gastrinomas and other pancreatic endocrine tumors can be stimulated to release hormones by administration of calcium into the arterial supply. Selective venous sampling can then localize the tumor to the area of highest stimulated hormone excretion, even if no mass is visible on other imaging.

Immunology

✧ Antibodies to thyroid peroxidase (antithyroid microsomal antibodies) or thyroglobulin are found in most patients with Graves' disease and those with Hashimoto's thyroiditis.
✧ Thyrotrophin-receptor antibodies (TRAb) are found in almost all patients with Graves' disease.
✧ Other autoantibodies such as thyroid-stimulating antibodies (TSA) and thyroid-stimulating immunoglobulin (TSI) are found in many patients with endocrine disease.

Genetic Tests

These are mainly used to screen first- and second-degree relatives of patients with multiple endocrine neoplasia (MEN) syndrome. MEN 1 is caused by an abnormality on the long arm of chromosome 11, while MEN 2 shows an abnormality on chromosome 10. Referral to a medical genetics department is essential, and pre-test and post-test counseling is an important part of the process.

Fine-Needle Aspiration

Fine-needle aspiration (FNA) is simple, safe and the most cost-effective method of assessing a thyroid mass. Results are always interpreted in combination with the clinical and imaging assessments.

Reports (e.g. following the Bethesda system for thyroid classification from the National Cancer Institute) may use terms such as malignant, benign, suspicious for malignancy, atypia of undetermined significance (AUS), neoplasm, and non-diagnostic. Results depend on the experience of the person performing the technique and that of the cytologist interpreting the result. Generally, inadequate FNA means the test must be repeated, always with ultrasound guidance in order to optimize the biopsy.

FNA provides a tissue diagnosis, and in thyroid disease can accurately diagnose colloid nodules, thyroiditis, papillary carcinoma, medullary carcinoma, anaplastic carcinoma and lymphoma.

Small numbers of cells are obtained. Follicular lesions on cytology cannot be separated into follicular adenomas and carcinomas, and thus usually require excisional biopsy (thyroid lobectomy); histology is required to identify capsular or vascular invasion.

Imaging Techniques
Ultrasound

This noninvasive technique is reliable (most sensitive) for differentiating cystic and solid lesions. It can detect solid nodules as small as 3 mm and cystic nodules that are even smaller. FNA should be performed under ultrasound guidance for cytologic examination or cyst aspiration for cytology, and ultrasound is also a critical part of the localization of parathyroid tumors.

Ultrasound is operator dependent and can be performed by radiologists or surgeons. It usually cannot definitively distinguish between benign and malignant disease, although there may be findings suggestive of thyroid malignancy (e.g. hypoechoic, irregular borders, internal vascularity, microcalcifications). New endeavors to increase diagnostic yields include the use of contrast agents, such as microbubbles, and elastography.

Thyroid Radionucleotide Scan

The most common agents used are iodine ^{123}I and technetium pertechnate ^{99m}Tc.
✧ ^{99m}Tc has a short half-life (6 hours) and thus delivers a very low dose of radiation.
✧ ^{123}I also has a relatively short half-life (13.3 hours), and is more reliable in imaging some cancers that are iodine-avid.

The technique can differentiate hot (functioning) from cold (non-functioning) nodules, but overall has a very limited role in thyroid cancer diagnosis. One to four percent of hot nodules contain malignant tumor versus about 20% of cold nodules (with ^{123}I scan).

Gallium ^{67}Ga is useful in detecting lymphomas.

Occasionally, detection of metastases in patients after total thyroidectomy for medullary carcinoma of the thyroid can be aided using ^{99m}Tc–pentavalent dimercaptosuccinic acid (^{99m}Tc-DMSA), ^{111}In-octreotide or ^{99m}Tc–methoxyisobutylisonitrile (^{99m}Tc-MIBI). These techniques alone have not proven sufficiently sensitive or specific to make a diagnosis of malignancy, but taken together or with other modalities, a positive result increases the likelihood of disease.

Parathyroid Isotope Scan

^{99m}Tc–sestamibi is one of the tests of choice in the pre-operative localization of parathyroid tumors. Sestamibi accumulates in the mitochondria of parathyroid cells and has a favorable emission spectrum, improving the sensitivity of the technique.

Single photon emission computed tomography (SPECT) is also possible with this technique, allowing better spatial resolution.

Adrenal Isotope Scan

✧ ^{131}I–meta-iodobenzylguanidine (^{131}I-MIBG) is taken-up by catecholamine granules and is used mainly for localizing pheochromocytomas in the adrenal gland and in extra-adrenal sites.
✧ Multiple gland involvement can be found in MEN syndromes.
✧ Therapeutic doses of ^{131}I-MIBG can be used to treat some lesions.
✧ ^{131}I-MIBG is very specific for catecholamine tumors, although false negatives occur in 5–10% of scans.

Computed Tomography Scans

Computed tomography (CT) utilizes ionizing radiation.

In terms of thyroid pathology, CT is particularly useful in the assessment of large retrosternal goiters for determining the gland's relationship to other structures, and with the evaluation of advanced and metastatic thyroid cancers (e.g. medullary). Consideration must be given to the use of intravenous contrast in patients with differentiated thyroid cancer, as adjuvant radio-iodine treatment might need to be delayed to allow for the excretion of the iodine. Thyroid-cancer-related lymphadenopathy and invasion of surrounding structures can be evaluated using this method, although it is not sensitive for delineating intrathyroidal masses.

High-resolution four-dimensional CT (4D CT) is emerging as an excellent modality for localizing parathyroid pathology, although data are still limited to single-institution series.

CT is the preferred method for imaging the adrenal glands and associated lesions, especially when a specific adrenal protocol is employed with fine cuts through the adrenal glands. Iodine-containing intravenous contrast should not be administered until pheochromocytoma has been ruled out, as the contrast can incite a pheochromocytoma crisis.

Magnetic Resonance Imaging Scan

Magnetic resonance imaging (MRI) is particularly useful in detecting pituitary, adrenal, and pancreatic lesions, and detecting metastases. T2-weighted series, in particular, are helpful for evaluating pheochromocytomas.

Like CT, MRI can be used for the evaluation of thyroid cancers and their metastases, but generally CT is preferred. MRI can be helpful for the evaluation of medullary thyroid cancer metastases to the liver, which are often miliary in pattern.

MRI can be used for locating parathyroid glands, but is generally thought to be less accurate than ultrasound, sestamibi (with or without SPECT), and 4D CT.

Selective Venous Sampling

This is utilized (occasionally) in parathyroid, adrenal, pituitary, and pancreatic diagnoses. The femoral vein is cannulated, and vascular catheters inserted and manipulated under radiologic guidance until positioned correctly. Samples of blood are withdrawn from the catheter and from a peripheral vein simultaneously, and the serum concentrations of hormone compared. Sometimes an injection of a substance such as calcium (at the pancreas) is used to stimulate hormone release. Selective venous sampling is used in difficult or recurrent cases to identify the site and side of secretion of a particular hormone.

The technique is expensive, time-consuming and invasive and has small but definite morbidity and mortality rates, so is usually confined to use in remedial surgical patients and some specific adrenal cases. For example:

✧ Arteriography and venous sampling are employed for localization of parathyroid tumors in the remedial setting, with blood samples taken for parathyroid hormone levels. A small risk of stroke and of hematoma are associated with the procedure.

✧ Adrenal vein sampling is employed for lateralization of small adrenal tumors, such as aldosteronomas.

Neck Masses

There are four main types of neck masses: salivary gland masses, thyroid masses, enlarged lymph nodes, and non-thyroid masses. The majority of thyroid masses can be palpated in the region of the thyroid gland and move upon swallowing, while non-thyroid masses are usually in other locations and do not move upon swallowing. Differentiating non-thyroid masses from lymph nodes requires knowledge of their different characteristics, and these are described below. If you are unsure of the origin of any of these masses, especially recurrent lesions or extensive primary lesions, a high-resolution ultrasound or CT scan is extremely helpful in making the diagnosis and assessing the mass for potential resectability.

Non-Thyroid-Related Neck Masses
Lymphangiomas

Lymphangiomas are abnormal collections of lymph-filled tissue. They occur as:

✧ *Lymphangioma simplex* (one-third occur in the floor of the mouth, e.g. as a ranula).
✧ *Cystic hygroma.*
✧ *Cavernous lymphangioma* (mainly affects the tongue).

Smaller lymphangiomas tend to occur in the lips and cheek, where the tissue planes are tighter, whereas cystic hygroma has more room to expand in the tissue planes of the neck. Two-thirds of lymphangiomas are noted at birth, and 90% before the end of the second year of life. They usually transilluminate. Cystic hygromas can recur in adulthood at the margins of previous surgical excision.

Midline Dermoid Tumors
These masses are caused by elements of one dermal layer being trapped in another, either congenitally or by trauma.
✧ *Epidermoid cysts* contain cheesy contents of squamous epithelium only.
✧ *True dermoid cysts* contain squamous epithelium and skin appendages, such as hair.
✧ *Teratoid cysts* contain endodermal, mesodermal and ectodermal elements, such as nails, teeth, brain, etc.

They tend to present as solid or cystic masses in the midline of the neck or lateral to the submandibular glands. Painless swelling is the only symptom, usually presenting in the second to third decades of life.

Thyroglossal Duct Cysts
These are a remnant from the descent of the thyroid from the base of the tongue, and can occur anywhere from the foramen cecum to the manubrial notch. They are found in patients aged 4.5 to 70 years; mean age at presentation is 5 years.

History
Most patients complain of a painless cystic mass. Some present with tenderness and rapidly increasing size due to infection, while others present with a fistula discharging fluid.

Examination
The mass is mobile, usually transilluminates, and moves on swallowing or protruding the tongue. The majority are midline, but 10–25% may be deviated to one side (usually the left). Suprahyoid cysts may be mistaken for submental adenitis or a dermoid cyst. Prehyoid cysts tend to be dumbbell- or bar-shaped, and if large, can push the tongue upwards causing dysarthria.

Diagnosis
This is usually a clinical diagnosis; in doubtful cases, ultrasound will confirm the cystic nature of the mass. FNA is usually unnecessary and can introduce infection, but may help in difficult cases.

Treatment
These cysts are prone to recurrent infection and are best treated by complete surgical excision along with the middle of the hyoid bone (Sistrunk procedure).

Follow-up
Patient should be seen at short intervals (1–4 weeks) until diagnosis is obtained. Arrange surgical excision promptly to prevent further episodes of infection.

Post-operative Follow-up

Review histology to confirm diagnosis and exclude the extremely rare thyroglossal duct carcinoma (see below). Examine for general complications of neck surgery (wound infection, abscess, nerve injury).

The most common specific complication is a thyroglossal fistula, which results from infection or failure to remove the whole cyst. It usually presents as an opening in the lower neck, discharging clear fluid. Treatment is further surgical excision.

Thyroglossal duct carcinoma: This is ectopic thyroid tissue with carcinoma, and while rare it should be excluded. It is always papillary. In 10% there are metastases. Treatment is local excision, thyroidectomy, radio-iodine therapy, and suppressive doses of levothyroxine.

Lingual Thyroid

A lingual thyroid results when an embryologic remnant of the thyroid fails to descend to the normal position in the neck. They may be asymptomatic and remain unnoticed unless enlargement of the thyroid tissue occurs. The lingual thyroid may be the patient's only thyroid tissue, so excision may render the patient hypothyroid or athyroid.

History

Patients may complain of a mass at the back of the tongue, respiratory or swallowing difficulties.

Examination

May be normal, or naso-oro-pharyngeal examination reveals the swelling.

Diagnosis

The diagnostic test is ^{123}I scan, which differentiates lingual thyroid from other causes.

Treatment

It is possible to shrink a simple enlarged lingual thyroid with thyroxine therapy. If this fails, therapeutic radioactive iodine (^{131}I) should be used. There is seldom any need to resort to surgery, unless cancer is found in the mass.

Follow-up

Follow-up is at short intervals (1–4 weeks) until diagnosis is obtained and relief of symptoms is achieved. Subsequently, intervals are increased (1–6 months) until the condition is stable and the patient is symptom-free.

Monitor thyroid function tests to ensure adequate T4 replacement and TSH suppression. The patient may then be discharged from the clinic, with advice to return if symptoms recur and for the primary care physician (PCP) to monitor thyroid function tests.

Branchial Cleft Cysts

These are thought to be remnants from non-obliterated embryonic branchial clefts. The cyst walls contain squamous or columnar epithelium, often with lymphoid infiltration, and may also contain cellular debris as well. The age range is 1–70 years, but symptomatology often occurs in early adulthood. The majority of cysts occur on the left side and appear anterior to the sternocleidomastoid muscle in the upper third of the neck.

History

Most patients complain of a continuous swelling or pressure sensation, although in some patients the swelling can be intermittent. Pain affects up to one-third of patients, but infection occurs in less than 15%.

Examination
Most feel smooth and cyst-like on palpation but do not transilluminate; approximately one-third are solid. They tend not to have any attached sinus or fistula track, as branchial fistulas are a separate condition.

Branchial fistulas extend from an internal opening in the tonsillar bed, through the carotid artery bifurcation to an external opening in the lower part of the anterior triangle of the neck. Sinuses have similar external openings but no internal ones. Fibrous tracts also can occur in these locations.

Diagnosis
CT/MRI may be needed to differentiate these cysts from a carotid body tumor if there is direct or transmitted pulsation and the lesion feels solid. If no pulsation is present, FNA can be performed and will reveal aspirates rich in cholesterol.

Treatment
Optimal treatment consists of primary excisional surgery, with stepladder incisions to dissect out affected tract. Surgical incision and drainage and/or antibiotic treatment for abscess or infection prior to definitive management is recommended.

Follow-up
Patients should be evaluated with complete diagnostic tests (within 1–2 months) and a decision then made on definitive management.

Post-operative Follow-up
Review the results of specimen histology (rarely, this may contain squamous carcinoma) to confirm the diagnosis. Examine for general complications of operation. Patients with uncomplicated cyst removal without signs of wound infection can be discharged from the clinic. If there is doubt about complete excision, patients are seen at 3- to 6-month intervals, as recurrence usually occurs within the first year.

Laryngocele
This is a rare air-containing sac arising from the laryngeal saccule that communicates with the larynx. It is congenital or results from prolonged, increased intralaryngeal pressure or, occasionally, trauma.

Incidence is 1 in 2.5 million people per year, with a male to female ratio of 5 : 1. Peak incidence is between 50 and 60 years of age. The laryngocele may be external, presenting through the thyrohyoid membrane, or internal (within the larynx). The most important causative factor to exclude is a coexistent carcinoma of the larynx.

History
Hoarseness, lateral neck swelling, stridor, dysphagia, sore throat, pain, cough. Ten percent become infected.

Examination
There is a large swelling over the thyrohyoid membrane which can easily be compressed. If infected, it can present as cervical inflammation – do not compress these.

Diagnosis
Soft-tissue neck X-ray shows an air-filled sac; CT can better elucidate the location in relationship to neighboring structures.

Treatment
Surgical excision; try to avoid emptying the sac before it is identified. Surgery is often handled by otolaryngology.

Follow-up
Review diagnostic test results. Once cancer is excluded, arrange excision if the patient is a suitable candidate for surgery.

Post-operative Follow-up
Histology should be reviewed and the patient examined to detect any general surgical complications, e.g. wound infection. Reassure and discharge from the clinic if the case is uncomplicated.

Carotid Body Tumors (Paragangliomas)
These are tumors of neural crest tissue that occur in the carotid body, the jugular bulb and the ganglion nodosum of the vagus nerve in the neck. *Carotid body tumors (see also Chapter 10, p. 305)* are rare, occuring in patients aged 35–50 years. Five percent are bilateral; 10% are malignant. There is a strong family history and they may be associated with pheochromocytomas.

Note that *glomus tumor (or glomus vagale tumor)*, a paraganglioma, is a rare cause of a mass at the angle of the jaw. Angiography may show abnormal circulation from the external carotid artery.

History
Long history of a painless mass (typically 4–7 years). Other symptoms include headache, neck pain, dizziness, hoarse voice and dysphagia caused by local invasion or cranial nerve compression. Occasionally, flushing, arrhythmias and hypertension are caused by neuroendocrine secretion by the tumor.

Examination
There is a mass up to 4–5 cm in size that moves laterally but not vertically. It exhibits a transmitted but not an expansile pulse. Bruit may be present and may reduce with carotid compression. Large tumors may involve cranial nerves IX, X, XI, and XII, and occasionally the sympathetic chain, causing an ipsilateral Horner's syndrome.

Diagnostic Tests
Duplex ultrasound and angiography show a splayed bifurcation and a "tumor blush" circulation. There may be a feeding vessel from the external carotid or vertebral artery. CT/MRI may be useful, especially if local invasion is suspected, to define the relationship of the tumor to other neighboring structures. Exclude bilateral tumors and pheochromocytoma.

Treatment
Surgical excision by an experienced vascular surgeon, since vascular reconstruction is usually required.

Follow-up
Patients should be seen at short intervals (1–3 weeks) until diagnosis is obtained.

Post-operative Follow-up
Review histology to confirm the diagnosis and the complete excision of the tumor. Patients should be examined to detect any complications of wound healing. Arrange for genetic counseling and screening if there is a strong family history suggestive of MEN or another genetic syndrome.

Enlarged Neck Lymph Nodes
The first objective is to determine whether the enlarged lymph node is due to a localized problem in the head and neck, or is part of a generalized lymphadenopathy. If the cause is localized to the head and neck, the second objective is to determine whether the cause of enlargement is non-malignant (e.g. acute or chronic infection) or malignant (i.e. metastatic from a head and neck carcinoma). Any patient over the age of 50 years presenting with a single enlarged lymph node in the upper part of the neck must have a full examination of the naso-, oro- and hypopharynx before biopsy of the neck node to exclude occult carcinoma in these areas.

History
Ask about local head and neck symptoms, nasal symptoms, voice change, cough, hoarseness, and dysphagia. Ask about recent bouts of sore throat or tonsillitis, which may have given rise to enlarged nodes in local drainage areas. Specific symptoms to ask about include weight loss, respiratory symptoms, abdominal/gastrointestinal (GI) symptoms, and night sweats.

Examination
Examine the mass, noting size, consistency, mobility, whether matted, etc. Try to determine whether the node is isolated or part of a generalized nodal enlargement.
   Site the node in one of the anatomical triangles of the neck:
✧ The *anterior triangle* is formed by the midline of the neck, the anterior border of sternocleidomastoid muscle, and the lower margin of the mandible.
✧ The *posterior triangle* is formed by the posterior border of the sternocleidomastoid, the anterior border of trapezius, and the upper border of the clavicle.

A thorough examination needs to be performed of the mouth, naso-, oro-, and hypopharynx.
   A thorough investigation should also be performed of the thyroid in particular, as well as the skin of the face and scalp (melanoma), breast, lung, abdomen (including spleen and liver), and upper extremities, as these are possible sites of primary tumors. This is especially true for enlarged nodes in the (left) supraclavicular fossa (Virchow's node).
   All other lymph node sites need to be examined (axillae, groins, mediastinum, and abdomen).

Diagnostic Tests
Laboratory tests should include fecal occult blood test (FOBT), complete blood count (CBC) (hematologic abnormalities), erythrocyte sedimentation rate (ESR), and monospot (mononucleosis).
   Perform FNA of a non-pulsatile mass for cytology. If lymphoma is a possibility in the differential diagnosis, ask the laboratory for advice regarding the transport of specimens for tumor markers and flow cytometry.

Imaging with ultrasonography is useful for the differentiation of solid and cystic masses, and for the diagnosis of vascular masses such as carotid artery aneurysms or carotid body tumors. FNA is also useful for potentially infected masses or lymph nodes; thus, a sample should also be sent for microbiology. If tuberculosis (TB) is suspected, a sample should be sent for Ziehl–Neelsen (ZN) stain and culture.

If above tests are non-diagnostic, core needle biopsy can be helpful, along with incisional versus excisional lymph node biopsy for the purposes of formal histology.

If no primary can be found in the head and neck for a malignant lymph node, then the search has to be continued into the chest and abdomen. A chest X-ray may indicate a bronchial neoplasm, TB or hilar/mediastinal pathology. Assessment of the gastrointestinal tract by upper and lower GI endoscopy may be indicated. Consider ultrasound of the abdomen or CT of the abdomen and retroperitoneum, and breast mammography for breast neoplasms.

Treatment

Management depends on the results of diagnostic tests.
- ✧ In children and young adults, once lymphoma has been excluded the causes are usually related to infectious episodes.
- ✧ Management of tubercular lymph nodes is the relevant chemotherapy and referral to an infectious disease specialist.
- ✧ For cases related to generalized lymphadenopathy (e.g. lymphoma/leukemia, mononucleosis, human immunodeficiency virus [HIV], sarcoidosis, Wegener's granulomatosis, etc.), management is of the underlying condition.
- ✧ For a single malignant lymph node presenting in the neck, a primary tumor will be found on examination in approximately one-third of cases. The primary sites in order of frequency are: nasopharynx, tonsil, base of tongue, thyroid gland, supraglottic larynx, floor of mouth, palate, pyriform fossa, bronchus, esophagus, breast, and stomach, although this will depend on the age and gender of the patient as well as on history of exposure.
- ✧ In a further third of patients, no primary is evident at the time of presentation but becomes apparent on follow-up in the following sites: oropharynx, nasopharynx, thyroid, hypopharynx, lung, abdomen, and miscellaneous (10%).
- ✧ For head and neck cancers, treatment is of the primary lesion with en bloc dissection of the relevant lymph node field, as indicated. If excisional biopsy is necessary, this should be performed by the surgeon who would perform the definitive head and neck surgery. FNA or core biopsy generally can avoid the need for surgical excision.

Follow-up

Follow-up intervals should be short until cancer has been excluded or the primary site identified.

Post-operative Follow-up

Patient should be seen 1–2 weeks after surgery, with the results of histology so that further treatment/oncology referral can be arranged if appropriate. Complications to look for include wound infection, abscess, seroma, and cranial nerve injury.

If lymph node resection reveals TB infection, refer to an infectious disease specialist.

Persistent lymph leak can occur, especially if the lymph node was neoplastic. Most will scar down over 4–6 weeks. Some persistent or copious leaks may be associated with neoplastic lymphatic obstruction, which may respond to local radiotherapy. Care should be taken to tie off lymphatics and to identify and formally ligate the thoracic duct on the left. If a lymphocele develops (based on identification of a high triglyceride content on drainage), a low-fat diet or NPO status can be employed to reduce ouput.

Salivary Gland Masses
Causes of salivary gland enlargement are divided into:
✧ *Enlargement of more than one gland* (mumps, echo, coxsackie viruses, Sjögren's).
✧ *Generalized enlargement of one gland* (sialectasis).
✧ *Localized enlargement of part of one gland*:
    ∝ Benign tumors – pleomorphic adenomas, monomorphic adenomas (Warthin's), oncocytoma
    ∝ Malignant tumors – adenoid cystic carcinoma, adenocarcinoma, squamous carcinoma, malignant pleomorphic adenoma
    ∝ Potentially malignant tumors – mucoepidermoid, acinic cell (rare).

Twenty percent of parotid tumors are malignant; 45% of submandibular tumors are malignant; 65% of minor salivary gland tumors are malignant.

History
✧ Age: mumps is more common in children, but if it occurs twice it is likely to be congenital sialectasis.
✧ Does the swelling affect one gland or more? Tumors are usually unilateral (Warthin's is occasionally bilateral).
✧ Is swelling related to eating? If so, consider calculous disease secondary to sialectasis.
✧ Pain is generally due to duct obstruction from calculous disease. Occasionally, adenoid cystic carcinoma with nerve involvement will be the cause of pain.
✧ Systemic disorders which can cause painless salivary gland enlargement include myxedema, diabetes, Cushing's, cirrhosis, gout, alcohol abuse, sarcoidosis, and TB.
✧ Certain drugs, such as thiouracil and high-estrogen pills, may be causes.

Examination
Examine all salivary glands.
✧ Is only one gland affected, or more than one?
✧ Is enlargement due to a localized mass within the gland or a generalized enlargement of the gland?
✧ Is there skin involvement? Is there facial muscle weakness?
✧ Is the lesion solid or cystic? Is the lesion irregular with regard to its borders and relationship to neighboring structures? (Benign pleomorphic adenomas are often irregular.)
✧ Is it fixed or mobile? Benign tumors are usually mobile.

Diagnostic Tests
If indicated by the absence of a discrete mass, laboratory tests should include those to exclude myxedema, diabetes, Cushing's, and rheumatoid arthritis. If sarcoidosis is suspected, a biopsy is needed. FOBT and ESR should be performed.

Plain X-rays: If calculous disease is suspected, intraoral films may be required. Parotid stones are radiolucent, while submandibular stones are radiopaque.

Sialography (cannulation of the salivary duct and injection of contrast) is useful for a diagnosis of sialectasis. Congenital saccular sialectasis gives a "snowstorm" appearance. Advanced cystic disease shows large collections of dye. Pure duct stenosis is nearly always an iatrogenic artifact caused by traumatic cannulation.

CT is useful for determining the extent of spread of malignant salivary tumors and for planning the surgical approach.

FNA for cytology is mandatory in every case. Avoid excisional biopsies unless there is diffuse enlargement of the gland and no diagnosis has been reached by other methods.

Diagnosis of minor salivary gland tumors is by incisional biopsy performed by the surgeon who will eventually remove the lesion.

Treatment

✧ *Benign parotid tumors* are treated by superficial parotidectomy if the tumor is located in the superficial part of the gland, which occurs in 80% of cases.

✧ *Benign submandibular tumors* are rare, and treatment is removal of the whole gland.

✧ *Minor salivary gland tumors* are diagnosed by incisional biopsy and then excised.

✧ *Malignant parotid tumors* are treated by total parotidectomy. If the facial nerve is involved this is also excised, and a decision made at operation regarding nerve grafting. If neck nodes are palpable, total parotidectomy is combined with a radical neck dissection. Post-operatively, radiotherapy is given if resection margins are in doubt.

✧ *Malignant submandibular tumors* are treated by excision of the gland and, if necessary, the mandible, skin, and adjacent nerves. Reconstruction is possible. Post-operative radiotherapy is recommended if resection margins are microscopically positive or concerning.

✧ *Malignant minor salivary gland tumors* are treated by wide excision and reconstruction of the oral cavity.

✧ *Mucoepidermoid and acinic cell tumors* are often diagnosed on post-operative histology after excision of an apparently benign mass. Tumors are graded as either high grade or low grade, and prognosis is determined by the grade. Low grade has 90% five-year survival; high grade 20% five-year survival. Many surgeons give immediate post-operative radiotherapy. Some surgeons prefer to follow up patients monthly/bi-monthly for 4–5 years to detect recurrence and then treat by wide field excision and post-operative radiotherapy. Refer for an oncology opinion in every case.

✧ *Sialectasis* with mild/infrequent symptoms – advise finishing each meal with a citrus drink and massaging the duct to expel debris from it. Many patients have no further trouble after the diagnostic sialogram, which flushes the ducts.

✧ *Submandibular stones* – duct stones are treated by surgical removal via the intraoral route and duct marsupialization; stones in the body of the gland are treated by removal of the whole gland.

✧ *Parotid duct stones* are removed intraorally. Persistent severe symptoms are treated by total parotidectomy (superficial parotidectomy is often insufficient).

Follow-up

✧ Follow-up intervals are short (1–2 weeks) until cancer has been excluded.

✧ Generalized causes of salivary gland enlargement are referred to the relevant specialist otolaryngology/head and neck surgery.

✧ Mild sialectasis can be discharged with the relevant treatment advice and a plan to return if symptoms progress. Patients with more severe cases can be seen at 3-month intervals, or prn when symptoms return, until the patient and surgeon feel that surgery is indicated.

Post-operative Follow-up:

The success of surgery is determined by histology, healing of the wound and absence of complications. Review the histology report to ensure that presumed benign conditions were indeed benign. If the operation was performed for malignant disease, confirm that the resection margins were clear of the tumor. If not, or if the resection margins were very close to the tumor, refer for an oncology opinion regarding radiotherapy.

Complications of Parotidectomy
✧ *Frey's syndrome* consists of discomfort, sweating, and redness of the skin over the parotid area, during and after eating. This is caused when the severed ends of parasympathetic secretomotor nerve fibers in scar tissue are stimulated and cause vasodilatation and sweating. Spontaneous resolution within 6 months is usual. Treatment for severe persistent cases is an ipsilateral tympanic neurectomy to divide the parasympathetic pathways.
✧ *Facial nerve injury* causes facial muscle weakness; it may respond to rehabilitation. Occasionally tarsorrhaphy, fascial sling procedures, nerve grafting, or a unilateral face lift are required.
✧ *Salivary fistula* tends to occur where a sialectatic deep lobe is left in situ with a cut surface. Most cases resolve with time. Anticholinergic drugs may help, as may radiotherapy for persistent cases. Alternatively, further surgery to remove the deep lobe is indicated.

Thyroid Masses
Causes of thyroid disease can be divided into: diffuse enlargement of the thyroid gland such as physiologic goiter (pregnancy, menarche); endemic goiter (iodine deficiency, Derbyshire neck); sporadic goiter (goitrogens, e.g. cabbage, p-aminosalicylic acid (PAS), and lithium drugs); bleeding into a pre-existing pathology; autoimmune (Graves' disease, Hashimoto's thyroiditis); and focal masses in the thyroid (non-toxic nodular goiters, adenomas, carcinomas, and lymphomas).

History
History of the presence of the mass and of thyroid symptoms are required. Most patients give a history of painless enlargement. Ask about:
✧ Rate of growth and whether there has been sudden recent enlargement.
✧ Hyperthyroid symptoms – diaphoresis, palpitations, heat intolerance, menstrual irregularities, weight loss, anxiety, diarrhea, muscle weakness, tremulousness.
✧ Hypothyroid symptoms – fatigue, weakness, weight gain, constipation, cold intolerance, depression.
✧ Pain – painful enlargement of the gland may indicate Hashimoto's thyroiditis.
✧ Voice change.
✧ Symptoms of tracheal compression (inspiratory stridor).
✧ Dysphagia.
✧ Anterior neck pressure or dyspnea, particularly when lying flat.

Examination
Examination of the Mass
✧ Inspect to see if the enlargement is visible and, if so, whether it moves on swallowing or protrusion of the tongue.
✧ Palpate to determine firmness, and whether the whole gland is enlarged or just part of it. Is the enlargement confined to one lobe?
✧ Does the gland feel regular (Graves' disease) or irregular (nodular goiter)?
✧ Are nearby draining lymph nodes enlarged?

Thyroid swelling that is firm to palpation, either diffusely or unilaterally in a post-menopausal female, usually raises the suspicion of Hashimoto's.

Undifferentiated and poorly differentiated thyroid cancers, primary thyroid lymphoma, and medullary cancers can present with a rapidly enlarging neck mass involving other neck structures (e.g. recurrent laryngeal nerve). Laryngoscopy may be required if recurrent laryngeal nerve palsy is suspected, or if the patient has a history of prior anterior neck surgery, including thyroidectomy, parathyroidectomy, anterior cervical fusion, or cardiac/thoracic surgery.

Examination of the Thyroid Status
✧ Overactivity is indicated by hand tremor, palmar sweating, restlessness, tachycardia, brisk reflexes, and a thrill/bruit over a hypervascular thyroid gland.
✧ Underactivity is indicated by slow pulse, hoarse voice, and slow-relaxing tendon reflexes.
✧ Features of severe Graves' disease may include exophthalmos, lid lag, lid retraction, and pretibial myxedema.

Destruction of the thyroid tissue by the autoimmune process in Hashimoto's thyroiditis usually renders patients hypothyroid eventually, although they may be thyrotoxic in the early stages.

Diagnostic Tests
✧ As with masses in other body sites, thyroid masses should undergo clinical assessment combined with imaging and FNA cytology, and biochemical assessment of thyroid status (in this case T4, T3, and TSH; TSH is probably the single best biochemical marker of hyperthyroidism).
✧ Thyroglobulin is available as a tumor marker for differentiated thyroid cancers (e.g. papillary, follicular, and Hürthle cell cancers), but is only of use after total thyroidectomy with or without radio-iodine, when it should fall to undetectable levels in the absence of metastases.
✧ Ultrasound examination of the thyroid will determine whether the primary mass is solid or cystic, and whether the mass is single (suspicious) or multiple (e.g. part of a multinodular goiter). Papillary thyroid cancer is multifocal in 25–75% of patients. Size, echogenicity, vascularity, borders, and extension are important criteria for determining whether the lesion is likely to be malignant.
✧ ^{123}I isotope scanning can identify thyroid tissue and determine whether nodules are hot or cold, but this is rarely useful except in the hyperthyroid patient (i.e. to determine whether the patient has Graves' disease or a toxic adenoma/multinodular goiter).
✧ CT (or MRI) of the neck and upper chest can identify size, local extension/invasion of a mass, and tracheal deviation; however, delivery of intravenous contrast implies an iodine load that can delay the delivery of radio-iodine in the adjuvant setting.
✧ FNA for cytology should be performed in every case of a thyroid nodule that is suspicious in appearance or over 1–1.5 cm in size.
✧ If medullary carcinoma is suspected, serum calcitonin and CEA levels are usually high and can be used as a tumor marker. These stains also should be ordered to facilitate pathologic examination of the biopsy. A rise in levels after treatment may indicate recurrence.
✧ If medullary thyroid carcinoma is confirmed, patients should be screened for coexisting parathyroid adenoma (calcium, phosphate, and serum intact parathyroid hormone [iPTH]) and pheochromocytoma (24-hour urinary catecholamine levels), and undergo

genetic testing for the rearranged-during-transfection (RET) proto-oncogene.
✧ Thyroid autoantibody tests are performed if Hashimoto's thyroiditis is suspected, and also can confirm a diagnosis of Graves' disease.

Specific Test Results
✧ *Diffusely enlarged gland, euthyroid* – physiologic and endemic goiter.
✧ *Diffusely enlarged gland, hyperthyroid* – Graves' disease. The early stages of Hashimoto's may also give this appearance, but this is rare. In contrast to Graves', Hashimoto's does not demonstrate increased uptake on a radio-isotope scan.
✧ *Focally enlarged gland, euthyroid* – diagnosis includes simple cysts, a single dominant nodule in a multinodular goiter, benign adenomas, and malignant tumors. Malignant tumors can be classified as papillary, follicular, Hürthle cell, medullary, poorly differentiated, and anaplastic thyroid cancers. FNA cannot differentiate between follicular adenomas and carcinomas, as this depends on the histologic identification of vascular and/or capsular invasion. Therefore, follicular neoplasms should be regarded as potentially malignant (generally 20–25%).
✧ *Focally enlarged gland, hyperthyroid* – thyrotoxic adenoma, thyrotoxic nodule in a multinodular goiter.

Treatment
All suspicious and malignant masses require surgical excision. Cystic masses (sometimes seen with papillary thyroid cancers), which are identified as malignant, are >4 cm in size (due to concern about sampling error), contain blood, or recur after two to three aspirations, also require surgery. Most retrosternal or substernal goiters require surgery due to the inability to monitor them for malignancy using FNA. Practice guidelines from many professional/specialty societies and associations now exist to guide diagnosis, treatment, and surveillance practice. Referral should be made to a high-volume surgeon, as surgeon experience is closely associated with patient outcome.

Benign Masses
✧ *Benign cysts* should be aspirated and reviewed at 6 weeks. This can be repeated on two to three occasions. If cyst recurs after two aspirations, excision is required as recurrence is inevitable. If there is no recurrence, the patient should be seen at 6 months and then as required for any concern regarding recurrence of symptoms, or can be followed up by the PCP.
✧ *Solitary thyroid nodule, euthyroid, benign* – surgery is only required for treatment of compression symptoms or because of patient preference. FNA is repeated once or twice over the next 12 months and, if there is no change in cytology, the patient can then be discharged from the clinic.
✧ *Solitary thyroid nodule, hyperthyroid, benign* – if <3 cm in size, this can be treated by radio-iodine or surgery; if >3 cm, surgical excision is favored.
✧ *Multinodular goiter, euthyroid* – if there is no dominant nodule and no compressive symptoms are present, patients should be observed for 12–18 months and then discharged with the recommendation to return if new symptoms develop, and to follow up regularly with their PCP or endocrinologist. Surgery is usually indicated for very large lesions or if the patient is worried by the cosmetic appearance and they are a good surgical candidate.
✧ *Multinodular goiter, euthyroid, dominant nodule* – if nodule is benign on FNA and there are no pressure symptoms, regular observation is acceptable. If the dominant nodule is suspicious or malignant, then surgery is indicated.

✧ *Multinodular goiter, hyperthyroid* – small glands can be treated with antithyroid medications, ^{131}I, or surgery; large glands are treated with anti-thyroid drugs and surgery.

Malignant Thyroid Tumors

These can be classified as papillary, follicular, Hürthle cell, medullary, poorly differentiated, anaplastic thyroid cancer, or primary thyroid lymphoma.

✧ *Differentiated thyroid cancer* (papillary, follicular, and Hürthle cell) – prognosis is determined by stage, and is worse if there is a history of prior neck irradiation. The American Joint Commission on Cancer (AJCC, 7th edition) upstages patients at the age of 45 years, because older patients tend to experience more aggressive disease.

  ∝ Treatment generally consists of near-total or total thyroidectomy. Papillary thyroid cancer is frequently multifocal on final histology, and this approach is associated with decreased rates of local recurrence and improved survival, and allows post-operative treatment with ^{131}I and monitoring of thyroglobulin levels. Hürthle cell cancer is less responsive to radio-iodine, but this treatment should still be given to the minority of patients who do respond.

  ∝ The role of prophylactic central (level 6) lymph node dissection is controversial for patients with clinical N0 disease.

  ∝ Locally enlarged lymph nodes also should be excised, followed by radio-iodine ablation and suppressive doses of levothyroxine. Lateral compartment neck dissection consists of compartmental extirpation of lymph nodes in levels 2, 3, 4, and 5 with a modified radical neck dissection.

  ∝ The patient is then monitored for recurrence using ultrasound, uptake scans, and measurement of thyroglobulin levels. Loss of iodine avidity on uptake scan suggests a more aggressive transformation of the tumor, and PET scanning should be used.

  ∝ Metastases are treated with remedial surgery if biopsy-proven recurrence can be identified, and/or with therapeutic doses of radio-iodine.

  ∝ Treatment of low-risk microcarcinomas (<1 cm) by near-total or total thyroidectomy or thyroid lobectomy is adequate, followed by TSH-suppressive doses of thyroxine.

  ∝ BRAF (V600E) mutation analysis is being employed increasingly to help establish the diagnosis of papillary thyroid cancer in suspicious/indeterminate lesions and the prognosis in patients with papillary thyroid cancer. The presence of the mutation portends a more aggressive behavior of the tumor.

  ∝ ^{131}I is used to treat differentiated thyroid cancer after surgical intervention, to eliminate any residual disease. It is also used to ablate the thyroid in patients with hyperthyroidism from Graves' disease, toxic adenomas, and toxic multinodular goiters. For use in differentiated thyroid cancer, the patient must have stopped thyroxine replacement some weeks beforehand (withdrawal) or be administered recombinant human thyroid-stimulating hormone (rhTSH). Detected metastases then can be treated with a therapeutic dose (150–200 mCi) of ^{131}I.

✧ *Anaplastic thyroid cancer* – frequently, symptoms of rapid swelling, voice changes, and stridor may require palliative thyroidectomy to relieve or prevent respiratory obstruction, but prognosis is grave. Adjuvant chemotherapy and/or radiotherapy can be given but is poorly effective.

✧ *Medullary carcinoma of the thyroid (MTC)* – this tumor arises from parafollicular (or C) cells. Calcitonin levels are elevated and can be used as a tumor marker, along with CEA levels. MTC is sporadic in 80% of patients, but 20% have familial medullary thyroid cancer or MEN 2 syndrome. MEN 2A syndrome is associated with pheochromocytoma and primary hyperparathyroidism, while MEN 2B syndrome is associated with pheochromocytoma, Marfanoid habitus, and neurilemmomas (benign tumors of the myelin sheath) but not primary hyperparathyroidism. Genetic testing should be performed (inherited forms of the disease are more commonly associated with multifocal tumors), and mutational analysis can suggest prognosis as well as the likelihood of the associated diseases. In particular, biochemical testing should be performed before thyroid surgery to exclude pheochromocytoma.

- ∝ Treatment consists of total thyroidectomy and excision of central compartment lymph nodes at the very least, with or without excision of ipsilateral lateral compartment lymph nodes. The decision is based on physical examination, pre-operative calcitonin levels, imaging (ultrasound), and FNA proof of disease. This tumor is not responsive to radiotherapy, chemotherapy, radio-iodine, or TSH suppression, so levothyroxine is given in replacement dosing.
- ∝ Evidence-based guidelines from the American Thyroid Association and other professional societies guide the extent of resection based on the criteria described above.

- ✧ *Lymphoma* – primary thyroid lymphoma is rare, usually of the non-Hodgkins B cell type, and tends to complicate cases of Hashimoto's thyroiditis of 10–15 years' duration.
  - ∝ Lymphoma responds well to radiotherapy and chemotherapy, and if diagnosed sufficiently early, thyroidectomy can be avoided.
  - ∝ Surgery is reserved for tracheal decompression. Stridor can sometimes be successfully managed with dexamethasone and radiotherapy.

Other Thyroid Conditions

- ✧ *Autoimmune thyroiditis* – in practice, this is Hashimoto's, since other variants (such as Reidel's and de Quervain's) are extremely rare. Surgical intervention is avoided, and the condition responds well to T3/T4 therapy to suppress TSH-stimulated enlargement of the gland.
- ✧ *Graves' disease* – three treatment options are available, but choice depends on individual circumstances and patient preference.
  - ∝ *Antithyroid drugs* such as carbimazole or methimazole (propylthiouracil should be used only with great caution and for select indications, given recent data demonstrating an association with liver failure) can be given for 18 months, which cures fewer than 50% of patients. Nearly 45% relapse in the first year after stopping the drugs, and 20% of the remaining patients relapse in each of the subsequent five years. Drug toxicity is not uncommon. Beta blockade can also be used for control of symptoms and is especially useful in patients being prepared for surgery, in combination with an antithyroid drug. Lugol's solution can also be employed, particularly in the pre-operative setting to reduce vascularity of the thyroid and intra-operative blood loss.
  - ∝ *Radio-iodine treatment* ablates the thyroid tissue and will cure most patients, although repeat doses may be needed. More than 60% of patients will become hypothyroid in the first year. ^{131}I ablation is the favored method of treatment due to its high cure rate, but is not suitable in women of childbearing age who wish to become pregnant in the near future, or those who are pregnant or breastfeeding, or those with young children in the home. It is contraindicated in patients with severe Graves' ophthalmopathy, and should be accompanied by steroids in patients with moderate eye disease. In patients with symptoms of compression or possible coincident thyroid cancer, surgery would be a better choice. Some patients simply prefer to avoid radiation exposure and opt for surgery.

∞ *Surgery* – near-total or total thyroidectomy is generally the recommended procedure, as subtotal thyroidectomy (leaving a small amount of tissue on each side) is difficult to judge successfully, and may result in persistence or recurrence. The patient should be rendered euthyroid before surgery, so antithyroid drugs are continued up to the day of surgery. Indications for surgery include patients with recurrence of thyrotoxicosis after medical therapy; patient preference; symptoms of compression in the neck; coincident thyroid malignancy; the presence of very large goiters; and where there are contraindications to radio-iodine and/ or medical therapy.

Follow-up

In the diagnostic phase, follow-up intervals should be short (1–2 weeks) until malignant causes have been excluded. Similarly, any thyrotoxic patient should be reviewed within 1–2 weeks with the results of thyroid function tests, and at 2–4 week intervals to assess the effect of any antithyroid drug therapy.

Patients with medullary thyroid cancer, poorly differentiated cancers and anaplastic thyroid cancers should undergo surgery rapidly due to the aggressive behavior of these tumors; those with differentiated thyroid cancers can undergo elective surgery.

Post-operative Follow-up

The histology report should be reviewed to confirm the diagnosis and adequate excision, and the patient should be examined to detect any complications of thyroidectomy (wound infection, recurrent laryngeal nerve injury, hypocalcemia). Serum calcium levels traditionally fall to a nadir 72 hours post-operatively; in anticipation, strategies for management include checking post-operative intact parathyroid hormone or serum calcium levels, to triage which patients should be discharged on calcium with or without vitamin D (calcitriol) supplementation. Some data support discharging all patients on a self-limited course of calcium with or without vitamin D. All thyroid cancer patients should be referred to a multidisciplinary team/endocrinologist for further assessment and management.

Differentiated Thyroid Cancer

For those patients who have undergone near-total or total thyroidectomy, surveillance for recurrence is required using regular estimations of serum thyroglobulin levels, ultrasound, or uptake scans, or a combination of these.

If tumor size is greater than 1–1.5 cm, then consideration should be given to adjuvant treatment. Prior to administration, the patient can undergo ^{131}I or ^{123}I total body scintiscan 4–6 weeks post-operatively. If there is evidence of uptake in the neck or elsewhere, then therapeutic radio-iodine is administered. In different countries, this is done variously in inpatient and outpatient settings. In preparation for ^{131}I scanning, patients can be prepared by withdrawal of thyroid hormone or with rhTSH. A low-iodine diet is recommended. Radiation precautions need to be discussed with the patient, and enforced. The scintiscan can be repeated every 6 months for the first two years, then annually for the next five years.

In the absence of metastases or persistent disease in the central neck (e.g. positive resection margins from locally advanced disease), thyroglobulin levels should fall to an undetectable level after total thyroidectomy. Any rise post-operatively is an indicator of functional thyroid tissue, either as a local recurrence or distant metastases, which will require ablation with radio-iodine if toxic doses have not been reached.

All patients receive TSH-suppressing doses of thyroxine.

Anaplastic Thyroid Cancer
All patients receive TSH-suppressing doses of thyroxine. Patients should be referred to an oncologist for consideration of adjuvant chemotherapy or radiation therapy and/or for consideration for enrollment in a clinical trial.

Medullary Carcinoma
There is a 90% five-year survival rate in the absence of lymph node involvement; 45% if lymph nodes are involved. Regional lymph node involvement is commonly seen, even with small tumors.

Patients are monitored for recurrence by regular measurement of calcitonin and CEA levels. A rise can indicate recurrence, which can be detected by cervical ultrasound, CT or MRI. Recurrences can be treated by re-operation when they occur in the neck, or radiotherapy, but response rates are poor.

Vandetanib is a tyrosine kinase inhibitor that has recently been approved for use in the US for select patients with locally advanced or metastatic disease.

Genetic counseling is employed for those patients with inherited forms of the disease, to guide screening of other family members.

Complications Related to Surgery
✧ Voice change due to inadvertent damage to the recurrent laryngeal nerve occurs in fewer than 1% of cases in the hands of experienced surgeons.
  ∝ Damage to the external branch of the superior laryngeal nerve supplying the cricothyroid muscle causes difficulty in tensing the vocal cords and affects the quality of the voice (high pitch and volume), which may be particularly significant to singers.
  ∝ Damage to the internal laryngeal nerves – usually during mobilizing of the upper pole – desensitizes the appropriate side of the larynx and causes spilling-over of liquids, causing aspiration, coughing, or dysphagia. Referral for an otolaryngology opinion is appropriate.
✧ Hypoparathyroidism occurs in approximately 1% of cases among high-volume surgeons.
✧ Temporary hypocalcemia is common in the first few days due to parathyroid injury or ischemia.
✧ Long-term treatment may be necessary with vitamin D and calcium if hypocalcemia does not resolve.
✧ Other problems include wound hematoma formation, keloid formation, and suture granuloma.
  ∝ Hematomas are uncommon but can be life-threatening. It is important to recognize that sudden respiratory difficulty after thyroid surgery may be due to hematoma formation. Most minor hematomas detected in outpatients can be handled conservatively.
  ∝ Keloid scars can be excised after a year, but can recur.
  ∝ Sutures should be removed in the ward or in a procedure/recovery room to evacuate the clot, including deep sutures. Suture granulomas respond to removal of the suture.

Parathyroids and Disorders of Calcium Metabolism
The dominant hormone regulating calcium metabolism is parathyroid hormone (PTH); calcitonin has little effect on calcium homeostasis. A fall in serum calcium levels stimulates an increase in PTH secretion, as does a fall in magnesium or an increase in phosphate.

PTH increases serum calcium concentrations by increasing resorption of bone, decreasing excretion by the kidney, and increasing absorption from the intestine. PTH mediates the production of the active 1,25 dihydroxycholecalciferol from vitamin D precursors at the kidney. The effects of PTH on the bones and intestine do not occur in cases of vitamin D deficiency.

Hypercalcemia

Causes of hypercalcemia include bone metastases, excess vitamin D ingestion, milk–alkali syndrome, hyperthyroidism, multiple myeloma, reticuloses, leukemias, sarcoidosis, Addison's disease, Paget's disease of bone, renal failure, ectopic secretion of PTH, thiazide diuretics, and, of particular interest to surgeons, hyperparathyroidism.

History

Classic symptoms are anecdotally referred to as "bones, moans, stones, and groans." Ask about lithium, salicylate, or thiazide diuretic medications and vitamin D ingestion as exogenous sources of hypercalcemia.

There may be a family history of hypercalcemia; this may be related to either MEN syndrome, familial hyperparathyroidism, or familial hypercalcemic hypocalciuria (FHH). FHH is due to a reset of the sensitivity of the calcium receptor, and is unrelated to parathyroid disease. A low level of urinary calcium excretion combined with a family history should alert the clinician to this condition. If it is identified, parathyroid surgery should not be performed.

Patients often report vague symptoms of fatigue, lethargy, arthralgias, and muscle pain; there may be a change in mood, especially anxiety or depression.

GI symptoms include dyspepsia/peptic ulceration, pancreatitis and/or constipation. Urinary symptoms include polyuria, nocturia or polydipsia; the patient may report a history of renal stones. Symptoms are related to the possible underlying causes.

Note that the majority of patients diagnosed with primary hyperparathyroidism are asymptomatic.

Examination

A full physical examination is performed, looking for signs suggesting possible causes of hypercalcemia, e.g. Paget's, malignancy, or sarcoidosis.

Hypercalcemia, unless severe, usually does not produce physical signs. Severe hypercalcemia can cause signs of dehydration, lethargy, hyperreflexia/tongue fasciculations, and proximal muscle weakness. Parathyroid adenomas (or even carcinomas) rarely produce masses in the neck that are large enough to palpate.

Diagnostic Tests

Confirm the hypercalcemia by measuring repeat serum calcium levels (correct for serum albumin level or perform an ionized calcium level test), vitamin D, iPTH, alkaline phosphate, and 24-hour urinary calcium excretion.

A low serum phosphate with elevated alkaline phosphatase and chloride suggests a parathyroid cause.

When combined, a chest X-ray (CXR), complete blood count (CBC), and basic chemistries will exclude many non-parathyroid cases. An elevated or inappropriately high normal iPTH level in the setting of hypercalcemia is indicative of the diagnosis.

Normocalcemic hyperparathyroidism is a relatively new phenomenon; patients present with high normal serum calcium levels, elevated iPTH levels, and osteoporosis. Many of these patients will go on to develop hypercalcemia and primary hyperparathyroidism, so early surgical intervention may be indicated.

Treatment (of Hypercalcemia)

✧ *Mild hypercalcemia* is initially treated with patient self-hydration and a low-calcium diet until the underlying cause is addressed.
✧ *Moderate to severe hypercalcemia*, depending on the severity of symptoms, is treated with IV hydration with Normal saline, and administration of loop diuretics. Other treatments include calcitonin, cinacalcet (a calcimimetic agent) and bisphosphonate medications. Diagnostic tests and surgical therapy (if indicated) should be expedited.

Follow-up

✧ *Mild hypercalcemia*: Calcium levels should be checked at short intervals (1–4 weeks) to monitor response to treatment and to establish the diagnosis.
✧ *More severe hypercalcemia* may require admission to hospital for further acute management.

Hypocalcemia

Causes include uremic osteodystrophy, post-operative parathyroid and thyroid surgery, and vitamin D deficiency.

Uremic osteodystophy occurs in chronic renal failure when calcium is excreted (and thus not reabsorbed) by the kidneys and phosphate is not secreted, leading to accumulation in the bloodstream. These changes in electrolytes lead to increased PTH secretion, and the parathyroid glands become hyperplastic. The increased PTH levels cause calcium resorption from bones, leading to osteitis fibrosa cystica. This is also called secondary hyperparathyroidism.

History

✧ Most commonly, significant hypocalcemia causes muscle cramps/spasms (tetany) and tingling or numbness of the fingertips and circumorally. It is life-threatening.
✧ Long-term hypocalcemia leads to cataracts, dry skin or psoriasis, brittle nails, poor dentition, dysphagia, and intestinal colic.
✧ Acute, severe hypocalcemia can cause syncope, congestive heart failure, angina (QTc prolongation), and seizures, as well as bronchospasm and stridor.

Ask about history of recent neck surgery, and medications (estrogen, bisphosphonates, loop diuretics, recent radiocontrast, antibiotics, or antiepileptics, etc.).

Patients may have a history of an inadequate diet, e.g. one that is poor in fat-soluble vitamins. Religious clothing preventing adequate exposure to sunlight can occasionally contribute to the condition. Patients who live far from the equator (at high latitudes) also have reduced sun exposure and higher rates of vitamin D deficiency.

Examination

✧ Classic signs of hypocalcemia are: Chvostek's sign (a tap at the facial nerve causes facial muscle twitch) and Trousseau's sign (inflation of blood presure cuff on arm causes carpal spasm).
✧ Long-term hypocalcemia leads to the development of cataracts, dry skin, and papilledema.
✧ Psychologic symptoms include irritability, confusion, hallucinations, and dementia.
✧ Look for signs of recent neck surgery and chronic renal failure.

Diagnostic Tests
Test for serum calcium, vitamin D, albumin, basic chemistries/electrolytes, and iPTH levels. Perform liver function tests and a renal ultrasound.

Treatment
✧ *Uremic osteodystrophy* – initally, correction of hypocalcemia; then subtotal parathyroidectomy (three and a half glands) or total parathyroidectomy (with heterotopic autotransplantation and, when possible, cryopreservation).
✧ *Osteomalacia and rickets* – vitamin D (1-α-cholecalciferol).
✧ *Post-surgical hypocalcemia* – temporary hypocalcemia is not uncommon after total thyroidectomy, usually due to parathyroid injury or ischemia.
  ∝ In the acute setting, intravenous injection of 10 mL of calcium gluconate or calcium chloride via a central line can be administered, followed by intravenous calcium infusion. Inpatients should be monitored with telemetry to ensure that there is no attendant cardiac irritability.
  ∝ These patients can generally be managed with a combination of oral calcium supplements and 1-α-cholecalciferol.
  ∝ Regular serum calcium and iPTH checks, along with magnesium, are essential, as parathyroid recovery may lead to iatrogenic hypercalcemia.

Hyperparathyroidism
✧ *Primary hyperparathyroidism* is due to a parathyroid adenoma (85%) or, rarely, a double parathyroid adenoma (5%) or four-gland hyperplasia (10%); carcinoma is rare (<1%).
✧ *Secondary hyperparathyroidism* is caused by reactive hyperplasia of the glands in response to chronic calcium-losing states such as malabsorption or chronic renal failure.
✧ *Tertiary hyperparathyroidism* occurs when a secondary hyperplastic gland becomes functionally autonomous.

Keep in mind that, in all cases, you must exclude other associated neoplasms (MEN 1, MEN 2).

History
Secondary and tertiary causes can be excluded if there is no history of malabsorption or chronic renal failure. A family history of other endocrine neoplasms should raise the possibility of the MEN syndromes.

Examination
Look for evidence of hypercalcemia (as above). Also look for malnutrition (malabsorption) or chronic renal failure (uremia, etc.).

Diagnostic Tests
There are inappropriately high normal or elevated iPTH levels in the presence of hypercalcemia.
  Once the diagnosis has been made and the patient has a safe calcium level, an attempt should be made to localize the tumor in order to potentially allow for minimally invasive surgery. High-resolution ultrasound and sestamibi scanning (preferably with SPECT) will find the affected gland in about 75–80% of cases. Four-dimensional CT is a new technology that appears promising.

For redo cases, other imaging (CT, MRI, or angiography with selective venous sampling) is often required. Two concordant localization studies are suggested in the remedial setting.

Treatment

✧ If the tumor has been localized with a sestamibi scan, then a focused exploration is indicated, removing only the affected gland.

✧ If the tumor is not localized or hyperplasia is suspected, then surgical exploration of all glands is undertaken and the abnormal gland(s) removed.

✧ Intra-operative frozen section can be used to confirm that the appropriate tissue has been removed. Other intra-operative adjuncts include the gamma probe and the rapid intra-operative PTH assay.

✧ Intra-operative PTH measurement is very useful if available – a reduction of pre-operative, or baseline, PTH 50% and into the normal range is sufficient to indicate that the appropriate gland(s) has been removed.

Primary Parathyroid Adenoma
Surgical excision of the affected gland by a minimally invasive approach is preferred. If not possible, then perform four-gland exploration with excision of the adenomatous gland.

Secondary Parathyroid Hyperplasia (Four-gland)
Perform excision of all four glands (least desired), or excision of three and a half glands (the last half being left marked with a titanium clip), or four-gland excision with heterotopic autotransplantation (usually to the brachioradialis muscle in the non-dominant forearm) with cryopreservation if possible.

Tertiary Hyperparathyroidism (Autonomously Functioning Hyperplastic or Adenomatous Gland)
The recommendation is either subtotal parathyroidectomy, including resection of the dominant gland, or total parathyroidectomy with heterotopic autotransplantation of gland fragments into the brachioradialis muscle of the forearm.

Parathyroid Carcinoma
If recognized pre- or intra-operatively, it is treated by parathyroidectomy, ipsilateral thyroid lobectomy, and central lymph node dissection (if nodes present), followed by surveillance with measurement of calcium and iPTH levels. If not recognized pre/intra-operatively, re-operation may be necessary.

Medical therapies currently do not aid survival of these patients; surgery is currently the best option, with medical management of hypercalcemia. Cinacalcet also can be used for metastatic disease not amenable to surgery.

Follow-up
Bone disease caused by excess reabsorption of calcium by hyperparathyroidism (osteitis fibrosa cystica) is particularly severe with secondary and tertiary hyperparathyroidism, and will require calcium and vitamin D therapy and serum monitoring for months, including after surgical intervention.

Post-operative Follow-up
Review histology to confirm the diagnosis. Confirm the biochemical success of the operation (serum calcium and iPTH levels).

✧ *Persistent hyperparathyroidism* is diagnosed if hypercalcemia persists or recurs within six months of the operation. The most common cause of persistent hyperparathyroidism is unrecognized multiple gland disease.

✧ *Recurrent hyperparathyroidism* occurs after six months.

The source of persistent or recurrent tumor can be re-localized with a combination of the imaging studies described above. Re-operation is indicated, but can be very technically difficult. Laryngoscopy should be performed prior to re-exploration to assure that no injury occurred to the recurrent laryngeal nerve(s) at the time of the initial exploration.

Parathyroid carcinoma is monitored with frequent estimations of serum calcium and iPTH levels to detect recurrence or metastases. Recurrence in the neck is treated by en bloc resection if possible; otherwise, medical palliation of hypercalcemia with calcimimetics and hydration can be employed.

Multiple Endocrine Neoplasia Syndromes

Multiple endocrine neoplasia (MEN) syndromes are rare, but screening for tumors and for the known genetic abnormalities in family members of suspected cases can lead to much improved outcomes. Family members without the genetic defect do not need to be screened for tumors.

MEN 1

MEN 1 is an autosomal dominant disease consisting of hyperparathyroidism, pituitary tumors and pancreatic neuroendocrine tumors. It is caused by a defect on the long arm of chromosome 11 (the MEN 1 gene).

✧ Hyperparathyroidism occurs in 90% of patients, characteristically hyperplasia.

✧ Pancreatic islet cell tumors occur in 30–75% of patients, and tend to be multiple.

✧ Gastrinomas occur in 30–60% and insulinomas in 35% of patients; glucagonomas and vasoactive intestinal peptide tumors (VIPomas) are rare.

✧ Pituitary adenomas occur in 15–40% of patients.

✧ Prolactinomas are the most common, with growth hormone tumors (causing acromegaly) and ACTH-producing tumors (causing Cushing's syndrome) less so.

✧ Carcinoid tumors and thymic neoplasms are more common than in the general population, and adrenocortical adenomas, which tend to be non-functional, are also found.

Diagnostic Tests

✧ Screening of affected family members consists of genetic testing, biochemical testing for specific diseases, and imaging.

✧ In family members carrying the defective gene on chromosome 11, biochemical screening is performed yearly after puberty, with measurement of serum calcium, iPTH, prolactin and gut hormone levels every 1–3 years.

✧ Suspected insulinomas are investigated by measuring serum glucose, insulin and pro-insulin levels during symptomatic episodes.

✧ MRI scans of the pituitary are performed every five years, combined with estimations of serum prolactin levels.

Treatment

✧ *Hyperparathyroidism* – total parathyroidectomy with heterotopic autotransplantation.

✧ *Gastrinomas* – medical therapy is effective, but is lifelong. Enucleation is performed for accessible lesions in the head of the pancreas or duodenum. Distal pancreatectomy is performed for lesions in the body or tail. Recurrent or metastatic disease occurs in 50% of patients and is treated symptomatically.

✧ *Insulinoma* – enucleation is performed for suitable lesions. Inoperable disease is treated with diazoxide and chemotherapy. Octreotide is also effective.

✧ *Pituitary lesions* – hypophysectomy and external beam radiation. Bromocriptine and its derivatives are effective for treatment of prolactinomas and acromegaly.

MEN 2

This is an autosomal dominant condition with a chromosomal defect in the RET proto-oncogene on chromosome 10. Three forms exist:

✧ *MEN 2A*: Represents approximately 90% of cases of MEN 2, consisting of medullary carcinoma of thyroid (MTC), pheochromocytoma (50%), and parathyroid hyperplasia (20–30%).

✧ *MEN 2B*: Represents ~5% of MEN 2 cases, consisting of MTC, pheochromocytomas (often bilateral, 50%), a Marfanoid body habitus, pruitis of upper back, mucosal and eyelid neuromas, and GI ganglioneuromas (which can cause constipation or diarrhea).

✧ *Familial MTC (FMTC)*: patients with inherited MTC but no other endocrine abnormalities.

Diagnostic Tests

Genetic screening is performed for all first- and second-degree relatives. Affected individuals undergo yearly biochemical screening consisting of calcitonin and CEA levels, urinary chatecholamines (epinephrine, norepinephrine, dopamine, VMA, metanephrines, and normetanephrines), or serum metanephrines/normetanephrines for pheochromocytoma, and serum calcium, albumin and iPTH for hyperparathyroidism.

Treatment

Total thyroidectomy is performed in all affected children at the latest between the ages of 5 and 7 years, in order to prevent the development of metastatic medullary carcinoma. Identification of the specific mutation underlying the syndrome should then be used to determine the timing of the thyroidectomy. Thyroidectomy *should* be done as early as possible in genetic carriers, as MTC can occur as early as the first months of life. Parathyroid glands are examined at the same time and removed if enlarged. Pheochromocytomas are treated appropriately if they are detected by screening laboratory tests.

The Adrenal Gland

Disorders of the adrenal gland requiring surgical intervention include Cushing's syndrome and Conn's syndrome (affecting the adrenal cortex), and pheochromocytoma (affecting the adrenal medulla).

Cushing's Syndrome

Excess amounts of cortisol lead to the characteristic features of Cushing's syndrome. The diagnosis is suspected in patients with characteristic clinical features and is confirmed by finding inappropriately elevated serum and urinary cortisol levels.

When the elevation in cortisol is discovered, it must be determined whether this is due to a pituitary lesion, an adrenal lesion (adenoma or carcinoma), or to ectopic production of ACTH by oat-cell carcinoma of the bronchus, bronchial carcinoid tumor, thymic tumor, islet-cell tumor, or pheochromocytoma (among others). If an adrenal lesion is implicated, it needs to be localized.

The most common cause of Cushing's syndrome is exogenous administration of glu-cocorticoids. True Cushing's disease is adrenocortical hyperplasia caused by a pituitary lesion.

History and Physical Examination
✧ *Physical appearance*: Obesity of the face and trunk with thin extremities, buffalo hump, moon facies, hirsutism, edema and striae. In ectopic ACTH syndrome, the clinical appearance may be dominated by the effects of malignancy.
✧ *Biochemical/physical/psychologic features*: Glucose intolerance, proximal muscle weakness, easy bruising, menstrual irregularities, osteoporosis, depression, emotional lability, symptoms of diabetes mellitus (including polyuria), and hypertension.

Diagnostic Tests
Initial screening tests are CBC and chemistries. Cushing's syndrome is associated with an elevated white blood-cell count (WBC), hyperglycemia, and hypokalemic metabolic alkalosis.

For definitive diagnosis, the patient generally needs more extensive biochemical testing, which may require hospitalization:
✧ *24-hour urine free cortisol*: Cortisol levels three to four times normal are highly suggestive of Cushing's syndrome.
✧ *Low-dose dexamethasone suppression test*: 1 mg dexamethasone is administered at night and serum cortisol is measured in the morning; cortisol levels >1.8 mcg/dL are highly suggestive of Cushing's syndrome.
✧ *Late night (11pm–12am) serum/salivary cortisol levels*: <50 nmol/L (serum) or <1.3–1.5 mcg/dL (saliva) excludes the diagnosis because normal nocturnal cortisol suppression would be lost in Cushing's syndrome.
✧ *Dexamethasone–CRH test*: Distinguishes pseudo-Cushing's syndrome from Cushing's syndrome.
   ∝ *Pseudo-Cushing's syndrome*: Involves high cortisol levels without progressive effects. It is found in patients with depression/anxiety, alcoholism, severe diabetes, and severe obesity.
   ∝ Low–dose dexamethasone (0.5 mg) is given every 6 hours for 8 doses, followed by CRH administration. ACTH and plasma cortisol levels are tested for 1 hour following CRH. Cortisol levels >50 nmol/L suggest Cushing's syndrome.

Localization
Localization is required to determine the etiology of diagnosed Cushing's syndrome.
✧ Undectable ACTH levels (<5 pg/mL) with elevated serum cortisol levels are diagnostic for an ACTH-dependent source of cortisol; that is, an adrenal adenoma or carcinoma (after exogenous sources of glucocorticoids are excluded).
✧ If carcinoma is suspected, serum DHEAS and 24-hour urine 17-ketosteroids may also be measured.
✧ ACTH levels >10–20 pg/mL with elevated cortisol levels are diagnostic of ACTH-dependent Cushing's syndrome.
✧ Equivocal ACTH levels require a high-dose dexamethasone suppression test (overnight or 48 hours): High-dose dexamethasone is given, with prior and subsequent measurements of serum or urine 8am cortisol levels. A >50% decrease in levels the morning after drug administration suggests a pituitary source of the ACTH rather than an ectopic or adrenal one.

CRH Test

This is used to distinguish ectopic from pituitary sources. CRH is administered, and subsequently cortisol and ACTH levels are tested. A >20% rise in cortisol and a >50% rise in ACTH levels are consistent with a pituitary source. Ectopic production is not affected by CRH.

Inferior Petrosal Sinus Sampling

This can also be used to distinguish ectopic from pituitary sources. ACTH levels are tested at bilateral sinuses and periphery after administration of CRH. Sinus to peripheral ratio is calculated and evaluated.

Imaging

After biochemical evaluation, imaging studies may be performed to confirm the source.
✦ CT or MRI of the brain or abdomen is used to localize pituitary or adrenal tumor(s).
✦ CXR may reveal a bronchial lesion or a widened mediastinum caused by a thymic tumor.
✦ MRI or CT of the chest for ectopic sources may also be useful.
✦ Octreoscan and PET scan can be used to search for underlying malignancy that can serve as the occult cause of ectopic ACTH production.

Treatment
✦ *Cushing's Disease* – transphenoidal hypophysectomy or transphenoidal hemihypophysectomy (based on inferior petrosal venous sampling). There is a 60–80% cure rate.
  ∝ If unsuccessful, pituitary irradiation may help (rate of cure 45% in adults, 8% in children).
  ∝ If radiation is unsuccessful, then bilateral laparoscopic vs open adrenalectomy may be considered.
✦ *Autonomous functional adrenal tumor* – surgical excision (laparoscopic approach preferable). Due to suppression of the normal gland function, post-operative steroid replacement therapy may be necessary for up to 2 years. Testing of the hypothalamic–pituitary–adrenal axis (ACTH stimulation test) at regular intervals over this period is indicated to assess remaining gland function.
✦ *Ectopic ACTH* – surgical excision of resectable primary tumors, as indicated by specific pathology, i.e:
  ∝ Oat-cell (small cell) lung cancer – palliation.
  ∝ Carcinoids – resect if possible. If not, bilateral adrenalectomy may be necessary to control symptoms in suitable candidates.
✦ *Adrenocortical carcinoma* (<10% of adrenal tumors) – often presents late with large tumor burden and pulmonary metastases. Treatment is surgical debulking of the tumor and/or control of metastatic disease with mitotane. Partial remission can be obtained with chemotherapy (5FU, doxorubicin, cisplatin).

Follow-up

Patients should be seen at short intervals (1–2 weeks) until diagnosis is made. In many cases, admission to hospital is planned to perform the necessary diagnostic tests in consultation with an endocrinologist.

Post-operative Follow-up
✦ Review histology to confirm the diagnosis and complete excision of tumor margins.

✧ Patients should be seen and examined for possible physical complications of surgery (wound infection, abscess).

✧ Patients should be questioned about symptoms and basic laboratory tests repeated in order to exclude adrenal insufficiency and to confirm adequate cortisol replacement, under co-management with an endocrinologist.

✧ A combination of hydrocortisone and fludrocortisone is required after bilateral adrenalectomy.

✧ Counsel the patient regarding the need for increased steroid therapy during illness or further surgical procedures. A medical alert bracelet should be worn.

✧ Patients receiving chemotherapy may also become hypothyroid and require thyroxine.

✧ Cushing's syndrome should gradually improve over the year following surgery. Scaly desquamation of the scalp is a sign of improvement. Weight loss occurs, muscle strength improves, and diabetes often resolves.

Conn's Syndrome

This consists of primary hyperaldosteronism resulting in hypertension and hypokalemia.

✧ Primary causes of hyperaldosteronism are functional adrenocortical lesions (that secrete aldosterone). Approximately 60% of cases are due to a benign adrenal adenoma (APA, aldosterone-producing adenoma), and 40% due to bilateral hyperplasia (IHA, idiopathic hyperaldosteronism). Occasional cases are due to adrenocortical carcinoma.

✧ Secondary causes of hyperaldosteronism include stimulation by angiotensin in response to decreased circulating volume. This may be caused by cirrhosis, nephrotic syndrome, diuretic therapy, and cardiac failure.

✧ Other causes include renal artery stenosis or a renin-secreting tumor.

History

Patients usually present with new-onset hypertension that is resistant to treatment or is associated with accompanying symptoms of muscle weakness, tetany, polyuria, nocturia, or polydipsia. The history may include congestive heart failure (CHF) and/or stroke.

Examination

Patients may be normal or there may be hypertension, with evidence of muscle weakness and tetany.

Diagnostic Tests

✧ Serum chemistries: hypokalemia, alkalosis. One-third of Conn's patients have a normal potassium level.

✧ Potassium excretion in the urine is inappropriately high.

✧ Hypernatremia is typical of primary aldosteronism. Hyponatremia is more commonly found in secondary hyperaldosteronism.

✧ Morning plasma renin (PRA) and aldosterone (PA) levels are measured from a blood sample taken from arm vein between 9am and 10am after fasting from 11pm the night before. Ideally, the patient should have been off all medications for four weeks prior to the blood test. This provides the PA : PRA ratio, which is helpful in diagnosis.
    ∝ Conn's is diagnosed by an elevated PA level in the presence of a low PRA level.
    ∝ High PA levels are not suppressed by increased intake of sodium chloride.

✧ Glucocorticoid levels should be normal.

✧ Secondary hyperaldosteronism is characterized by high PRA levels with hypertension and often renal disease or sodium depletion.

Localization

CT, sometimes along with 131-iodine-6-beta-iodomethyl-19-norcholesterol (NP59) scintigraphy, can localize masses and distinguish between adenoma and hyperplasia. Occasionally, MRI and/or adrenal vein sampling are useful in difficult cases, as aldosterone-secreting adenomas are often small.

Treatment

✧ *Adrenal tumor* – unilateral laparoscopic adrenalectomy. Precede surgery by 1–6 weeks of spironolactone to return serum potassium to normal.
✧ *Adrenal hyperplasia* – medical therapy is to treat hypertension with spironolactone 100 mg/day rising to 400 mg/day until potassium returns to normal, then reduce the dose. Resistant hyperplasia is treated by total or subtotal adrenalectomy.

Follow-up

Patients should be seen at short intervals (1–2 weeks) until diagnosis is obtained, hypertension is controlled, and potassium returns to normal. Admission to hospital is often required.

Spironolactone can cause gynecomastia, decreased libido, impotence, menstrual irregularities, and not control the patient's hypertension. Second-line therapy with amiloride or triamterene may be required.

Post-operative Follow-up

Review histology to confirm the diagnosis and the tumor margins. Patients should be examined to detect any general post-operative complications. Confirm a biochemical return to normalcy. Adrenal insufficiency is rare in the post-operative setting.

A reduction in the number and doses of antihypertensives, along with potassium supplementation, is anticipated post-operatively, starting with spironolactone. Often, however, patients on multiple blood pressure drugs will not come off all of them because of underlying essential hypertension.

Pheochromocytoma

Of these, 10% are malignant, 10% are bilateral, and 10% occur extra-adrenally, anywhere along the sympathetic chain from the neck to the pelvis.

Pheochromocytomas may be familial, either inherited in isolation (mutations in the *SDHB*, *SDHC*, or *SDHD* genes) or as paraganglioma [PGL] syndromes), or associated with other tumors, such as neurofibromatosis (NF1, 10%), acoustic neuroma, meningioma, glioma, astrocytoma, cerebellar hemangioma (14%), and von Hippel–Lindau (VHL) syndrome.

In MEN 2, pheochromocytoma is associated with medullary carcinoma of thyroid and parathyroid tumors (for MEN 2A).

History

✧ Palpitations, headaches, anxiety, facial flushing, abdominal symptoms such as nausea and vomiting, diarrhea and weight loss, glucose intolerance, and cardiac failure.
✧ Sudden episodes of hypertension, headaches, nausea/vomiting, chest and abdominal pain, anxiety, pallor, sweating, and palpitations lasting a few minutes to several hours can occur.

Examination

Hypertension can be sustained or paroxysmal, with periods of normotension or hypotension, so single blood pressure readings can be normal. If the pheochromocytoma secretes norepinephrine or dopamine, hypotension can be the presenting sign.

Examine for tachycardia and palpitations, evidence of cardiac failure, dehydration, and recent weight loss.

Diagnostic Tests

✧ Measure catecholamines and metanephrines in a 24-hour urine collection (90% sensitive); these include epinephrine, norepinephrine, VMA, metanephrines, normetanephrines, and dopamine.
✧ Plasma catecholamine levels are elevated, but levels can be rendered inaccurate by calcium channel blockers, monoamine oxidase inhibitors (MAOIs), phenothiazines, tricyclic antidepressants and beta-blockers, or epinephrine-containing medicines, including those used for allergies and nasal congestion.
✧ Extra-adrenal and malignant pheochromocytomas tend to secrete norepinephrine, while benign adrenal pheochromocytomas tend to secrete epinephrine. The majority of pheochromocytomas secrete norepinephrine.
✧ Biopsy should *never* be performed. Indeed, biopsy of adrenal lesions is only indicated in the rare setting of lesions that are believed to be metastases of other primaries and when pheochomocytoma has absolutely been excluded.

Localization

Most tumors can be detected by CT of adrenal, para-aortic and pelvic areas. Intravenous contrast should only be administered if a pheochromocytoma has been excluded, as the contrast material can incite a pheochromocytoma crisis. If not, then a non-contrast CT must be performed. In this setting, MRI is more useful; gadolinium can be administered, and pheochromocytomas are seen to "light up" on T2-weighted images. Adrenal-specific protocols for CT and MRI allow for fine cuts through the adrenal glands to enhance resolution and the ability to see small pathologic lesions.

[131]MIBG (meta-iodobenzylguanidine) is taken up by catacholamine granules and is extremely useful in confirming the site of the tumor in diagnosing extra-adrenal and bilateral pheochromocytomas. It also can be used therapeutically for treatment of metastases.

Treatment

Phenoxybenzamine (or any other alpha-blocker) should be started at the time of diagnosis and continued for at least two weeks prior to surgery (or longer in the presence of ECG abnormalities). Additional therapy with beta-blockers (after the alpha-blocker has been started) can be used to control continued tachycardia. Labetalol (an alpha- and beta-blocker) can also be utilized. Metyrosine is particularly useful in highly functional tumors.

Once hypertension is controlled, unilateral laparoscopic adrenalectomy is performed. Cortical-sparing procedures can be used; they are associated with a greater chance of local recurrence but can be useful in patients with bilateral disease (MEN 2 patients).

Follow-up

Patients should be seen at short intervals (1–2 weeks) until diagnosis is achieved, or should be admitted to hospital for control of acute symptoms.

There is a clinical association with MEN 2; therefore, medullary carcinoma of the thyroid and hyperparathyroidism should be excluded in all cases of pheochromocytoma.

Post-operative Follow-up

Seventy percent of patients are cured of hypertension by surgery. Review histology to confirm diagnosis and excisional margins. Patients should be examined to detect any general complications of surgery.

Patients with malignancy should be followed-up long term to detect recurrence. Because of the chance of bilateral disease, patients are surveilled with 24-hour urinary catecholamine collections. Recurrence is suspected by return of symptoms or biochemical abnormalities.

Metastases are localized by MIBG scan or MRI/CT; MIBG also can be given in therapeutic doses. Malignant pheochromocytomas that recur can also be treated by surgical debulking. Chemotherapy has been used, with a 50% response rate; clinical trials also are ongoing.

Childhood Adrenal Tumors

These include neuroblastoma, ganglioneuroma, and neurofibroma; these conditions are beyond the scope of this book.

Adrenal Incidentalomas

With the rise in use of abdominal CT, asymptomatic adrenal masses are increasingly being referred for surgical opinion. Over 50% are metastases from a known primary; 30% are cortical adenomas with potential endocrine symptoms (pheochromocytoma, Cushing's, Conn's); 5% are metastases from an occult primary; and 5% are adrenal malignancies. Other causes include cysts, hematomas, angiomyelolipomas, and myelolipomas.

History and Physical Examination

History taking should include specific questions to elicit symptoms of functional adrenal conditions, and patients should be examined for relevant clinical signs. In particular, determine any known primary malignancy.

Diagnostic Tests

Often the mass on the initial CT scan has a diagnostic appearance or is suggestive of malignancy due to an irregular outline, invasion of adjacent structures, or lymph node metastases.

If CT does not provide diagnosis, perform biochemical tests for pheochromocytoma, Cushing's and Conn's syndromes, e.g. 24-hour urinary catecholamines, serum potassium, renin, and ACTH levels, and 24-hour urinary cortisol estimation (or low-dose dexamethasone suppression test).

If the tumors are non-functional and small, they are amenable to surveillance with CT or MRI at regular intervals to ensure that they do not change in appearance or increase in size.

Treatment

- ✧ Adrenal masses greater than 4 cm should be considered for surgical excision because of malignant potential.
- ✧ For metastatic masses, surgical excision may also be justified (depending on invasion and presence of a known primary).
- ✧ Cysts are very rarely malignant and do not require surgery unless very large. Pheochromocytomas can be cystic.
- ✧ Hematomas may occur spontaneously and resolve over time, but can occur within primary or metastatic tumors.

✧ Myelolipomas are benign and have a classic appearance on body imaging; surgery is only indicated if they become large or symptomatic (i.e. early satiety with large left-sided lesions that compress the stomach).

Follow-up
Patients should be seen at short intervals (1–3 weeks) until diagnosis is achieved. If all diagnostic tests are normal and surgery is not indicated because of size or other features, serial imaging observation performed every 6 months initially is acceptable.

Post-operative Follow-up
Review histology to confirm diagnosis and excisional margins and to detect any general complications of surgery. Follow-up for specific lesions is described under their relevant sections.

Hirsutism/Virilization
Most patients have congenital adrenal hyperplasia, which may present as virilization in male and female children. Laboratory abnormalities are dependent on the particular enzyme deficiency, which results in increased hormone precursors and their urinary metabolites. Testosterone and other sex hormones may be elevated in the presence of a virilizing adrenal tumor, but may also be elevated in other virilizing syndromes such as ovarian tumor.

History
Determine the onset of hirsutism. Patients may complain of oily skin, acne and increasing facial and other body hair. The voice may deepen. There may be menstrual irregularities or amenorrhea.

Examination
Perform a full physical examination. In females, examine for male pattern of body hair and acne. Abdominal examination may reveal an abdominal or a pelvic mass. Rectal and vaginal examination may reveal an ovarian mass or abnormal genitalia.

Diagnostic Tests
Adrenal imaging by CT or MRI is essential. Simultaneous imaging of the ovaries is also helpful.

Measure plasma testosterone, 17-hydroxyprogesterone, 11-deoxycortisol, and/or other steroid precursors. Serum ACTH levels are high in congenital adrenal hyperplasia.

Treatment
✧ Simple benign adrenal tumors are treated by surgical excision; this improves acne and restores menstruation, ovulation, and fertility. Hirsutism usually persists. Malignant tumors may require chemotherapy.
✧ Congenital adrenal hyperplasia is treated by replacement of deficient adrenal steroids to reduce the stimulation of the adrenals and the production of virilizing byproducts by high levels of ACTH.

Follow-up
Patients should be seen at short intervals (1–3 weeks) until adrenal or ovarian tumors are excluded. Monitor the effect of hormone replacement in collaboration with an endocrinologist. Gynecologic referral is indicated for treatment of ovarian tumors.

Post-operative Follow-up
Review histology to confirm diagnosis and excisional margins and to detect any general complications of surgery. Exclude adrenal insufficiency.

Surgical Management of Obesity

Determine whether the patient is clinically obese, exclude underlying metabolic disorder, detect complications of obesity, and select appropriate patients for surgery (based on presumed psychosocial capability to comply with complex medical needs post-operatively). Surgery should be considered as prophylactic in young adults or middle-aged patients.

History
Patients usually report abnormal eating or binge eating. Discuss types of diets attempted, the impact of obesity on life, and any psychologic upsets. Document trials of medical therapy, including medications, both prescribed and over-the-counter, as well as exercise regimens.

Examination
✧ Determine the body mass index (BMI) = weight in kg ÷ height^2 in m^2. A BMI of 20–25 indicates desirable weight. Morbid obesity is defined as a BMI >40–45, or more than 100 lbs (45 kg) overweight.
✧ Examine for conditions caused by obesity, including cardiovascular disease, diabetes mellitus, osteoarthritis, and respiratory disease.
✧ Examine for underlying metabolic conditions which can cause obesity, including Cushing's syndrome and hypothyroidism. Excess weight gain can also be associated with fluid retention secondary to cardiac, renal, or hepatic disease.

Diagnostic Tests
Height, weight, BMI, blood pressure, electrocardiography (ECG), complete blood count (CBC), lipid levels, CXR, spirometry, blood gases, glucose tolerance test, ultrasound gall bladder, and thyroid function tests.

Treatment
Criteria for selection of patients suitable for surgery are:
✧ Presence of morbid obesity for five years or more, BMI >40–45 kg/m^2.
✧ Patient has made serious attempts at weight loss through diet.
✧ Increasing immobility or obesity-related health problems.
✧ Patient is intelligent and hard-working, strongly motivated, and mentally stable, and has no history of alcoholism, drug addiction, or attempted suicide. Patient is not a high operative risk.

Relative indications include hypertension, hyperlipidemia, non-insulin dependent diabetes mellitus, and osteoarthritis.

Contraindications include unwilling patient, unfit for general anesthesia, psychologic instability, unable to lose any weight on dieting.

The team will include the anesthesiologist, surgeon, dietitian, and physical therapist. Surgical procedures include laparoscopic banding, vertical banded gastroplasty, sleeve gastrectomy, and gastric bypass with Roux en Y reconstruction leaving a 15–30 mL reservoir. Patients are fed a diet of solid food requiring chewing. Exercise is highly encouraged.

Operative mortality is approximately 2%. Morbidity consists mainly of pulmonary atelectasis, venous thrombosis, and wound infection. Laparoscopic bands can slip and be overinflated, causing dysphagia and requiring immediate decompression. Staple lines can leak, causing peritonitis, which may be particularly difficult to detect in these patients.

Reducing BMI to <35 is successful in 40–70% of vertical gastric stapling procedures.

Follow-up
Patients should be seen at regular intervals (every 4 weeks) until underlying metabolic disorder is excluded and the need for surgery determined.

Post-operative Follow-up
Patients should be seen 1–2 weeks after surgery to detect any general post-operative complications. Thereafter, regular visits should be scheduled every 3 months, then 6 months, then yearly, to determine continued success in terms of weight reduction and nutritional status.

Questions and Answers

Q1　Diagnostic evaluation of a patient with an incidentally identified adrenal mass does NOT routinely include:
   A　24-hr urine collection for catecholamines.
   B　Low-dose dexamethasone suppression test.
   C　PRA (plasma renin to aldosterone ratio).
   D　Biopsy of the mass.
   E　Serum potassium level.

A1　D: Biochemical evaluation should evaluate the mass for functionality, since the mass should be removed if it is producing aldosterone, cortisol, or is a pheochromocytoma. Biopsy is rarely required and should only be performed AFTER a pheochromocytoma has been excluded, as biopsy of a catecholamine-producing tumor can lead to pheochromocytoma crisis.

Q2　Routine evaluation of a thyroid nodule for potential thyroid cancer includes all of the following EXCEPT:
   A　Ultrasound.
   B　Thyroid radionucleotide scan.
   C　Biopsy.
   D　Thyroid function tests.
   E　History and physical examination.

A2　B: Thyroid radionucleotide scan should only be used in the setting of hyperthyroidism, to help clarify whether a patient has Graves' disease, toxic adenoma, toxic multinodular goiter, etc. It should not be a routine component of evaluating a mass for a potential malignancy, as "cold" and "hot" nodules both can represent thyroid cancer.

Q3   A patient who presents with medullary thyroid cancer should be screened for
a potential association with:
   A   Primary hyperparathyroidism.
   B   Prolactinoma.
   C   Insulinoma.
   D   Gastrinoma.
   E   Jaw tumors.

A3   A: If a patient has medullary thyroid cancer, it is important to exclude MEN 2A
and MEN 2B syndromes. Prolactinoma and gastrinoma are potentially components of MEN 1 syndrome, and jaw tumors can be seen with familial forms of
hyperparathyroidism.

Q4   All of the following are essential components of evaluation of a patient with
primary hyperparathyroidism EXCEPT:
   A   Serum intact parathyroid hormone level.
   B   Serum calcium level.
   C   Serum creatinine level.
   D   24-hour urine collection for calcium.
   E   Serum phosphate level.

A4   E: It is important in a patient potentially with primary hyperparathyroidism to
identify a high or inappropriately high normal PTH level, a high calcium level,
a normal creatinine level (to exclude secondary hyperparathyroidism), and a
24-hour collection for calcium (to exclude benign familial hypocalciuric hypercalcemia). A serum phosphate level is not essential.

Q5   A patient with an aldosteronoma typically presents with hypertension and
the associated biochemical abnormality of:
   A   Low sodium.
   B   High phosphate.
   C   Low potassium.
   D   High potassium.
   E   Suppressed aldosterone level (<10 ng/dl) after saline infusion test.

A5   C: Low potassium/hypokalemia. These patients typically are hypertensive and
often require multiple antihypertensive agents. They also usually have hypokalemia requiring potassium supplements. For challenging cases of diagnosis, a 2L
Normal saline infusion can be delivered; patients with Conn's syndrome will not
suppress their aldosterone <10 ng/dl after infusion.

Esophagus

Lynn S. Model and Malcolm V. Brock

FOUR

Potential Consultations

✧ Hiatal hernia.
✧ Congenital diaphragmatic hernia.
✧ Traumatic diaphragmatic hernia.
✧ Reflux esophagitis.
✧ Non-reflux esophagitis.
✧ Benign esophageal stricture.
✧ Achalasia.
✧ Vigorous achalasia.
✧ Diffuse esophageal spasm.
✧ Nutcracker esophagus.
✧ Pharyngeal pouch.
✧ Motility disorders secondary to systemic disease.
✧ Esophageal cancer.

The Esophagus

On a basic level, the esophagus is a muscular tube whose function is to transport food from the mouth through the chest and diaphragm and into the stomach. Successful completion of this task requires the coordinated function of the brain, the nervous system, voluntary and involuntary muscles, and the esophageal mucosa. Thus, disorders affecting any of these systems can result in esophageal pathology.

A particular diagnostic difficulty you will be confronted with is the differential diagnosis of "chest" pain that, at times, presents similarly whether of cardiac or esophageal origin. Cardiac pain may represent a potentially immediate life-threatening event, hence investigation of the cardiovascular system may take priority over esophageal assessment in these situations.

Abnormalities in gastric function, such as acid hypersecretion, may first present with esophageal reflux rather than gastric symptoms. Therefore, the assessment of esophageal symptoms may require the consideration of a number of different body systems to arrive at the correct diagnosis.

Esophageal History

Start with a general gastrointestinal (GI) function history. When the responses indicate a possible esophageal problem, a more detailed esophageal history is required to differentiate esophageal problems from cardiac or pulmonary disorders or gastric problems.

Dysphagia

> "It is difficult to swallow (liquids/solids)."

This strongly suggests an esophageal problem, and can be due to mechanical or motility disorders. The dysphagia should then be further defined as being to solids or liquids.
✧ Dysphagia to solids suggests a mechanical cause.
✧ Dysphagia to only liquids suggests a motility disorder.

Important questions to ask are:

✧ Approximate site along the esophagus where food gets "stuck."
✧ Time course after food intake to start of symptoms; time to resolution.
✧ Are symptoms intermittent, and helped by sipping fluids or repeated swallowing (motility), or persistent and progressive suggesting a mechanical stricture of the lumen, e.g. carcinoma?

Regurgitation

> "I've been coughing up pieces of food."

Patients often complain of a sour taste in the mouth; this may occur mostly at night and the patient finds that in the morning, regurgitated fluid has stained the pillow.

Important questions to ask are:

✧ Any postural symptoms? Is it worse after large meals? With postural regurgitation, symptoms are increased by a supine posture or are worse after large meals.
✧ Timing of symptoms: Increased symptoms at night? Do they cause coughing? This may be due to a constricting lesion, but is more common in motility disorders, e.g. achalasia.
✧ Concomitant heartburn symptoms?
✧ Be sure to ask questions to elucidate the atypical symptoms of regurgitation, including laryngitis or hoarseness, chronic throat clearing, sore or burning throat, worsening asthma symptoms after eating a big meal, or a globus sensation (a feeling of a lump in the throat, more common between meals with resolution thereafter).

Odynophagia

> "It hurts to swallow (liquids/solids)."

Important questions to ask are:

✧ Questions to localize the pain.
✧ Type of pain: is it burning?
✧ Are symptoms immediate after eating? Only after certain foods/liquids? Symptoms that occur after swallowing hot drinks suggest organic disease, e.g. esophagitis.

Heartburn

> "I have a burning sensation in my chest after I eat."

This is due to gastro-esophageal reflux causing chemical inflammation of the esophageal mucosa.

Important questions to ask are:

✧ Questions regarding localization/character/timing of pain.
✧ Is there pain radiation?
✧ Cardiac history (heartburn can also be a symptom of ischemic heart disease).

Esophageal Causes of Anterior Chest Pain

This is an angina-type pain, which can radiate to the back, jaw, and arm, and is often relieved by nitrates. It is seen in both reflux and motility disorders, and can be precipitated by meals, emotion, and exercise.

Water Brash

Excess secretion of saliva which tastes salty, often experienced in reflux disease.

Other Atypical Presentations of Esophageal Pathology
✧ Anemia.
✧ Hematemesis.
✧ Classic cardiac-type chest pain: 20–40% of patients with chest pain and normal angiograms actually have esophageal pain.

Esophageal Examination
Perform a full physical examination. In particular, look for:
✧ Signs of weight loss: sagging skin, facial bony prominence.
✧ Pallor due to anemia: face, conjunctiva, nail beds.
✧ Neck swelling (e.g. pharyngeal pouch).
✧ Enlarged lymph nodes: e.g. in the left supraclavicular fossa, this may represent metastatic spread from a GI malignancy.

Carry out:
✧ Percussion and auscultation of the lungs, to detect aspiration pneumonia.
✧ Abdominal exam: The presence of an epigastric mass and/or hepatomegaly may represent the presence of advanced malignant disease.
✧ Cardiovascular exam – to help detect any underlying cardiac disease that may be the cause of chest symptoms.

Diagnostic Tests for Esophageal Disorders
Specific Laboratory Tests of Interest
Hematology
✧ Fecal occult blood test (FOBT) may indicate microcytic anemia.
✧ Leukocytosis may suggest infection.

Biochemistry
Abnormal liver function tests (LFTs) may indicate liver metastases in malignancy.

Microbiology
Candidiasis of the mouth/esophagus.

Cytology/Histology
Cytology of brushings or histology of biopsies taken at endoscopy.

Imaging Tests
Chest X-ray
All patients who have esophageal symptoms should have a chest X-ray (CXR), to look for:
✧ Aspiration pneumonia.
✧ Mediastinal widening due to lymph node metastases.
✧ Suspicious soft-tissue shadows (infection or metastatic disease).
✧ Fluid/gas levels (large hiatal hernia with intrathoracic stomach, dilated esophagus in achalasia).

Esophago-Gastro-Duodenoscopy
Esophago-gastro-duodenoscopy (EGD) should be the first investigation in all patients with esophageal symptoms, except for suspected Zenker's diverticulum or suspected perforation (where water-soluble or barium swallow study is best for diagnosis). EGD allows direct visualization of mechanical obstructions and enables biopsies to be taken

for histologic diagnosis. It also allows visualization of conditions such as esophagitis, ulcerations, varices, etc., and for certain therapeutic maneuvers to be performed, e.g. dilatation of benign strictures.

Negatives are:
✧ It is an invasive procedure.
✧ Cannot diagnose early motility disorders (requires esophageal manometry).
✧ Despite sedation, some patients may find it unpleasant and are unable to swallow the scope.

Complications:
✧ Aspiration.
✧ Trauma to the esophagus, stomach, and duodenum which may cause bleeding, pain, or occasionally perforation.

Barium Swallow (Liquid or Solid)
This is the first-line investigation if esophageal web, esophageal motility disorders, esophageal perforation, or esophageal pouches are suspected. It is the second-line investigation if EGD fails to provide a diagnosis. Barium swallow is also useful after esophageal or gastric surgery in patients with esophageal symptoms, to exclude a mechanical cause (i.e. stricture) or leak.

It is especially good at diagnosing:
✧ Hiatal hernia.
✧ Esophageal perforations (use water-soluble contrast, e.g. gastrograffin).
✧ Abnormalities of the upper esophageal sphincter and coordinated swallowing mechanism.

Double contrast (barium–air) barium meals are useful for the evaluation of esophageal cancer, especially the length of the lesion which may correlate with depth of invasion and ability to resect.

Barium swallow is not reliable in the diagnosis of reflux. Approximately 20% of people without gastro-esophageal reflux disease (GERD) exhibit reflux in the Trendelenburg position; only reflux that is demonstrated in the upright position is clinically significant.

Computed Tomography
Computed tomography (CT) is used in staging esophageal malignancy to demonstrate:
✧ Extent of mural invasion.
✧ Involvement of adjacent structures.
✧ Mediastinal lymph node involvement.
✧ Distant metastases.

Negatives are:
✧ CT tends to underestimate early mediastinal spread and lymph node metastases.
✧ It is not reliable in differentiating direct metastatic spread from reactive inflammation surrounding a tumor.

Ultrasound
✧ *Endoluminal ultrasound* is a specialized technique where an ultrasound probe is placed into the esophagus to provide images of the esophageal wall and adjacent lymph nodes (the best way to determine intramural spread, tumor size [T stage], and lymph node involvement).

✧ *Laparoscopic ultrasound* is another specialized technique which utilizes an ultrasound probe inserted into the abdomen at laparoscopy, and may be applied directly to organs, e.g. the liver, to look for nodal or solid organ metastases and sometimes determine their resectability.

The technique is operator dependent, and CT is required to confirm findings.

Esophageal Scintigraphy
This technique is used to assess lower esophageal sphincter (LES) incompetence in patients with reflux and to evaluate the transit of liquid or solid boluses in motility disorders.
     The process is as follows:
✧ The patient swallows 99m-technetium-labeled liquid or solid (e.g. eggs).
✧ Swallowing is recorded by a gamma-counting camera to detect radioactivity.

This provides useful visualization of esophageal function, particularly in the investigation of achalasia.

Physiologic Tests
Esophageal Manometry
A soft, plastic, multilumen tube connected to a pressure transduction system is passed orally or nasally into the esophagus and positioned at the desired point in the stomach or esophagus. Static measurements can be made at different positions to determine the pressure profile of peristalsis, the upper esophageal sphincter (UES) and the LES.
     The technique is useful for assessment of motility disorders, dysphagia, and the complications of antireflux surgery. Ambulatory manometry is now available for investigation of infrequent esophageal spasm.
     Negatives are:
✧ Low sensitivity for reflux diagnosis.
✧ Can be uncomfortable for patients.

High-Resolution Manometry and Impedance
This is a novel technique that not only provides a more precise assessment of esophageal motility than conventional manometry, but is also simpler and faster to perform. It measures pressure and impedance events simultaneously along the entire length of the esophagus without the need for catheter-pullback maneuvers. Advances in software have resulted in spatiotemporal plots that are intuitively easier to interpret.
     Early clinical experience shows that high-resolution manometry is better able to assess the abnormal transport of a bolus along the esophagus. For example, in achalasia three distinct patterns of aperistalsis are observed with high-resolution manometry, each with its own clinical characteristics and responsiveness to medical and surgical therapies.

24-Hour pH Monitoring
The conventional method of pH assessment; patients are assessed after having been off all antacid or proton-pump inhibitor (PPI) medications for 10 days.
     A twin micro-pH probe is passed orally or nasally. The esophageal transducer is positioned 5 cm above the high-pressure zone in the lower esophagus (as determined by manometry), and the gastric transducer is positioned in the stomach. pH in both the esophagus and the stomach is monitored for 24 hours. The patient can press an event marker when symptoms are experienced, and this can be correlated with pH recordings.
     The process tends to be uncomfortable, and requires patient compliance.

Hiatal Hernia
Esophageal hiatus in the diaphragm becomes enlarged, allowing part of the stomach to pass through into the chest. There are four types:
✧ Type I (70–80% of cases) – sliding.
✧ Type II (8–10%) – para-esophageal.
✧ Type III – mixed.
✧ Type IV – other abdominal organs hernia also.

History
✧ Take a general and esophageal history (as above).
✧ Take a cardiac history to differentiate esophageal symptoms from atypical angina.

Type I patients may have symptoms of reflux esophagitis, chronic blood loss or stricture, but are often asymptomatic.
   In type II:
✧ The patient may complain of a pressure-like sensation when the stomach is distended with gas or food.
✧ There may be pain, dyspnea and tightness in the chest that is precipitated by food intake, bending or stooping positions.
✧ Pain is usually sharp, located under the lower sternum and radiates to the back; it is often accompanied by a bloated sensation, anxiety, palpitations, and dyspnea.
✧ Pain is often relieved by belching or vomiting.
✧ There may be symptoms of anemia associated with ulcer within the hiatal hernia (Cameron's ulcer).
✧ Dysphagia is also present in 20% of patients.

Examination
Perform a full physical examination, with special attention to:
✧ Signs of anemia.
✧ Chest exam for evidence of effusions or infection.
✧ Supraclavicular fossae for evidence of lymph node spread of malignant disease.
✧ Abdomen for epigastric masses or evidence of liver enlargement.

No abnormalities on physical examination makes the diagnosis of hiatal hernia *more* likely.
   Perform a cardiovascular examination to help rule out a cardiac cause for chest symptoms.

Diagnostic Tests
✧ CXR may show a soft-tissue mass or an air–fluid level behind the heart.
✧ EGD demonstrates reduced distance from incisors to gastro-esophageal junction (GEJ), and may be used to detect the hernia via specific maneuvers required to pass the scope and visualize the entire stomach.
✧ Barium swallow is usually diagnostic in cases not detected by EGD.
✧ FOBT may show iron-deficiency anemia.
✧ Cardiac tests are performed as indicated by the presence of atypical chest pain symptoms.

Treatment
Type I:
✧ Symptoms of reflux esophagitis can be controlled medically with PPIs, diet and life-style behavioral modifications.

✧ If symptoms are severe enough to merit intervention and the patient is a good operative risk, surgery can be considered – hernia reduction and antireflux surgery (open or laparoscopic).

Type II carries significant (~5%) risk of incarceration, and thus should be surgically repaired if the patient is of reasonable operative risk. Repair of diaphragmatic defect is open or laparoscopic, with or without antireflux surgery. An infarcted or strangulated type II hernia may need a thoracotomy or thoraco-abdominal approach for better access to the hernia sack.

Types III and IV – surgical reduction with or without antireflux procedure.

Follow-up

Most patients with esophageal reflux secondary to hiatal hernia are treated by gastroenterologists, who refer patients with uncontrolled or recurrent symptoms on medical therapy, or with newly diagnosed type II hernias, for surgery.

Patients with pressure symptoms in the chest may be referred to a surgeon directly by their primary care physician (PCP). Diagnostic tests should be scheduled promptly, especially if a cardiac cause cannot be excluded immediately by history and physical exam.

Post-operative Follow-up

In routine cases, patients are seen for follow-up approximately 2–3 weeks post-operatively. Review the operative note to determine whether there were any complications during the procedure; early complications to look for include wound infection and incisional hernia. Determine whether the operation has been successful in relieving the original symptoms.

Special complications are:

✧ Tight wrap – patients may complain of dysphagia or bloating if the fundal wrap is too tight. Usually the symptoms are relatively mild, and will resolve within 3 months with observation.

✧ Severe or persistent cases beyond 3 months require further investigation with a barium swallow, EGD, or esophageal manometry.

✧ Treatment options include endoscopic balloon dilatation (often successful) or remedial surgery.

✧ Slipped Nissen – the Nissen wrap either slips down the stomach, causing an hourglass deformity and presenting as dysphagia and abdominal discomfort, or the wrap slips up between the crura into the chest with accompanying dysphagia.

   ∝ Diagnosed by a barium meal.

   ∝ Requires prompt revision surgery.

Congenital Diaphragmatic Hernia

Congenital diaphragmatic hernia (CDH) is often diagnosed and treated shortly after birth, but a patient may be asymptomatic in youth and present with symptoms later in life.

Bochdalek (90% of CDH cases):

✧ 90% are left-sided.

✧ Persistent pleuroperitoneal canal leads to posterolateral defect.

✧ Present in the neonatal period, with respiratory distress due to pulmonary hypoplasia on the affected side.

Morgagni (5–10% of CDH cases):

✧ Parasternal, anterior hernia; 90% are right-sided.

✧ Present in adult life, with episodes of pain and tenderness in the subcostal region and intermittent obstructive symptoms. Often associated with intestinal malrotation.

Central tendon defect/Congenital hiatal hernia (rare):
✧ Stomach herniates through an esophageal hiatus.
✧ May be associated with defect in pericardium (intestine herniates into pericardium).

History
Take a general esophageal and gastrointestinal history. In particular, note any history of intermittent subcostal pain or dysphagia.

Examination
Perform a full physical examination; this is often normal in adults. Patients may have tenderness and/or fullness in the subcostal region.

Diagnostic Tests
✧ CXR-PA (chest X-ray, posterior anterior view) shows a round gas-containing shadow to the right of the cardiac outline (left-sided defect). Lateral CXR shows a gas-containing shadow behind the sternum.
✧ Barium swallow is usually diagnostic.
✧ For right-sided defects, ultrasound may be needed to differentiate diaphragmatic neoplasm (rare) from herniated liver parenchyma.

Treatment
Symptomatic patients are considered for surgical reduction and prosthetic mesh repair. Right-sided abnormalities usually require no treatment, while left-sided and central hernias require surgical repair.

Follow-up
Follow-up is at short intervals (1–4 weeks) until diagnosis is made. Mild cases can be observed at gradually increasing intervals (1–6 months).

Post-operative Follow-up
Determine whether the operation has relieved the symptoms and whether there are any general complications associated with abdominal and thoracic surgery, including wound infection, abscess, residual pleural effusion, etc.

Recurrence of symptoms may indicate recurrence of the hernia – investigate as for primary cases.

Traumatic Diaphragmatic Hernia
This may present months or years after the trauma event, e.g. a seat-belt injury from a motor vehicle accident. Generally, all traumatic hernias should be repaired immediately if the patient's condition allows.

History
Take a general history, focusing on GI symptoms. Symptoms tend to be related to the size of the herniated contents and to the onset of mechanical complications such as intestinal obstruction, strangulation, hemorrhage or progressive cardiorespiratory insufficiency.

Examination
Perform a full physical examination. Examine the chest for evidence of respiratory insufficiency, bowel sounds, or infection.

Diagnostic Tests

✧ CXR demonstrates a space-occupying lesion; if spleen or omentum is herniated, this appears as a solid mass.
✧ Barium swallow may confirm the diagnosis.
✧ Ultrasound or CT can be helpful to determine chest contents.

Treatment

Surgical repair through the abdominal or thoracic approach.

Follow-up

Severe cases need prompt investigation and treatment. Persistence of a diaphragmatic hernia can lead to bowel obstruction or strangulation, and thus to dire outcomes.

Post-operative Follow-up

Determine whether the operation has relieved the symptoms and if there are any complications of the thoracic or abdominal procedure. Recurrence of symptoms may mean recurrence of the hernia.

Reflux Esophagitis

Reflus esophagitis is caused by the abnormal retrograde movement of gastric contents into the esophagus. The normal mechanisms to clear the esophagus of any refluxed gastric contents are overwhelmed, so that gastric contents remain in the lower esophagus and inflammation of the mucosa occurs.

Esophagitis occurs due to acid reflux as well as the presence of bile salts, trypsin and lysolecithin in the reflux; this is especially problematic after partial gastrectomy.

Complications of reflux esophagitis include chronic blood loss, deep ulceration with periesophagitis, and the formation of strictures and webs.

The presence of columnar mucosal change indicates the development of Barrett's esophagus.

✧ Barrett's esophagus may lead to stricture, ulceration and the development of adenocarcinoma.
✧ The risk of developing cancer is relatively low (approximately 1% per year), but is higher in those that develop simple mucosal dysplasia.

History

✧ Heartburn, regurgitation, and dysphagia (constant or intermittent).
✧ May have wheezing, coughing, or hoarseness of voice.
✧ Symptoms are aggravated by supine posture; worse at night and after large meals or with the patient bending over forward.
✧ Persistent dysphagia usually suggests stricture formation.
✧ Other presentations include odynophagia, waterbrash, atypical chest pain, or asthma (due to aspiration).

Examination

✧ Perform a full physical examination (this is often normal).
✧ Examine for anemia, weight loss, etc.
✧ Examine the chest for signs of effusion or infection.
✧ Examine the abdomen for epigastric mass or liver enlargement.

Diagnostic Tests
✧ EGD and biopsy for histology.
✧ Barium swallow – demonstrate presence of hiatal hernia.
✧ 24-hour pH monitoring and manometry.
✧ Radionucleotide assessment of gastric emptying.
✧ FOBT may reveal anemia.

Treatment
Uncomplicated Disease
✧ Lifestyle changes: Weight loss; avoidance of alcohol, citrus, tomato, and chocolate; raising the head of the bed; stopping smoking; avoidance of large meals and lying down within 3 hours of meals.
✧ Antacids, H2-receptor antagonists (H2 blockers), PPIs and prokinetics if symptoms do not improve with lifestyle changes.
   ∝ PPIs are the most powerful pharmacologic treatment for GERD (8 weeks of therapy).
   ∝ Prokinetics are particularly useful for relief of nausea, fullness, regurgitation, belching and odynophagia.
✧ For neutral/alkali reflux after post-operative gastric surgery, a bile salt binding agent such as cholestyramine is useful.

Eighty percent of patients will be cured with lifestyle/pharmacologic therapy.

Complicated Disease
✧ Barrett's esophagus with low-grade dysplasia – confirm the diagnosis with two endoscopic biopsies 3 months apart, after an 8-week course of PPIs. Confirmed cases may require antireflux surgery, acid suppression therapy and continued EGD surveillance (columnar change reverses in approximately 10% of patients, but all cases need continued surveillance).
✧ High-grade dysplasia may represent carcinoma in situ and, if confirmed, is an indication for esophageal resection. Upon resection, 30–40% of patients are found to have invasive carcinoma in the histologic specimen.

Indications for Surgical Treatment
✧ Failure of medical therapy: persistent symptoms, intractable esophagitis.
✧ Development of complications such as stricture or Barrett's esophagus.
✧ Reflux associated with motility disorders or esophageal chest pain.
✧ Reflux in children persisting beyond the age of 2 years.
✧ Reflux after upper abdominal surgery: acid or bile.

Surgical Treatment
Nissen fundoplication: 360° stomach wrap around esophagus; this may be laparoscopic or open. The thoracic approach is preferred in patients with severe esophagitis, stricture formation, peri-esophagitis or esophageal shortening. Post-operative "gas bloat" can occur in 2–5% of patients, but is usually self-limited. With a properly constructed loose Nissen fundoplication, dysphagia is rarely encountered.

Follow-up
✧ The majority of patients with esophageal reflux are treated by gastroenterologists, who refer patients with uncontrolled or recurrent symptoms on medical therapy for surgery.

✧ Different clinics have their own policies regarding Barrett's esophagus patients and whether regular endoscopy monitoring to detect malignant change is performed in all patients or selected patients. At present, there is no conclusive evidence to suggest that routine follow-up of Barrett's esophagus is justified in any patient other than those with dysplastic change.

Post-operative Follow-up

Look for wound/infectious complications, and recurrence of symptoms (5–10% of Nissen fundoplications come undone).

Persistent heartburn occurs in approximately 5–8% of patients. This may be due to delayed gastric emptying resulting from unrecognized distal peptic ulcer disease or disruption of the fundal wrap. Investigate with EGD, barium swallow and/or esophageal manometry.

Non-reflux Esophagitis

All types of non-reflux esophagitis produce a mixture of strictures, motility disorders, hiatal hernias, and occasional cancers. These patients can become acutely ill very quickly; thus they are treated as inpatients at first.

Non-reflux esophagitis may be caused by ingestion of corrosive substances, infections, radiation, or may be drug induced. Specific disorders are Behçet's syndrome, Crohn's disease, and scleroderma.

History

Take a history of esophageal symptoms as well as a general medical history, if the patient's condition allows. History will usually be suggestive of the underlying disorder and there will be progressive dysphagia from liquids to solids.

If esophagitis is due to acute ingestion of a corrosive substance, note the substance ingested, the amount, and the time course.

Examination

Perform a full physical examination with particular focus on face/oropharynx, chest, and abdomen. Look for other evidence of an underlying systemic disorder.

Diagnostic Tests

✧ EGD, barium swallow, motility and pH studies.
✧ If Crohn's is suspected, a small bowel follow-through study may be helpful.

Treatment

Mild cases are treated medically as appropriate:
✧ Antibiotics for infectious causes.
✧ Steroid treatment for cardiovascular disease, Behçet's, Crohn's, etc.
✧ Medication cessation for drug-induced causes.

More severe cases may be considered for surgery:
✧ Extensive persistent stricture(s), need for frequent dilatations.
✧ Presence of high strictures or late bronchotracheo-esophageal fistulas.
✧ Late esophageal shortening with reflux esophagitis.
✧ Severe dysplasia, carcinoma in situ, or invasive carcinoma.

Extensive scarring may require total esophagectomy with colonic, isoperistaltic jejunum, or stomach interposition.

There may be a "frozen mediastinum," where scarring is such that manually dissecting out the esophagus in the mediastium is not possible; in these cases, the esophagus is left in place and an extra-anatomic bypass is performed.

Follow-up
Follow-up is long-term, as complications often develop. If symptoms are non-existent or mild and stable, discharge patient from clinic with plans to return if symptoms worsen.

Post-operative Follow-up
✧ Follow-up is long-term.
✧ Initially, determine the success of the procedure and look for any complications associated with abdominal and thoracic procedures.
✧ Monitor nutrition at regular intervals (weight, skin-fold thickness, routine blood work); dietary and vitamin supplements may be necessary.
✧ Monitor function of bypass with regular barium swallows.
✧ Endoscopic dilatation of strictures may be necessary.

Benign Esophageal Strictures
All strictures need urgent EGD and multiple biopsies to exclude cancer.

History
Take a general medical and esophageal symptom history. Note particularly any history of reflux esophagitis, or caustic fluid ingestion in the past. Generally, dysphagia symptoms will be of slow onset and progress from solids to liquids.

Examination
✧ Perform a full physical examination, with particular focus on oropharynx and chest.
✧ Look for evidence of weight loss, anemia, and sepsis.
✧ Examine the chest for respiratory and cardiovascular disease.
✧ Examine the abdomen for other gastrointestinal disease.
✧ Examination can often be normal.

Diagnostic Tests
✧ Diagnosis is usually by a combination of EGD and biopsies for histologic examination.
✧ If surgery is considered, add studies of esophageal motility (barium swallow).
✧ A CT scan, to detect scarring in the mediastinum, can be performed to help in planning surgical intervention.

Treatment
✧ *Endoscopic dilatation*: EGD is performed to visualize the stricture; simple bougie, wire-guided bougie, or balloon-dilator dilatations are performed. Some centers prefer to perform the procedure under fluoroscopic guidance. All patients should remain nil by mouth (NPO) after dilatation for a short period of observation to rule out any obvious perforations. Some centers routinely perform a CXR to exclude perforation before allowing the patient to eat.
   ∝ Complications include hemorrhage, perforation, and septicemia.
   ∝ Subsequent treatments: Following a course of dilatation, 20–50% of patients remain symptom free. Twenty percent require frequent dilatation; and in these cases, surgery or insertion of a self-expanding metal stent should be considered.
   ∝ Patients often must remain on lifelong treatment if the stricture is not to recur.

✧ *Inhibition of reflux*: An equally important aspect of the management of benign strictures is inhibition of acid reflux, usually with a PPI, and lifestyle changes (as described in the GERD section). If bile reflux is a problem, revision surgery (Roux-en-Y gastric bypass) may be necessary.

Indications for Surgery
✧ Young patients with reflux strictures.
✧ Frequent and increasingly difficult dilatations.
✧ Intractable/impassable strictures.
✧ Stricture associated with Barrett's esophagus (dysplasia confers risk of adenocarcinoma).

Surgery
✧ Resection of affected segment or total esophagectomy.
✧ For GERD-associated disease, antireflux surgery: Perform thoracotomy and intraoperative dilatation, then return to the abdomen and perform Nissen's. If the esophagus is too short, also perform a Collis gastroplasty.

Follow-up
✧ Intervals should be short (1–2 weeks) until cancer is excluded.
✧ If a repeated course of dilatation is indicated, the patient should be seen in the clinic 2–4 weeks after completion of the course for any recurrent symptoms to be detected. Thereafter, follow-up intervals can be lengthened (1–6 months). If the condition remains stable, the patient may be discharged from the clinic with advice to return if the symptoms reappear.
✧ GERD patients are advised that they must remain on lifelong antireflux treatment (PPIs) if the stricture is not to recur.

Post-operative Follow-up
Following surgery, the patient should be evaluated to determine whether the procedure has relieved the original symptoms and to detect any complications. Complications include wound infection, incisional hernia, and pleural effusions.

GERD patients are advised that they must remain on lifelong antireflux treatment if the stricture is not to recur.

Motility Disorders
Most motility disorders can be classified as:
✧ Primary – achalasia, diffuse esophageal spasm, nutcracker esophagus, hypertensive LES.
✧ Secondary – neurologic disorders (poliomyelitis, pseudobulbar palsy), myopathies (dermatomyositis), systemic disease (scleroderma, diabetes, alcohol-related, psychiatric disorders), parasitic infections (Chagas disease).

Achalasia
Achalasia is the absence of peristaltic contractions within the esophageal body and incomplete relaxation of the lower esophageal sphincter. This is caused by the progressive loss of inhibitory ganglion cells at the LES, progressing cranially. It is most common in patients aged 25–60 years old.

History
✧ Take a general medical and esophageal-motility history.
✧ Commonly reported symptoms include: dysphagia, undigested food regurgitation,

chest pain, heartburn, and weight loss. Typically, dysphagia is for solids *and* liquids, with progressively worsening symptoms. As esophageal dilatation increases, pain and dysphagia decrease and regurgitation symptoms increase. Patients may also complain of regurgitation, of foamy, mucoid saliva.

✧ Halitosis and belching of foul air may be described. Patients may report coughing when lying in a horizontal position.

✧ Advanced achalasia leads to massive dilatation of the esophagus, causing severe dysphagia, weight loss, anemia, and respiratory complications due to aspiration, fever, sweating, and breathlessness.

Examination
✧ Perform a full physical examination (this may be normal).
✧ Look for evidence of weight loss, anemia, and sepsis.
✧ Specifically examine the oropharanx; halitosis may be noticed.
✧ Examine the chest for evidence of infection or effusion.
✧ Examine the abdomen for other gastrointestinal pathology.

Diagnostic Tests
✧ CXR may show a convex shadow to the right of the vena cava and right atrium, with or without a fluid level within the shadow (representing a massively dilated esophagus). The lungs should also be assessed for pneumonia.

✧ Barium swallow may show dilatation of the esophagus and the characteristic "bird's beak" appearance. Slow emptying of contrast into the stomach is also often noted.

✧ EGD should be performed to exclude peptic stricture or carcinoma of the esophagus.

✧ Esophageal manometry may or may not have classic findings: Absence of propulsive peristalsis in esophageal body, elevated LES resting pressure (>40 mmHg), absence of LES relaxation.

   ∝ High amplitude (>60 mmHg) simultaneous contractions of the esophageal body are referred to as "vigorous achalasia." This may be part of early-stage achalasia.

   ∝ In early or doubtful cases, esophageal manometry may demonstrate no relaxation of the lower esophageal sphincter with swallowing.

✧ Edrophonium (an acetylcholinesterase inhibitor) injection decreases LES pressure while atropine (muscarinic antagonist) injection increases LES pressure, respectively.

Treatment
✧ In early achalasia, some patients (~10%) benefit from long-acting nitrites (isosorbide) or calcium-channel blockers.

✧ After endoscopic intrasphincteric injection of botulinum toxin, 30% of patients are symptom-free 1 year after the procedure; a good treatment for elderly patients who may not tolerate surgery or dilatation.

✧ Endoscopic pneumatic balloon dilatation. Repeat dilatations are often required.

   ∝ 70–80% successful, ~5% perforation rate, ~25% rate of GERD post-procedure.

   ∝ Usually does not help in cases of vigorous achalasia. Surgical myotomy is the preferred treatment in this group.

✧ Surgical myotomy (Heller's), usually with partial fundoplication (the laproscopic route is preferable), is indicated for:

   ∝ Advanced disease with dilatation and esophagitis, in younger patients and when there is coexistent pathology requiring surgical treatment, e.g. hiatal hernia, phrenic diverticulum.

   ∝ Failure of repeated dilatation/recurrence of symptoms.

✧ Severe achalasia with a huge, tortuous megaesophagus may require subtotal esophagectomy with gastric pull-through and cervical anastomosis.

Follow-up
Severe cases need prompt assessment and treatment. Mild cases may respond to nitrates and be seen in the clinic at 2–3 month intervals to gauge response.

Patients requiring short-interval endoscopic dilatations should be seen in the clinic as soon as symptoms recur.

Post-operative Follow-up
✧ Patients are generally seen for follow-up 2–3 weeks after the procedure.
✧ Early complications to look for include: esophageal obstructive symptoms, wound infection, and pleural effusion or other respiratory complications if a thoracotomy was performed.
✧ Recurrence of symptoms can be treated with further endoscopic dilatation if persistent.
✧ Esophagectomy can be complicated by recurrent laryngeal nerve palsy, gastric outlet obstruction, gastro-esophageal reflux, and dumping (see esophageal cancer).

Diffuse Esophageal Spasm and Nutcracker Esophagus
Diffuse esophageal spasm (DES) is uncoordinated esophageal contractions, while nutcracker esophagus consists of coordinated contractions of the esophagus of an excessive amplitude. Patients with nutcracker esophagus often have associated psychiatric disorders such as anxiety, depression, and somatization disorder.

History
✧ Take a general medical history, with a focus on esophageal motility. Also take a psychiatric history.
✧ Typical symptoms are: chest pain (can be similar to anginal pain), radiating to back, neck and jaw; odynophagia and dysphagia (affecting solids and liquids equally); food regurgitation; globus; heartburn.
✧ Often diagnosed after normal coronary angiography.

Examination
✧ Perform a full physical examination (this is often normal). Focus on the oropharynx.
✧ Look for evidence of weight loss and anemia.
✧ Examine the chest for any respiratory or cardiovascular abnormalities.

Diagnostic Tests
✧ Barium swallow shows corkscrew appearance in DES, but is non-diagnostic in nutcracker esophagus.
✧ CT shows muscular hypertrophy of esophagus (>3 mm thick).
✧ EGD is performed to exclude organic disease, with or without intraluminal ultrasound.
✧ Consider cardiology assessment if cardiac disease is suspected.
✧ Manometry (best for DES):
   ∝ *DES*: >2 uncoordinated contractions during 10 wet swallows, with >1 peristaltic contraction. Or >20% simultaneous contractions in stationary motility testing, all with normal amplitude.
   ∝ *Nutcracker*: Orderly, progressive esophageal contractions with amplitude >2 standard deviations above normal.

✧ Radionuclide scan shows oscillatory movement of isotope-labeled bolus and marked delay in transit time in some patients.
✧ 24-hr pH monitoring often detects concomitant GERD.

Treatment
✧ Conservative/medical:
  ∝ Long-acting nitrites, tricyclic antidepressants (TCAs) (imipramine), calcium-channel blockers (especially for nutcracker esophagus).
  ∝ Botulinum toxin injection into the LES.
  ∝ Trial of PPIs.
  ∝ Pureed diet.
✧ Endoscopic pneumatic dilatation – although the reason for its effectiveness is unknown, small trials have shown some improvement in symptoms for DES and nutcracker esophagus.
✧ Surgery is indicated in fit patients in whom conservative therapy has failed.
  ∝ For DES – thoracoscopic/open long myotomy of entire involved segment (as determined by manometry) through the LES, and partial or full fundoplication. This *does not work* for nutcracker esophagus, and may actually worsen symptoms as peristaltic wave effectiveness is decreased.
  ∝ Esophagectomy (last resort).

Follow-up
Severe cases are investigated and treated promptly. Less severe cases can be assessed at longer intervals (1–2 months) to determine the effect of individual therapeutic agents or procedures. Assess the need for endoscopic dilatation or, in severe cases and in suitable patients, the need for surgery.

Post-operative Follow-up
✧ Assess for common thoracic surgical complications: wound infection, pleural effusion, atelectasis, pneumonia, empyema, etc.
✧ Some centers recommend a barium swallow at six months to assess the effect of surgical myotomy (for DES).
✧ Recurrence may respond to further endoscopic balloon dilatation.

Motility Disorders Secondary to Systemic Disease
The most common systemic disorder causing esophageal motility symptoms is systemic sclerosis (SS, scleroderma). Nearly all patients with SS and esophageal involvement have symptoms of esophageal reflux, often severe. Less common conditions with esophageal symptoms are mixed connective tissue disorder, Sjögren's syndrome, systemic lupus erythematosus (SLE), rheumatoid arthritis (RA), diabetes, thyrotoxicosis, myxedema, Allgrove syndrome, Chagas disease, paraneoplastic syndromes, amyloidosis, and sarcoidosis.

   Common pathophysiologic defects consist of LES incompetence and complete loss of peristaltic activity in the lower two thirds of the esophagus.

History
✧ Take a general medical and esophageal motility history.
✧ Look for symptoms of esophagitis and dysphagia in association with specific symptoms of the underlying disorder.
✧ For scleroderma: Raynaud's, fingertip ulcers, telangiectasias, dyspnea, persistent cough, arthralgias/myalgias, muscle weakness, congestive heart failure (CHF),

hypertension, chronic renal insufficiency (CRI), sicca syndrome, hypothyroidism, fatigue, weight loss.

Examination
Perform a full physical examination. Look for evidence of underlying disorder:
- ✧ For RA, look for rheumatoid joints.
- ✧ For scleroderma, look for telangiectasias, hyper- or hypo-pigmentation, edematous/ sclerotic skin, xerostomia, Raynaud's, pulmonary rales, etc.

Diagnostic Tests
- ✧ Depending on etiology: barium swallow, EGD, manometry and pH studies have different effectiveness in diagnosis.
- ✧ Scleroderma: manometry is the best test, as it shows lack of peristalsis and low/absent LES pressure.
- ✧ Video swallow study is best for thyrotoxicosis-related symptoms.
- ✧ Biopsy is best for amyloidosis/sarcoidosis.
- ✧ As history and physical exam information dictates, perform serum studies for markers of underlying systemic disease.

Treatment
- ✧ Mainly medical, using drugs which increase esophageal motility (cisapride and metaclopramide are used, but with inconsistent results).
- ✧ Motility agents generally do not work in scleroderma.
- ✧ Treat reflux aggressively with standard medical regimes (usually PPIs).
- ✧ Any peptic strictures are treated by endoscopic dilatation.
- ✧ Antireflux surgeries are very rarely recommended, and often worsen patient dysphagia.
- ✧ Immunosuppressors/immunomodulators and anti-inflammatory drugs are used to treat underlying disorder, where appropriate.

Follow-up
- ✧ Follow-up is long-term for treatment of motility disorder and the underlying condition.
- ✧ Assess for development of strictures and diverticulae.
- ✧ Treat as appropriate with medications, regular endoscopic dilatation, etc., as per the specific condition.

Chagas Disease
In Chagas disease, *Trypanosoma cruzi* infection destroys the myenteric plexus of the esophagus, and causes dilatation and muscular hypertrophy (also known as megaesophagus). It occurs mainly in the southern and southwest US, in Latin America and South America.
- ✧ Histology shows inflammatory lesions with lymphocytic infiltrates.
- ✧ Chagas simulates achalasia both radiologically and manometrically:
  - ∝ Early symptoms include dysphagia, odynophagia, and chest pain.
  - ∝ Late symptoms include weight loss, pneumonitis, and erosive esophagitis.
- ✧ Cardiac disease is common, and thus patients are often in poor medical health; therefore, they are usually best treated by endoscopic dilatation.
- ✧ In severe cases or for those patients who can tolerate surgery, esophagocardiomyectomy (of the GEJ), laproscopic myotomy, or partial esophagectomy can be performed.

Esophageal Diverticula

There are two forms:

✧ *Pulsion diverticula* from high intraluminal pressure at an area of weakness. Includes Zenker's diverticulum and epiphrenic diverticulum.

✧ *Traction diverticula* from pulling forces outside the esophagus, such as an inflammatory process or mass.

True diverticula contain all layers of the esophageal wall; false (pseudo-) diverticula contain mucosa and submucosa that is herniated through the muscular layers of the esophageal wall.

Zenker's diverticulum is the most common symptomatic esophageal diverticulum:

✧ Most common in those aged from 70 years to the 80s.

✧ Involves a false, pulsion diverticulum which occurs through Killian's triangle of the posterior hypopharynx.

✧ Usually lies to the left side of the esophagus.

✧ Caused by motility defect (failure of relaxation of cricopharyngeus, causing increased intraluminal pressure against a closed UES).

Epiphrenic diverticulum, at the distal 6–10 cm of the esophagus, is relatively rare.

✧ Can be caused by motility disorders (DES, achalasia, hypertensive LES) that lead to increased intraluminal pressure against a closed LES (pulsion).

✧ Mid- or distal-esophageal diverticula can also be traction diverticula due to inflammation from mediastinal lymphadenopathy secondary to tuberculosis (TB) or histoplasmosis infections, as well as carcinomas, iatrogenic surgical injury, and Ehlers–Danlos syndrome.

History

Take a general medical history, along with an esophageal motility history.

Zenker's diverticulum:

✧ Oropharyngeal dysphagia, usually to solids and liquids.

✧ Regurgitation of undigested food. This may cause throat irritation, gurgling noises during swallowing, chronic cough and recurrent aspiration pneumonia.

✧ Compression of the esophagus causes the dysphagia and attacks of spluttering and coughing with each meal.

Mid and distal esophageal diverticula:

✧ Often asymptomatic.

✧ Patient may have dysphagia, regurgitation, and aspiration, but these are often related to underlying motility disorder and not the diverticulum.

Examination

✧ Perform a full physical examination (which may be normal), with focus on the neck and oropharynx.

✧ Features specific to Zenker's diveritculum are:

   ∝ Occasionally, a lump may be palpable in the left side of the neck.

   ∝ Gurgling may be detected on palpation of the left side of the neck at the level of the cricoids; performed after the patient is asked to swallow several gulps of air.

   ∝ Halitosis.

✧ Examine the chest for evidence of respiratory or cardiovascular disease.

✧ Examine for abdominal pathology.

Diagnostic Tests

✧ CXR for chest complications (pneumonia), also CT scan of the chest: may be seen as fluid or air-filled pockets.
✧ Barium swallow and meal: usually best for diagnosis.
  ∝ Defines structural appearance and location of diverticula.
  ∝ Often demonstrates esophageal motility disorder as the cause of diverticula, or diagnoses another cause of symptoms, such as hiatal hernia.
✧ EGD is indicated with dysphagia, odynophagia, or acute onset of symptoms.
✧ Manometry is especially helpful in evaluating the presence of other motility disorders of the esophagus.
✧ FOBT for anemia.

Treatment

Asymptomatic diverticula of the esophageal body usually do not require intervention. If diverticula are due to an underlying motility disorder, treat this disorder.

Surgical Treatment

In general, diverticulectomy (laproscopic or open) should be performed for any diverticula which cause aspiration. Zenker's diverticula commonly cause aspiration.

For Zenker's – perform diverticulectomy with cricopharyngeal myotomy, diverticulopexy with myotomy, or cricopharyngeal myotomy alone.
  ∝ Any defect in cricopharyngeal function is not improved by diverticulectomy alone, thus addition of myotomy is necessary.
  ∝ Endoscopic techniques (cutting or stapling the common wall between the diverticulum and orpharynx) are increasingly being utilized, especially in eldery patients unsuitable for surgery.

Follow-up

Severe cases should be investigated and treated promptly. Less severe cases can be assessed at longer intervals and treated if symptoms worsen, e.g. if aspiration occurs.

Post-operative Follow-up

✧ Patients are commonly assessed as outpatients 2–3 weeks post-operatively. They may have had a post-procedure gastrograffin swallow to evaluate for leak before initial discharge from hospital.
✧ Determine if the operation has relieved the symptoms.
✧ Assess for post-operative complications: wound infection, fistula, or recurrence. Recurrence is more frequently encountered in endoscopically repaired diverticulae.

Esophageal Cancer

More than 95% of esophageal cancers are either squamous cell or adenocarcinomas. Worldwide, 90–95% of esophageal cancers are squamous cell; while in the US, more than 50% are adenocarcinoma. Cancers at the GEJ and gastric cardia have been found to behave as if they were esophageal in origin, and are thus currently treated as esophageal cancers.

Overall, the five-year survival for esophageal cancer is poor (13–20%).

Risk factors are: male sex (3 : 1), old age (most commonly >65 years old), tobacco use (squamous cell cancer; somewhat reversible risk), alcohol consumption (proportional to intake; squamous cell cancer), obesity, a diet low in fruits/vegetables, exposure to dry-cleaning solvents, ingestion of lye (squamous cell cancer), achalasia, tylosis, esophageal webs (Plummer–Vinson syndrome), radiation to central chest (i.e. for non-Hodgkin's or Hodgkin's lymphoma), previous squamous cell cancer of head/neck.

GERD confers 2–16 times the risk and Barrett's esophagus 30–125 times risk of esophageal cancer (adenocarcinoma).

History
✧ Take a general medical and esophageal motility/symptom history. The typical history is of dysphagia over a period of months, usually progressively worsening and progressing from solids to liquids.
✧ There may be symptoms associated with anemia caused by bleeding from the tumor, e.g. fatigue, and signs such as melena.
✧ There may be history of unintentional weight loss.
✧ Odynophagia or mid-substernal chest pain may be reported.
✧ There may be hiccups, hoarseness, or pneumonia.

Examination
✧ Perform a full physical examination.
✧ Note signs of weight loss, sepsis, anemia (FOBT).
✧ Check for a palpable Virchow's node in the left supraclavicular fossa.
✧ Examine the chest for evidence of cardiovascular or respiratory disease.
✧ Examine for abdominal pathology, e.g. epigastric mass, liver metastases, etc.

Diagnostic Tests
✧ Urgent EGD and biopsy for high levels of suspicion.
✧ Barium swallow may be useful if patient is unable to pass the EGD scope. It can also define the length of lesions better; lesions longer than 5 cm are associated with deeper invasion levels, unresectability, and a worse prognosis.
✧ FOBT.
✧ Assess nutritional status (skin-fold, albumin, transferrin, Hb, iron, etc.).

Staging
Staging is required to establish the presence of inoperable disease, including mediastinal or subdiaphragmatic spread. Use the American Joint Commission on Cancer (AJCC) TMN staging classification (see below).
✧ Staging chest and abdominal CT, MRI, and/or positron emission tomography (PET).
✧ Esophageal ultrasound to stage the tumor (depth of invasion) and peri-esophageal nodal status.
✧ Bronchoscopy if there is evidence of tracheo-bronchial invasion.
✧ Staging laparoscopy for lower esophageal cancer: look for peritoneal disease or liver metastases.
✧ Vocal cord paralysis (ENT examination) and phrenic nerve paralysis (ultrasound screening) may indicate mediastinal spread.

AJCC Staging
TNM Classification
Tis: Carcinoma in situ/high-grade dysplasia
T1: Lamina propria or submucosa
T1a: Lamina propria or muscularis mucosae
T1b: Submucosa
T2: Muscularis propria

T3: Adventitia
T4: Adjacent structures
T4a: Pleura, pericardium, diaphragm, or adjacent peritoneum
T4b: Other adjacent structures (e.g. aorta, vertebral body, trachea)
N0: No regional lymph node metastasis
N1: 1–2 regional lymph nodes (N1 is site-dependent)
N2: 3–6 regional lymph nodes
N3: More than 6 regional lymph nodes
M1: Distant metastasis (M1a and M1b are site-dependent)

Grade
GX: The grade cannot be assessed (treated in stage grouping as G1).
G1: The cells are well differentiated.
G2: The cells are moderately differentiated.
G3: The cells are poorly differentiated.
G4: The cells are undifferentiated (not possible to tell if they are adenocarcinoma or
        squamous cell carcinoma).
For staging, G4 cancers are grouped with G3 squamous cell cancers.

Stage Grouping
Stage 0: Tis, N0, M0
Stage I: T1, N0, M0
Stage IIA: T2, N0, M0; or T3, N0, M0
Stage IIB: T1, N1, M0; or T2, N1, M0
Stage III: T3, N1, M0; or T4, any N, M0
Stage IV: Any T, any N, M1
Stage IVA: Any T, any N, M1a
Stage IVB: Any T, any N, M1b

Treatment
✧ Surgical resection alone for early-stage disease, or neoadjuvant chemoradiation (if
  patients are suitable candidates), followed by surgical resection for locally advanced-
  stage disease. Trans-hiatal and transthoracic esophagectomy have similar complication
  and mortality rates.
✧ Stenting, or laser or electro-coagulation for symptomatic relief of unresectable cancers. Treatment depends on stage and operative fitness, including nutritional state.
  Malnourished patients may require pre-operative nutrition (via J-tube) prior to major
  surgical intervention. Some surgeons routinely place J-tubes in anticipation of radiation esophagitis during neoadjuvant therapy.

Surgery
✧ The main objective is both the complete removal of cancer and the restoration of the
  ability to swallow.
✧ 30–40% of esophageal tumors are resectable.
✧ Operative mortality is 5–10%.
✧ Surgical resection of tumors of the lower two thirds of the esophagus is the treatment
  of choice when:
    ∝ The patient is considered fit for major surgical intervention.
    ∝ Pre-operative staging tests indicate that the tumor is resectable and there is no
      metastatic disease (pre-operative chemoradiation to attempt to shrink the tumor

is another possible approach).
✧ Tumors of the upper two thirds of the esophagus are treated using either chemoradiation or pharyngolaryngectomy.
✧ Malignant esophagotracheal fistulae are usually treated by endoscopic insertion of a covered esophageal stent.
✧ Other palliative options include laser or electro-fulguration.

Follow-up
✧ Intervals are short until diagnosis and staging is complete.
✧ If surgical intervention is planned, it should be performed 4–6 weeks after neoadjuvant therapy ends.
✧ Palliative procedures should be coordinated with surgical and oncologic services, with clear understanding of patient and family wishes.
✧ If symptoms are to be controlled with diathermy or laser fulguration, this treatment may need to be performed every 1–3 months to keep symptoms under control. Stenting may be considered as an alternative.
✧ After stent placement, patients need to be seen regularly (every 1–3 months) to detect problems with the stent, e.g. blockage or displacement.

Post-operative Follow-up
Long-term follow-up will be required. Goals of initial follow-up are:
✧ Assess the patient to determine whether the operation has been a success in relieving any symptoms and in completely removing the tumor.
✧ Maintain the nutritional requirements of the patient.
✧ Review the operation note and the histology report. Assess for general complications of abdominal surgery or thoracotomy.

Specific early complications include:
✧ Recurrent laryngeal nerve palsy caused during resection of the tumor; patients may complain of a hoarse voice and a weak cough. If only one vocal cord is affected, the other side may compensate. May be temporary and improve over several months. If the paralysis is permanent, improvement in the voice can be achieved by referral to ENT surgeons for teflon injection or formal thyroplasty.
✧ Gastric outlet obstruction – occurs if the stomach was mobilized and the vagus nerves cut without an adequate pyloroplasty. Diagnosed with barium meal. Remedial surgery may be necessary in severe cases, but usually endoscopic dilatation is sufficient.
✧ Gastro-esophageal reflux may occur if the stomach has been moved into the chest to establish continuity. Treatment is with PPIs and prokinetic drugs such as cisapride, metoclopramide, and erythromycin.
✧ Dumping symptoms are common after esophageal surgery, but usually dissipate after 12 months with conservative treatment.

Late complications include:
✧ Anastomotic stricture: can be treated with endoscopic balloon dilatation.
✧ Evidence of recurrence: untreatable by surgical intervention; may require palliation, including J-tube insertion for nutrition.

Questions and Answers

Q1   A 61-year-old Caucasian male is transferred to you for treatment of a resectable, well circumscribed cervical esophageal cancer that is <5cm from the cricopharyngeus. What is your approach?
A Three incision esophagectomy.
B Trans-hiatal esophagectomy.
C Local enucleation.
D Definitive chemoradiation therapy.

A1   D. In general, esophageal cancers in the cervical area respond well to chemoradiation therapy and there is no benefit of surgical resection. Cervical and cervicothoracic esophageal carcinomas that are <5cm from the cricopharyngeus should be treated with definitive chemoradiation therapy.

Q2   Which of the following is not a common risk factor for esophageal squamous cancer?
A Tylosis.
B Plummer–Vinson syndrome.
C Esophageal candidiasis.
D Chagas disease.

A2   C. Risk factors for esophageal squamous cancer include smoking and alcohol along with substances that irritate the esophagus such as lye ingestion, diets high in starch without fruits and vegetables, radiation therapy, etc. Also, certain diseases such as Chagas, tylosis, achalasia, and Plummer–Vinson syndrome all are risk factors.

Q3   In giving informed consent to a patient, what are the major and minor complication rates after a routine esophagectomy for esophageal cancer at an institution with a high volume of esophagectomies?
A <5%.
B <10%.
C 10–25%.
D >25%.

A3   D. In general, the average complication rates for routine esophagectomy are >25% regardless of the approach. Even minimal esophagectomy surgery at well-established centers has a rate of major and minor complications over 25%.

Q4 A 45-year-old healthy male presents acutely with an esophageal perforation that he has suffered while undergoing EGD for an obstructing distal esophageal cancer. The best treatment is:

A Primary repair of the perforation.
B Repair of the perforation with EGD and stenting.
C Esophagectomy.
D Emergent palliative radiation.

A4 C. Esophagectomy is the preferred treatment option here. If the perforation is less than 24 hours old and there is little spillage of intraluminal contents, then primary anastomosis in the esophageal bed can be performed during esophageal reconstruction.

Q5 A patient presents with a 5 cm polypoid distal esophageal cancer at the GE junction. The EUS reveals that the tumor has invaded the muscularis mucosae without any evidence of lymph node metastases. The correct treatment approach is:

A Neoadjuvant chemotherapy and then surgery.
B Combined modality chemoradiation and then surgery.
C Definitive chemoradiation therapy.
D Esophagectomy alone.

A5 D. Most esophageal cancers present as locally advanced staged malignancies with lymph nodes positive for disease on EUS and require combined modality therapy. This patient presents with an early, stage 1 esophageal cancer that can be treated with surgery alone.

Stomach and Duodenum
Clinton D. Protack and George A. Sarosi Jr.

FIVE

Potential Consultations
✧ Dyspepsia/epigastric pain.
✧ Dysphagia.
✧ Post gastric surgery/ potential complications.
✧ Gastric tumors.
✧ Gastric cancer.

A general surgical outpatient clinic will commonly have patients who have been sent up by their primary care physician (PCP) to discuss a *laparoscopic cholecystectomy* because an ultrasound scan has detected gallstones. However, there is a large overlap between biliary and gastro-duodenal symptoms and it is vital that a careful history is taken to avoid inappropriate biliary surgery when the patient has a duodenal ulcer. More specialized Upper GI (upper gastrointestinal) clinics will have large numbers of new and follow-up patients with very specific problems, some of which will be due to the disease process and some due to treatment they have received. Gastrointestinal surgeons should be just as competent at diagnosing and treating GI disease as their gastroenterology colleagues. Clearly the two specialties bring their own unique skills and experience to bear on a patient's problem, but should work closely together and refer freely between themselves as appropriate.

Assessment of Gastric and Duodenal Disorders
Gastric and Duodenal History
Pain
Pain is generally in the *epigastric* region and is caused by inflammation, ulceration, distension or tumor of the stomach.

Characteristics of pain due to peptic ulceration may vary according to the *site* of the ulcer.
✧ *Gastric ulcer pain*: May be exacerbated by food and may be relieved by vomiting. Consequently, the patient is afraid to eat and loses weight.
✧ *Duodenal ulcer pain*: Epigastric but may radiate through to the back, is typically relieved by eating and may sometimes wake the patient at night.
✧ *Pyloric stenosis*: Vomiting and weight loss are unusual and may suggest the development of pyloric stenosis. With the widespread use of acid-suppressing medication this is now a very rare complication in developed countries. Pain tends to be periodic, lasting 10–14 days every 3–4 months. Pain due to pyloric stenosis may cause abdominal distension, which is uncomfortable.
✧ *Gastric carcinoma*: Pain due to cancer of the stomach is common and cannot reliably be distinguished from benign inflammation. Worryingly, patients with gastric cancer will usually report relief of their burning epigastric pain soon after starting a proton-pump inhibitor (PPI). This falsely reassures both patient and physician that there is nothing sinister and delays the diagnostic endoscopy, which then is requested only when the pain returns or the patient loses weight.

Vomiting
Vomiting may be a feature of gastric ulcer disease with or without gastric outlet obstruction. Gastric outlet obstruction may also be caused by tumor. Patients may report vomiting food ingested several days before. Always take this symptom seriously and investigate it.

Waterbrash and Heartburn

Waterbrash is caused by excess secretion of saliva; it tastes salty and is an indicator of esophageal reflux. *Heartburn* is a much more common symptom and is often felt after meals, at night or when bending down. It can radiate into the neck and be very similar to cardiac chest pain. However, unlike the latter it is often quickly relieved by antacids or acid suppression.

Dysphagia

Primarily an esophageal symptom, but may also indicate a gastric problem – carcinoma of the cardia obstructing the gastroesophageal junction. *Always investigate dysphagia urgently.*

Fatigue, malaise

These non-specific symptoms may indicate anemia secondary to chronic blood loss from a peptic ulcer or tumor.

Drug History

The ingestion of certain medications may predispose to gastroduodenal ulceration, e.g. non-steroidal anti-inflammatory drugs (NSAIDs), steroids; or predispose to complications from ulceration, e.g. warfarin.

Past Medical History

Previous peptic ulceration or gastric surgery may be relevant.

Social History

Smoking and excess alcohol ingestion are associated with peptic ulceration.

Gastric and Duodenal Examination

◇ This will usually be entirely normal.
◇ Look for the signs of advanced upper GI malignancy – weight-loss, anemia, an abdominal mass, ascites and lymphadenopathy. These are *signs of incurability* and it is sad that they are still used as "alarm features" to guide PCPs to refer patients for investigation. *Curable* upper GI malignancy usually presents with *mild dyspepsia* only and unless an endoscopy and biopsy is done then, the chance of cure is often lost.
◇ Distension in the epigastrium and left hypochondrium may represent gastric distension secondary to gastric outlet obstruction. Auscultation in this region may reveal a sucussion splash in response to rocking the abdomen.
◇ Surgical scars may indicate previous gastric surgery.
◇ Always look for the signs of liver disease such as spider nevi, liver palms, hepatomegaly, jaundice, tremor, etc.

Investigation of Gastric and Duodenal Disorders
Laboratory Investigations

◇ *Hematology* – routine indications, e.g. complete blood count (CBC), may indicate anemia; leukocytosis may suggest infection and may be raised in inflammatory or malignant conditions.
◇ *Biochemistry* – routine indications, e.g. abnormal liver function tests (LFTs), may indicate liver metastases in malignancy. More specialized gastric acid secretion tests, or tests of vagal nerve integrity such as sham feeding, may be performed.
◇ *Immunology* – e.g. identification of serum antibodies to *Helicobacter pylori*, parietal cell antibodies in pernicious anemia.

⬦ *Cytology/Histology* – cytology of brushings or histology of biopsies taken at endoscopy.
⬦ Urea breath test or fecal antigen test for *H. pylori*. Urea containing radio-labeled carbon is consumed by the patient and, if *H. pylori* is present in their stomach, the urease enzyme produced by it will split the urea into radio-labeled carbon dioxide (CO_2) and ammonia. The CO_2 is exhaled and can be detected.
  ∝ Patients under the age of 55 years (some would argue 45) who present with simple dyspepsia should be tested for *H. pylori* and, when positive, undergo triple therapy eradication treatment with a combination of two antibiotics and a PPI (clarithromyin, amoxicillin and omeprazole is one example).
  ∝ Serum antibody testing for *H. pylori* is possible but will stay positive for many months after eradication and is less reliable than a urea breath test.
  ∝ Fecal antigen testing using antibodies specific for *H. pylori* is an alternative technique, but is not available in many institutions. A gastric biopsy taken at endoscopy can also be tested using a "CLO" test (see below) which works on the same principle as the urea breath test except that a color change is induced by the urease rather than CO_2.

Imaging Techniques
Esophago-Gastro-Duodenoscopy
Esophago-gastro-duodenoscopy (EGD) should be the *first investigation* in all patients with gastroduodenal symptoms.
⬦ *Results* – a written report of the procedure and findings is compiled by the endoscopist.
  ∝ The report will usually comment on the *esophagus, stomach, and duodenum*. Usually measurements will be given for the position of the esophago-gastric junction (38–40 cm), the presence of the Z-line (squamo-columnar junction), the presence of intestinal metaplasia, and the presence of a hiatal hernia. The first (D1) and second (D2) parts of the duodenum will be described. The site, size and character of any ulcers or other lesions will be described.
  ∝ If biopsies were taken, look for the histology report, which may also comment on the presence or absence of *H. pylori*.
  ∝ Recommendations for treatment are sometimes suggested.
⬦ *Advantages* – allows direct visualization of gastroduodenal lesions and enables biopsies to be taken for histologic diagnosis. Can visualize esophagitis, ulceration, varices, etc. Certain therapeutic maneuvers, including injection of bleeding ulcers or endoscopic excision of small masses, can be performed.
⬦ *Disadvantages* – it is an invasive procedure, unable to diagnose early motility disorders. Some patients may find it unpleasant and are unable to swallow the scope. Complications include aspiration, trauma to the esophagus, stomach and duodenum, which may cause bleeding, pain, or occasionally perforation. This is particularly a risk in an uncooperative patient. Linitis plastica can be difficult to diagnose with EGD. Patients who are unable to swallow the scope may be offered a general anesthetic.

CLO (Campylobacter-Like Organisms) Tests for Helicobacter pylori
⬦ *Technique* – this is performed in conjunction with EGD. Endoscopic gastric biopsies are taken under direct vision from the gastric antrum. The tissue is placed in indicator medium, which detects the presence of urease activity by *H. pylori*. The presence of *H. pylori* results in an indicator color change within a specified time period, e.g. 60 minutes. Color change after this time period is non-specific.
⬦ *Advantages* – quick result enabling eradication therapy to be immediately prescribed.

✧ *Disadvantages* – false negatives occur in 5–15% of cases; therefore, a negative result does not completely exclude the presence of *H. pylori*. PPI, bismuth and antibiotic use may interfere with the test and give a false-negative result.
✧ *Alternative tests for* H. pylori – *H. pylori* can also be detected from gastric biopsies sent for histology using immuno-histochemical stains.

Barium Swallow

This technique is used as a second-line investigation if EGD fails to provide a diagnosis.
✧ *Indications*:
  ∝ Dysphagia in a frail person not suitable for EGD.
  ∝ Dysphagia when patient refuses EGD.
  ∝ Provides anatomic detail in patients with prior surgery or suspected hiatal or paraesophageal hernia.
  ∝ To exclude a cricopharyngeal diverticulum if there is concern prior to endoscopy.
✧ *Advantages* – useful in the investigation of dysphagia where endoscopy has not detected a mechanical cause and a motility disorder of the esophagus or stomach is suspected. Double contrast (barium–air) barium meals are useful for the evaluation of suspected gastric cancer. Rigidity and absent peristalsis may occur at the site of a localized tumor while linitis plastica produces an abrupt circumferential narrowing of the stomach lumen.
✧ *Disadvantages* – irradiation is used. Simultaneous therapeutic procedures are not possible. Overall, the technique is not as sensitive as endoscopy for the detection of small lesions. The presence of barium in the stomach can damage the endoscope, so endoscopy cannot be performed until the barium is cleared from the stomach.

Ultrasound

✧ *Technique* – mainly used non-invasively, with the ultrasound probe applied to the outside of the body after applying acoustic water-based gel. Gallstones will often need to be excluded.
✧ *Advantages* – a cheap, quick, and safe way of imaging the liver; hence useful for screening for liver metastases.
✧ *Endoluminal ultrasound* (EUS) is a specialized technique where a specialized probe is placed in the stomach to provide images of the stomach wall and adjacent lymph nodes. EUS can:
  ∝ Help with diagnosis, i.e. gastric gastrointestinal stromal tumor (GIST).
  ∝ Stage tumors.
  ∝ Get tissue (EUS-directed fine-needle aspiration [FNA] and core biopsy).
✧ EUS is good for determining intramural spread and lymph node involvement. Combined laparoscopy and laparoscopic ultrasound is good for identifying transcoelomic spread and peritoneal seedlings, which can then be biopsied under direct vision. Laparoscopic ultrasound gives better images than external ultrasound of intra-abdominal organs, helping to detect smaller metastases which can then be biopsied.
✧ *Disadvantages* – limited application on its own. Confirmation of findings is needed by performing computed tomography (CT), so this tends to be preferred to ultrasound. Endoluminal ultrasound and laparoscopic ultrasound are not widely available.

Computed Tomography

CT is used in gastric malignancy to demonstrate the extent of mural invasion, involvement of adjacent structures, and liver and lymph node involvement. Sometimes CT is used as a "diagnostic fishing trip" when the clinician is worried that the patient has disseminated cancer but cannot find anything concrete on examination or blood tests.

✧ *Advantages* – invasion of the wall of the stomach is demonstrated as wall thickening (>5 mm). A thickness greater than 2 cm generally correlates with spread beyond the stomach. Lymph node metastases can be detected in about 70% of cases. CT is good for detecting liver metastases.

✧ *Disadvantages* – involves irradiation. Tends to underestimate early peritoneal spread and lymph node metastases. Not totally reliable in differentiating direct metastatic spread from reactive inflammation surrounding a tumor; therefore, tends to under-stage tumors.

Radio-isotope Techniques
The only test routinely in use is a two-phase gastric emptying study. This is to investigate patients with suspected functional problems with their stomachs (gastroparesis and gastric hurry).

Technetium-99m Hepatobiliary Iminodiacetic Acid (HIDA) Scan
This is used to detect and quantify enterogastric reflux and afferent loop obstruction after gastrojejunostomy reconstructions.

✧ *Technique* – intravenous injection of technetium-99m HIDA, which is secreted in the bile and concentrated in the gall bladder. The amount of radioactivity in the gall bladder is calculated and the gall bladder is stimulated to contract by admin-istration of cholecystokinin. This expels the radioactivity into the duodenum. The passage of the radioactivity along the small bowel can be traced and the obstruc-tion identified. Enterogastric reflux of radioactivity from the small bowel back into the stomach can be identified and quantified as a percentage of the total abdominal radioactivity.

✧ *Advantages* – provides quantitative assessment of the degree of enterogastric reflux and can detect afferent loop obstruction in gastrojejunostomy reconstructions.

✧ *Disadvantages* – involves use of radioactivity. Requires a functioning unobstructed biliary system.

Schilling Test
This test is used to assess a patient's ability to absorb vitamin B12.

✧ *Technique* – radioactive vitamin B12 is given by mouth and urine is collected for 24 hours.

✧ *Results* – a normal individual will excrete at least 10% of the original dose over this period. A patient with pernicious anemia will excrete less than 5%.

✧ *Advantages* – provides a quantifiable measure of the ability of the GI tract to absorb vitamin B12.

✧ *Disadvantages* – does not localize the disease to stomach or terminal ileum. Uses radioactivity.

Laparoscopy
Laparoscopy is increasingly used for diagnosis and staging of tumors. It is often combined with intra-operative ultrasound.

✧ *Technique* – performed in the operating room under general anesthetic. A laparoscopic port is inserted under direct vision and CO_2 insufflated to produce a pneumoperito-neum. May be combined with intra-operative ultrasound using a special laparoscopic ultrasound probe. Also enables biopsy of focal lesions under direct vision.

✧ *Results* – in the form of a written operation note and still photographs or video.
✧ *Advantages* – direct visualization of abdominal pathology. In gastric cancer, it may establish irresectability without subjecting the patient to a full laparotomy. Enables direct biopsy of small lesions, e.g. peritoneal deposits, small liver lesions.
✧ *Disadvantages* – an invasive procedure requiring general anesthetic.

Peptic Ulcer Disease
Chronic Duodenal Ulcer
Peak incidence occurs in the 40–60 age group. However these ulcers are now rare in developed countries due to effective treatment in the primary care setting.

Objectives
✧ Diagnose and differentiate from other causes of abdominal pain.
✧ Exclude gastric cancer, treat ulcer, and correct predisposing factors.

History
✧ Typically presents with recurrent episodes of epigastric pain.
✧ Exacerbations are associated with stress, dietary/alcoholic overindulgence and smoking. Symptoms increase during fasting (night pain) and are decreased by food, especially milk or alkalis.
✧ Pain radiating through to the back is typical of posterior ulceration.
✧ Vomiting is uncommon unless associated with edema/fibrosis around ulcer causing pyloric obstruction.
✧ There may be a history of aspirin/NSAID ingestion. Often the patient is referred to surgery with a long history of H2-receptor antagonist (H2RA) or PPI treatment with relapses.

Examination
✧ The patient may be overweight due to constant nibbling and there may be evidence of anemia.
✧ On abdominal examination there may be diffuse epigastric tenderness.
✧ In cases with a degree of gastric outlet obstruction a sucussion splash may be detected.
✧ Examination may otherwise be normal.

Chronic Gastric Ulcer
This is less common than duodenal ulcer. There are two distinct types:
✧ *Type I* – occur along the lesser curve of the stomach.
✧ *Type II* – two ulcers are present. One ulcer is present in the body of the stomach, while another is present in the duodenum.
✧ *Type III* – a prepyloric ulcer.
✧ *Type IV* – a gastric ulcer high on the lesser curve, near the gastroesophageal junction.
✧ *Type V* – a gastric ulcer induced by NSAIDs

The natural history, acid secretory profile and therapeutic response are the same as duodenal ulcers.

Type I may arise in normal mucosa or atrophic gastritis. These ulcers are not associated with hyperacidity and, in fact, hypoacidity may be found, tending to occur in older patients.

Objectives
Diagnose ulcer, exclude malignancy, differentiate from other causes of abdominal pain, identify underlying causes, treat ulcer, treat underlying cause.

History
✧ Gastric ulcer patients may describe discomfort and a sensation of fullness in the stomach.
✧ Eating increases the pain and is relieved by fasting; patients may be afraid to eat and lose weight.

These symptoms are the same as for gastric cancer, but cancer tends to be associated with more nausea and vomiting and pain is more constant.

Examination
✧ Examine for evidence of weight loss, anemia and epigastric tenderness.
✧ A palpable epigastric mass suggests carcinoma of the stomach but may represent an inflammatory mass.

Investigations for Ulcer Patients
✧ EGD and/or double contrast barium meal are used to investigate all dyspepsia patients.
✧ EGD combined with CLO-testing of gastric antrum biopsies will establish *H. pylori* status.
✧ If EGD indicates *duodenal ulcer*, then diagnosis and biopsy of gastric antrum are needed to detect *H. pylori*.
  ∝ Several biopsies will be performed, including one for the instant CLO test, and one for histologic examination.
  ∝ If either of the above biopsies are positive, the patient is started on *H. pylori* eradication therapy and medical ulcer healing therapy. EGD is repeated after medical therapy to check healing.
✧ If EGD indicates *gastric ulcer*, biopsy of the ulcer is mandatory to exclude gastric cancer, and biopsy of the antrum for *H. pylori* bacteria. If biopsy is benign, start patient on medical ulcer healing therapy and *H. pylori* eradication as indicated but repeat endoscopy after 2–3 months of medical therapy. If ulcer is then not healed, repeat the biopsy. Failure to heal even in the presence of negative biopsies may be an indication for surgical therapy.

Medical Treatment
✧ The *first step* is to eradicate *H. pylori* infection. Thereafter H2RAs – a therapeutic course lasting 2–3 months heals 90% of ulcers with symptom relief achieved within 2–3 days.
✧ *Resistant ulcers* – a double dose of H2RAs or a combination of H2RA and PPIs. Only PPIs heal all resistant ulcers. With *H. pylori* negative ulcers, relapse is universal unless maintenance therapy is continued indefinitely. Breakthrough ulceration on maintenance therapy is 16% on ranitidine and 26% on cimetidine over a five-year period.
✧ *PPIs* – heal both duodenal and gastric ulcers. Problems of long-term PPI therapy are achlorhydria, hypergastrinemia, and evidence from rat studies of proliferation of gastric fundal endocrine cells and G-cells with the development of carcinoid tumors.
✧ *Triple therapy* was originally bismuth, metronidazole and amoxicillin for 4 weeks. Current regimens consist of a PPI, clarithromycin and metronidazole for 1–2 weeks. The PPI is continued for 6 weeks. Permanent healing is achieved in all patients in

whom *H. pylori* infection is eradicated – approximately 90%. Patients undergo a urea breath test at 6–8 weeks to confirm eradication. If this fails, the original regimen is tried.

Refractory Ulcers
Criteria are:
✧ Duodenal ulcer – no healing after 8 weeks of therapy.
✧ Gastric ulcer – no healing after 12 weeks of therapy.

Perform EGD to differentiate a true refractory ulcer from those patients with persistent symptoms despite ulcer healing which requires investigation of alternative causes.
✧ If refractory ulcer is present, then successful *H. pylori* eradication should be confirmed by further biopsy for CLO test and histology.
✧ If *H. pylori* is still present, investigate non-compliance with eradication therapy and if indicated prescribe another regimen.
✧ If no *H. pylori* is detected, enquire regarding the presence of other ulcerogenic factors e.g. smoking (measure urinary nicotine levels), aspirin ingestion (measure blood salicylate levels).

True Resistant Ulcer
A true resistant ulcer fails to heal despite *H. pylori* eradication. A relapsed ulcer heals initially but then recurs.
✧ Perform EGD and take multiple biopsies for evidence of neoplasia, infection, and inflammation. Measure serum gastrin levels and if high investigate for Zollinger–Ellison syndrome.
✧ Where no cause can be found, the ulcer can be termed an idiopathic refractory ulcer. Prolonged drug treatment and EGD surveillance or surgery is indicated to exclude undetected malignancy.

Indications for Surgical Treatment of Peptic Ulcer Disease
✧ Failure to comply with maintenance regimen.
✧ Ulcers resistant to *H. pylori* eradication therapy.
✧ Gastric ulcers which remain unhealed after three months of treatment, irrespective of the biopsy findings.
✧ Complications associated with ulcers, e.g. pyloric obstruction, perforation, bleeding.

Follow-up
Follow up with medical therapy and follow-up EGD. Once ulcer is healed and *H. pylori* is eradicated, patient can be discharged.

Post-operative Follow-up
Follow-up is long-term to detect complications, which include recurrent ulceration, dumping, diarrhea, and adverse nutritional consequences. However, remedial surgery for most chronic conditions is usually delayed for at least 18 months as most symptoms improve.

Nutritional Consequences of Gastric Surgery
These are more common after gastrectomy, which results in:
✧ Decreased food intake.
✧ Malabsorption of fat or nitrogen.
✧ Decreased small bowel transit time.

Iron Deficiency Anemia

Iron deficiency is very common after vagotomy and drainage and gastric resections, especially in females. The incidence increases with time until it is 60–80% at 10–20 years. It is caused by altered handling of iron. All patients are treated prophylactically with oral iron after gastrectomy and vagotomy and drainage.

Macrocytic Anemia

This is caused by vitamin B12 deficiency and invariably occurs after total gastrectomy due to loss of intrinsic factor. Partial gastrectomy and truncal vagotomy and drainage result in lower levels of vitamin B12 due to lack of an acid environment. After partial gastrectomy, diagnosis is by an abnormal Schilling test.

Treat by 3-monthly injections of cyanocobalamin indefinitely. If the Schilling test is normal, treatment is with oral crystalline vitamin B12.

Bone Disease

✧ Develops several years after gastric resection with duodenal exclusion; the duodenum is the major site of calcium absorption. Many women develop osteomalacia 10–20 years after gastrectomy.
✧ May present with symptoms of generalized bone pain, weakness due to associated myopathy, and stress fractures. Investigations show a raised serum alkaline phosphatase and calcium and areas of bone rarefaction on X-rays.
✧ Calcium and alkaline phosphatase levels should be measured annually. After five years all patients should have a full assessment for metabolic bone disease.
✧ Treatment is with oral calcium and vitamin D. Post-menopausal women and all patients over 70 should take an oral calcium supplement, twice a day, for life.

Post-gastric Surgery Dumping and Reactive Hypoglycemia
Dumping

✧ Dumping is rapid gastric emptying – vasomotor symptoms occur within minutes of eating due to hypovolemia (decreased cardiac output and peripheral resistance) caused by outpouring of fluid into bowel to dilute hyperosmolar gastric contents.
✧ Treatment:
  ∝ Mild/moderate dumping – advise small dry meals, rich in protein and fat but low in carbohydrate. Methoxy-pectin or bran can be added to the diet to slow gastric emptying.
  ∝ Severe dumping – remedial surgery. The commonest cause of dumping after vagotomy procedures is the drainage procedure. Therefore, closure of the pyloroplasty can be performed and any resultant gastric stasis treated with motility-enhancing drugs, e.g. cisapride. Other surgical options include conversion of the procedure to a Roux-en-Y or, to slow down small bowel transit time, the formation of a 10–15 cm antiperistaltic segment of the jejunum.

Reactive Hypoglycemia

✧ Symptoms of sweating, tremor, etc. occur 2–3 hours after a meal due to hypoglycemia.
✧ Diagnosis is made by performing an extended glucose tolerance test as an inpatient. Following a meal this shows initial hyperglycemia provoking an exaggerated insulin release with increased plasma insulin and entero-glucagon levels. This results in the subsequent hypoglycemia and occurrence of symptoms.
✧ Treatment is mainly dietary, advising low carbohydrate/high protein meals.

Post-gastric Surgery Vomiting

Bilious vomiting is common after gastric surgery, and may indicate:

✧ Recurrent ulceration.
✧ Enterogastric reflux.
✧ Intermittent obstruction of the afferent or efferent loop of a gastroenterostomy.
✧ Cardio-esophageal incompetence.

Enterogastric Reflux/Reflux Gastritis

This consists of reflux of bile/pancreatic juice into the stomach, which causes a reflux erosive gastritis and bilious vomiting.

History

Epigastric pain, nausea, and vomiting in the early post-prandial period. The pain is a burning type aggravated by food and not relieved by antacids, and episodes culminate in the vomiting of bile-stained fluid 1–2 hours after a meal. Less commonly, vomiting occurs early in the morning after night pain. Iron deficiency anemia develops.

Investigations

Diagnosis is confirmed by EGD, which reveals gastritis and pooling of bile in the stomach.

Treatment

Bile-salt-binding agents such as cholestyramine combined with sulcralfate at night are often effective. If medical therapy fails to control symptoms, remedial surgery is indicated. Procedures similar to those for the treatment of dumping are performed.

Note that atrophic gastritis and intestinal metaplasia associated with enterogastric reflux has been implicated in the development of carcinoma and requires long-term follow-up with regular EGD assessment.

Extrinsic Loop Obstruction

This is rare. It occurs after truncal vagotomy and gastroenterostomy, usually affects the afferent loop, and is predisposed to by the formation of antecolic anastomoses and long loops (>20 cm). Causes include internal herniation, kinking of the anastomosis, volvulus, stenosis, jejunogastric intussusception and development of gastric cancer in the stomach remnant.

History

The patient reports usually intermittent feelings of fullness, a cramp-like pain and nausea within 1 hour of eating. Attacks culminate in vomiting of copious amounts of bile-stained fluid, which relieves the symptoms.

In acute cases there is no relief and the condition may be accompanied by development of acute pancreatitis, jaundice, and necrosis with perforation.

Examination

During pain-free episodes, examination may be normal. During attacks there may be upper abdominal distension and tenderness.

Investigations

✧ LFTs may be deranged and there may be a dilated small bowel loop visible on abdominal X-ray (AXR).
✧ Delayed emptying of the afferent loop may be demonstrated by HIDA scan.
✧ There may be failure of barium to enter afferent loop during a barium meal.

Treatment

Some cases are amenable to endoscopic pneumatic dilatation. Unresponsive cases require surgical correction.

Acute Jejunogastric Intussusception

This is characterized by severe epigastric pain, hematemesis, a palpable abdominal mass, and high small bowel obstruction. Diagnosis is by AXR, which shows a soft-tissue mass surrounded by air. Treatment is by surgery.

Gastro-esophageal Reflux/Esophagitis

Mobilization of the esophagus during surgery may cause cardio-esophageal incompetence. If associated with enterogastric reflux, this may lead to a severe neutral/alkaline esophagitis and stricture formation.

Post-gastric Surgery Diarrhea

Three patterns of diarrhea occur after gastric surgery:
1. Frequent loose motions.
2. Intermittent episodes of short-lived diarrhea.
3. Severe intractable diarrhea, which occurs in 2% of cases after truncal vagotomy and, unlike dumping, is often precipitated by small meals.

Diarrhea may be caused by malabsorption of bile salts and/or fatty acids, accelerated small bowel transit time or bacterial overgrowth.

History

Determine the pattern of the diarrhea and any precipitating or exacerbating factors. Estimate the severity of the symptoms.

Examination

Examine for anemia, weight loss, and dehydration.

Investigation

✧ Investigations are usually delayed until simple treatments have failed to control the symptoms.
✧ Investigations include fecal fat estimation, butter fat test, small bowel transit time, and ^{14}C glycocholate breath test for bacterial overgrowth.

Treatment

A diet low in animal fat is advised. Intestinal sedatives (codeine phosphate, lomotil) and bile-salt-binding agents (cholestyramine) usually provide short-term relief.

If symptoms are severe and fail to settle consider remedial surgery, e.g. reversed small bowel segment.

Post-gastric Surgery Decreased Appetite

A small stomach results after extensive gastrectomy and produces early satiety, which precludes adequate intake and can cause malnutrition.

History and Examination

✧ Determine the average dietary intake and whether this is associated with weight loss.
✧ Examine for evidence of anemia and weight loss.

Investigations
✧ Carry out CBC, electrolytes, and LFTs to estimate nutrition.
✧ Investigate serum iron, vitamin B12, and folate levels.
✧ Perform contrast studies to examine the gastric remnant.

Treatment
✧ Mild cases are treated with small, frequent meals with dietician input and high-calorie supplements.
✧ More severe cases may require elemental diets administered by enteral feeding tube.
✧ Eventually, surgical reconstruction to increase the gastric reservoir and restore duodenal continuity may be required.

Other Complications After Gastric Surgery
These include:
✧ Gallstones.
✧ Bezoars – balls of undigested vegetable/fruit matter in the stomach remnant.

History and Examination
These reveal nausea and vomiting, abdominal discomfort, halitosis, and early satiety leading to small bowel obstruction, severe gastritis, and ulceration.

Investigation
✧ EGD or barium meal.
✧ There is an increased risk of carcinoma in the gastric remnant at 15–20 years; therefore EGD should be performed in any patient with new upper abdominal symptoms after any previous ulcer surgery.

Treatment
Medical treatment is enzymic cellulose. If that fails, then surgery is indicated.

Gastric Volvulus
Usually a degree of gastric outlet obstruction develops, resulting in a dilated stomach which is prone to twist after a heavy meal.

History
This can present in the outpatient setting with chronic symptoms of episodes of epigastric distress and vomiting, or acutely with severe epigastric pain, ineffectual retching with distension, tenderness and signs of shock.

Examination
Examination may be normal if performed between episodes, or there may be evidence of epigastric distension and tenderness with a sucussion splash.

Investigations
AXR may show abnormal gastric shadow. Barium meal may demonstrate an abnormal, dilated stomach.

Treatment
Surgery to relieve obstruction and correct anatomy.

Follow-up
Follow-up is at short intervals until diagnosis is established.

Post-operative Follow-up
As for gastrectomy and gastric ulcer surgery.

Gastritis
✧ *Type A* – auto-immune, circulating parietal cell antibodies cause pernicious anemia with achlorhydria and absent intrinsic factor. The antrum is spared, so serum gastrin levels are high due to alkaline pH. There is a significantly increased risk of development of carcinoma, usually of the diffuse type.
✧ *Type B* – begins distally in the pyloric region due to *H. pylori* infection. Gastrin levels are normal. It is always present in duodenal ulceration.
✧ *Lymphocytic gastritis* – infiltration of gastric epithelium by T lymphocytes. EGD shows nodularity, erosions, and enlarged mucosal folds.
✧ *Erosive gastritis* – caused by NSAIDs and alcohol.
✧ *Other causes* – reflux, stress, granulomatous (tuberculosis, Crohn's disease) gastritis, cystica polyposa, AIDs gastritis, eosinophilic gastritis, Menetrier's disease, suppurative gastritis, emphysematous gastritis.

Objectives
Diagnose gastritis, differentiate different types, exclude cancer, treat cause, monitor for development of cancer.

History
Patients may complain of dyspepsia and abdominal pain. There may be a history of alcohol or NSAID ingestion.

Examination
Examination may be normal, or there may be evidence of anemia, weight loss, or of an underlying disorder.

Investigations
✧ EGD and biopsy for detection of dysplasia and *H. pylori*.
✧ Vitamin B12 and folate levels may be low; perform a Schilling test if atrophic gastritis is suspected.
✧ Measure serum gastrin levels.
✧ Carry out CBC for lymphocyte and eosinophil levels.

Treatment
Treatment depends on diagnosis and the effect of symptoms, and should be given in combination with anti-ulcer therapy if indicated.
✧ *Type A* – vitamin B12 injection every 3 months.
✧ *Type B* – *H. pylori* eradication.
✧ *Erosive gastritis* – NSAID or alcohol withdrawal.
✧ *Dysplasia* – if mild/moderate, can be monitored by regular EGD surveillance. Gastric resection is indicated for severe dysplasia.

Follow-up
If gastritis is accompanied by dysplasia, then surveillance by EGD is indicated. If dysplasia is severe then gastric resection is indicated.

Post-operative Follow-up
✧ Review histology.
✧ Refer to oncology if indicated.
✧ Follow-up for complications is the same as gastrectomy for peptic ulcer disease; follow-up is usually long-term.

Gastric Tumors
✧ Adenomas and other benign tumors are rare, accounting for 5% of benign gastric polyps. Many are found in the antrum; they may be single or multiple.
✧ Progression to cancer is possible. Adenomatous polyps *larger than 4 cm* are associated with 11% malignant change over a four-year follow-up period.
✧ The majority (75–95%) of gastric polyps are hyperplastic, which represent regeneration of the mucosa after mucosal damage. These also need to be observed because up to 4.5% may undergo malignant change; the risk increases with size.
✧ Polyps may also be associated with independent cancer elsewhere in the stomach (6.5–25%).

Objectives
Diagnose tumor, differentiate from cancer, treat tumor, and monitor to detect malignant change.

History
Patients usually present with the symptoms of dyspepsia, and the tumor itself is asymptomatic.

Examination
Examination may be normal, or there may be epigastric tenderness or a mass.

Treatment
✧ If small and found on endoscopy, endoscopic removal is advisable for histologic diagnosis. This is combined with multiple biopsies of the stomach with prophylactic anti-ulcer treatment.
✧ Endoscopic resection is associated with 40% recurrence of polyps.
✧ If polyps are too large for endoscopic resection, then surgical excision or partial gastrectomy is necessary.

Follow-up
Intervals should be short until the diagnosis is made and malignancy excluded. After treatment, long-term follow-up with EGD surveillance is indicated to detect recurrence or malignant change.

Post-operative Follow-up
Review histology to detect any evidence of malignancy. The complications are the same for gastrectomy as for peptic ulcer disease.

Non-neoplastic Gastric Polyps
✧ Regenerative polyps are inflammatory and associated with gastritis and peptic ulceration. All should be removed endoscopically for histology: 2% have areas of focal carcinoma, 4% dysplasia. Long-term follow-up with EGD surveillance is indicated.
✧ Other polyps:
  ∝ Inflammatory fibroid polyps – eosinophilic gastritis occurs in the pyloric antrum and duodenum and is caused by a gastrointestinal allergy.
  ∝ Myoepithelial hamartomas, Peutz–Jeghers syndrome, heterotopic pancreatic tissue in the antropyloric region.

Carcinoma of the Stomach
Five-year survival rates range from 90% for Stage IA to 10% for Stage IV. It is rarely seen before 40 years of age, most occur in the 70–80 year age range. The male to female ratio is 2 : 1.
✧ *Etiology* – spicy food, polycyclic hydrocarbons, inorganic dusts, high consumption of animal fat, high salt intake, tobacco smoking.
✧ *Risk factors* – atrophic gastritis, pernicious anemia, previous partial gastrectomy, adenomatous and regenerative polyps, familial polyposis, hypogammaglobulinemia, blood group A, type III intestinal metaplasia, severe dysplasia, long-standing infection with *H. pylori*.

Dysplasia
Dysplasia is the most important marker of gastric cancer.
✧ *Type A* – affects metaplastic gastric epithelium and can lead to the development of the intestinal type of gastric cancer.
✧ *Type B* – arises in the non-metaplastic gastric epithelium and predisposes to diffuse or intermediate gastric cancers.

Objectives
Diagnose dysplasia, grade severity, monitor for malignancy.

History
Most patients present with dyspepsia and dysplasia that is detected during routine investigation. Some cases are detected by screening.

Examination
A normal examination is a good sign. Look for evidence of malignancy, e.g. epigastric mass, weight loss.

Investigations
✧ Diagnose by EGD and biopsy for histology.
✧ Dysplasia is graded into mild, moderate and severe (carcinoma in situ).

Treatment
✧ *Mild/moderate* – regular EGD surveillance.
✧ *Severe* – a second EGD and biopsy is mandatory within a few weeks. If severe dysplasia is confirmed, then gastrectomy is advised. Histology of gastrectomy specimens shows that 40–50% have early invasive gastric cancer.

Follow-up
Short intervals initially (1–2 weeks) until neoplasia is excluded. Regular EGD surveillance is needed to detect development of neoplasia and to grade it.

Post-operative Follow-up
✧ Check histology to determine evidence of malignancy.
✧ Refer to oncologist for adjuvant therapy if appropriate.
✧ Check that excision was complete; further resection may be indicated.
✧ Complications of gastrectomy are as previously described.

Pathology of Gastric Cancer
The main classification of gastric cancers is into:
1. Intestinal type.
2. Diffuse type.
3. Others.

Each is then classified as *well differentiated, poorly differentiated,* or *undifferentiated.* Well-differentiated intestinal-type gastric cancers can be subdivided into *large gland, small gland,* and *colloid.* The undifferentiated diffuse type is equivalent to linitis plastica.

Early Gastric Cancer
Cancer limited to the mucosa and submucosa, treated by gastrectomy, has a five-year survival rate of 80%.

Endoscopic appearance may be *protruding, superficial,* or *excavated.* At time of diagnosis, 10–15% have already spread to the lymph nodes and represent early simulating advanced gastric carcinoma.

Advanced Gastric Cancer
The tumor involves the muscularis propria, and most have lymph node spread as well as peritoneal and liver spread. Borrman types 1 (polypoid) and 2 (limited ulceration) have a better prognosis. Types 3 (infiltration with ulceration) and 4 (diffuse infiltrating) are incurable.

Staging of Gastric Cancer
Staging involves the TNM system, depth of invasion of the stomach wall, lymph node spread, type (intestinal or diffuse), location (cardia is worse), histologic differentiation.

Spread
Once the muscular coat is invaded, cancer cells spread to lymph nodes on the lesser and greater curves. Spread is then to the celiac axis and its trifurcation, nodes in the splenic hilum, the root of the mesentery, retropancreatic nodes and common hepatic arteries, and paracolic nodes above and below the transverse colon. Cancer then spreads to the peritoneum, liver, omentum, transverse colon, and the left lobe of the liver.

Objectives
Diagnose cancer, determine surgical resectability, and treat cancer.

History
✧ Early intestinal cancer is asymptomatic.
✧ Early diffuse types may present as dyspepsia which may respond to and appear to heal with H2RAs.
✧ Other symptoms include malaise, early satiety, postprandial fullness, and loss of appetite. Weight loss usually indicates advanced disease.
✧ Cardia lesions may present with dysphagia; middle and pyloric antrum tumors with obstructive symptoms and vomiting after meals. Advanced cases may present with hematemesis and melena.

The most common presentation is *recent-onset dyspepsia in someone over the age of 50.* Therefore, all patients in this age group should have an EGD before starting ulcer treatment.

Examination
✧ No abnormal findings is a good sign.
✧ Anemia often presents at diagnosis.
✧ Signs of weight loss, an epigastric mass, and an enlarged left supraclavicular lymph node indicate late disease.
✧ Jaundice, hepatomegaly, or ascites indicate incurable disease.

Investigations
✧ EGD and multiple biopsies, brush cytology.
✧ CXR, LFT.
✧ CT or ultrasound of liver.
✧ CT of para-aortic nodes, endoscopic ultrasound of stomach to determine depth of involvement.
✧ Diagnostic laparoscopy can be performed to detect peritoneal spread.

Treatment
Treatment takes place in the setting of a multidisciplinary team.
✧ *Curative surgery*:
   ∝ Indications for curative resection are no peritoneal or hepatic disease, and resection margins free of tumor on histologic examination. The resection level should exceed the level of nodal involvement. The extent of lymphadenectomy is referred to as the "D-level":
      – D1 – lymph node clearance of cardia, greater and lesser curves, and juxtapylorus (i.e. excise the greater and lesser omentum).
      – D2 – lymph node clearance around the left gastric, celiac, common hepatic, splenic, retropancreatic and hilar lymph nodes (i.e. splenectomy, resection of body and tail of pancreas).
      – D3 – lymph node clearance from the porta hepatis, behind the head of the pancreas, the root of the mesentery, and middle colic and paracolic lymph nodes. Partial colectomy, hepatic lobectomy, subtotal pancreatectomy, pancreatico-duodenectomy.
✧ *Palliative treatment*:
   ∝ Can be partial or total gastrectomy.
   ∝ Indications for palliative surgical treatment are pain, vomiting, dysphagia, bleeding, and malaise. Dysphagia due to inoperable lesion of the cardia is treated by intubation.

✧ *Chemotherapy* – EAP (etoposide, adriamycin, cisplatin) has a 40% response in advanced cancer, with a complete objective response in 15–20% of cases. It often results in downgrading of the tumor for subsequent curative resection. In good-risk patients, neoadjuvant chemotherapy has been shown to increase overall survival and progression-free survival.

✧ *Radiotherapy* – has little role but is useful in some cases.

Follow-up
Diagnosis and curative treatment should be performed promptly. Palliative management requires long-term regular follow-up to detect worsening symptoms or complications with intubation, etc.

Post-operative Follow-up
✧ Check histology to confirm complete excision and correct resection level.
✧ Arrange oncology referral if appropriate.
✧ Follow-up for complications of gastric surgery is as previously described.

Other Tumors
✧ These include mesenchymal tumors, now called gastrointestinal stromal tumors (GIST), and previously called leiomyoma (benign) and leiomyosarcoma (malignant).
✧ Submucosal and intramuscular tumors occur in the upper and middle third of the stomach.
✧ Ulceration and/or bleeding is a common presentation.
✧ Treatment is by wedge resection if the tumor is small or partial gastrectomy if the tumor is large.

Gastric Lymphomas (2–5%)
These are mainly *B-cell non-Hodgkin's lymphomas* arising in the mucosa-associated lymphoid tissue (MALT). They are slow growing and remain localized until late, and are less aggressive than non-Hodgkin's. They infiltrate the wall, producing mucosal thickening, and may present with ulceration and bleeding. Lymph node spread occurs late and tends to remain in regional lymph nodes.

Objectives
Diagnose lymphoma, differentiate from other tumors, stage tumor, treat tumor.

History
✧ These are the usual dyspeptic symptoms, but nausea, vomiting, and weight loss are more common. Diarrhea is often present.
✧ Some patients will present as emergencies with perforation or hematemesis.
✧ Pain, fever, and anorexia may also be features.

Examination
A palpable epigastric mass may be present in 20% of patients and does not indicate inoperability. However, hepatomegaly and/or splenomegaly suggest a diffuse process with a worse prognosis, as does general lymphadenopathy.

Investigations
✧ Fecal occult blood tests (FOBTs) are positive in 50% of cases.
✧ ESR is usually grossly elevated.

✧ Diagnosis is by EGD – cobblestone mucosal appearance and rugal hypertrophy, and multiple tumor nodules.
✧ Biopsies for histology are taken but may be negative in a large proportion of cases due to the submucosal location of the tumor. Therefore, in the presence of a typical appearance a negative histology result does not rule out the diagnosis. Repeat EGD and deeper biopsies may be indicated.
✧ Endoscopic ultrasound is useful.

Criteria for Establishing a Primary Gastric Lymphoma
✧ Absence of superficial lymphadenopathy.
✧ Absence of splenomegaly.
✧ Normal chest.
✧ No hepatic involvement.
✧ Appropriate histology with primary site in the stomach.
✧ Normal CXR and white cell count.

Staging
✧ Ann Arbor or TNM for gastric lymphoma.
✧ CT of the chest and abdomen is performed to detect spread.
✧ Bone marrow aspirate and biopsy may demonstrate diffuse disease.
✧ Laparoscopy is useful for stage III and IV and to distinguish between primary gastric lymphoma and advanced primary nodal disease.

Treatment
The management of primary gastric lymphoma is controversial. In diffuse primary gastric lymphoma, surgery with adjuvant chemotherapy using CHOP (cyclophosphamide, vincristine, doxorubicin and prednisone), and primary chemotherapy alone both produce high rates of overall survival with low relapse rates. In patients treated with primary surgical resection, complete tumor resection followed by adjuvant chemotherapy is necessary to achieve low relapse rates.

Follow-up
Follow-up is at short intervals until diagnosis and resectability are determined. Preoperative hematology and oncology opinions are required.

Post-operative Follow-up
✧ Check histology to determine complete resection and re-stage the tumor.
✧ Refer for chemotherapy in almost all cases.

Gastric Carcinoids
These are associated with atrophic gastritis (type A) and chronic hypergastrinemia of pernicious anemia. The incidence in pernicious anemia patients is 2–9%.

More recently, fundal enterochromaffin tumors in Zollinger–Ellison patients are treated with omeprazole.

The tumors produce gastrin, somatostatin, serotonin, and vasoactive invasive peptide. They are generally slow-growing and indolent, but can metastasize if they exhibit abnormal cytology and are larger than 2.0 cm.

Objectives
Diagnose carcinoid, differentiate from other tumors, treat carcinoid.

History
✧ Rarely symptomatic; usually diagnosed on endoscopy as investigation for dyspepsia.
✧ Other presentations include abdominal pain or evidence of gastrointestinal bleeding.
✧ The carcinoid syndrome can be produced by gastric carcinoids, but this is usually endocrinologically silent unless associated with liver metastases. Typically, gastric carcinoid produces bright red geographic blushing.

Examination
This may be normal, but examine for evidence of tumor and spread. An epigastric mass and liver enlargement are late signs.

Investigations
✧ EGD with biopsy is usually diagnostic.
✧ Investigate for carcinoid syndrome if suspected.

Treatment
✧ Local (or endoscopic) resection followed by endoscopic surveillance.
✧ Larger tumors require surgical excision.
✧ If not suitable for resection, chemotherapy can be administered.

Follow-up
✧ Follow-up is at short intervals until diagnosis and treatment is performed.
✧ Tumors treated by endoscopic resection require long-term endoscopic follow-up to detect recurrence.
✧ Irresectable lesions require oncology referral for chemotherapy and if necessary treatment of the carcinoid syndrome.

Post-operative Follow-up
Check histology for resection. Complications of gastrectomy are as previously described.

Questions and Answers

Q1 Pain caused by a chronic duodenal ulcer classically:
  A Is worsened by food and often relieved by vomiting.
  B Is episodic in pattern with a frequency of 10–14 days.
  C Is relieved by food intake, and often wakes the patient up in the night-time.
  D Radiates to the right scapula.
  E Is associated with abdominal distension and dysphagia.

A1 C: Improves with eating and often occurs at night 2–4 hours after eating.

Q2 The appropriate role of a barium swallow in the evaluation of gastric and duodenal pathology is:
  A To exclude *H. pylori* infection in a patient with suspected peptic ulcer disease.
  B To provide precise anatomic detail in a patient with suspected gastric or esophageal pathology.
  C To confirm obstruction immediately prior to EGD in a patient with suspected gastric outlet obstruction.
  D As a lower-cost replacement for EGD in the diagnosis of dyspepsia and heartburn.
  E As the primary staging evaluation in a patient with biopsy-proven gastric cancer.

A2 B: Barium swallow is most useful for providing anatomic detail in a patient with hiatal or paraesophageal hernia, or in a post-operative patient. It should not be used if an EGD is planned in short order as the barium in the stomach can destroy the endoscope.

Q3 An appropriate indication for elective surgery in a patient with peptic ulcer disease is:
  A A gastric ulcer that does not heal despite 12 weeks of appropriate medical therapy.
  B A duodenal ulcer which recurs after 6 weeks of treatment with a PPI alone.
  C As primary ulcer therapy for a patient who is chronically taking NSAIDs for osteoarthritis.
  D As the initial management of all duodenal ulcers.
  E As the initial management of all *H. pylori* positive patients with duodenal ulcers.

A3 A: Elective ulcer surgery is reserved for patients who are noncompliant with medical therapy, or fail medical therapy, or have a gastric ulcer which fails to heal after 12 weeks of appropriate medical therapy to exclude the risk of a gastric malignancy.

Q4 The primary treatment of a gastric adenocarcinoma of the gastric antrum without evidence of lymphatic spread on staging evaluation is:
A Definitive chemotherapy and radiation therapy.
B Endoscopic excision and aggressive anti-ulcer therapy.
C Surgical wedge excision of the tumor with a close margin.
D Subtotal gastrectomy with appropriate lymphadenectomy.
E Subtotal gastrectomy alone.

A4 D: A patient with gastric cancer should undergo partial or total gastrectomy with 6 cm margins and an appropriate lymphadenectomy. Depending on the depth of tumor invasion and degree of nodal involvement, a D1 or D2 lymph node dissection should be performed. In a fit patient with Stage II or higher disease, neoadjuvant chemotherapy may improve survival.

Q5 The initial management of dumping syndrome after vagotomy and pyloro-plasty is:
A Early operation and formation of an antiperistaltic jejunal segment.
B Medical therapy with cholestyramine and sucralfate.
C Dietary modification with dry, high protein, and high-fat meals.
D Dietary modification with high-carbohydrate liquid meals.
E Use of antimotility agents such as narcotics.

A5 C: Dumping is caused by rapid emptying of concentrated carbohydrates into the small bowel after destruction or bypass of the pylorus. Dry, high-protein, and high-fat meals slow gastric emptying, and provide calories without a large carbohydrate load. Liquids usually empty more quickly, and liquid carbohydrates are the worst food for a patient with dumping.

The Small Intestine and Vermiform Appendix
Clinton D. Protack and Jason S. Gold

The basic functions of the small bowel are digestion and absorption. Chronic disorders of the small bowel are often managed by gastroenterologists with referral to surgeons if surgery is indicated. However, some knowledge of these disorders is necessary for the surgeon, especially of inflammatory bowel disease (IBD), small bowel tumors, and the investigation of weight loss and diarrhea.

Assessment of Small Bowel Disorders
Small Bowel History
Take a general gastrointestinal (GI) history. There are no symptoms which exclusively indicate small bowel disease, but small bowel disorders should be considered in patients presenting with intermittent, colicky central abdominal pain. These symptoms may be accompanied by diarrhea, changes in the consistency and texture of stool, and weight loss. Patients may also complain of symptoms typical of anemia. As adhesions secondary to abdominal surgery are a frequent cause of small bowel pathology, patients should be questioned about previous operations. Patients may complain of nausea, bloating, or vomiting, typically 1–2 hours after meals.

Small Bowel Examination
- ✧ Perform a general examination focused on the abdomen.
- ✧ Examine for anemia and weight loss.
- ✧ Examine the mouth and pharynx for ulcers.
- ✧ Abdominal examination may reveal distension, scars from previous surgery, tenderness or a mass.
- ✧ Rectal examination and sigmoidoscopy and biopsy, if indicated, completes the examination.

Diagnostic Tests
Laboratory Investigations
- ✧ *Complete blood count*: May reveal anemia due to GI bleeding or chronic disease. Abnormal white blood-cell count (WBC) may indicate infection, inflammation, or lymphoma. Erythrocyte sedimentation rate (ESR), and C-reactive protein (CRP) may indicate active inflammatory bowel disease.
- ✧ *Biochemistry*:
    - ∝ *Urinalysis* – raised urinary levels of 5-HIAA may indicate carcinoid syndrome.
    - ∝ *Serum biochemistry* – routine indications. Abnormalities of serum albumin, transferrin, urea and electrolytes including calcium may occur in small bowel disease.
    - ∝ *Liver function tests* – abnormal LFTs may be associated with inflammatory bowel disease.
    - ∝ *Blood glucose* – may reveal diabetes mellitus.
    - ∝ *Estimation of fecal fat* – 3 to 5-day collection of stool on a standard diet containing 80–100g of fat. Normal excretion is less than 6.0 g/day (18mmol triglyceride). This is a non-invasive screening test for malabsorption.
- ✧ *Microbiology*: Stool cultures are useful in various small bowel infections, e.g. *Yersinia*.
- ✧ *Cytology/Histology*:

∝ *Jejunal mucosal biopsy* – used for diagnosis of celiac disease, Whipple's disease, parasites and amyloidosis. Biopsies are often obtained endoscopically. Biopsies can also be obtained using Crosby suction, where the patient swallows a capsule at the end of a fine-bore catheter and time is allowed to elapse for the capsule to be propelled into the jejunum. This is confirmed by plain AXR. The capsule is opened and suction applied via the catheter. The capsule is then closed, taking a jejunal mucosa biopsy, and the capsule removed.

Imaging Techniques

✧ *Abdominal X-ray*: May identify dilated small bowel loops in obstruction or thickened bowel loops in inflammatory disorders.

✧ *Contrast computed tomography (CT)*: The patient drinks, or is instilled through a nasogastric tube, a special radiologic contrast solution to opacify the intestine. The patient is then passed through the CT body scanner. This is useful to detect thickening of bowel wall and presence of enterocolic and enterovesical fistulas. It provides detailed information of the small and large bowel, but is expensive, time-consuming, and uses ionizing radiation. CT enterography is a specially protocoled examination using large volumes of ingested enteric contrast material that improves the assessment of the mucosa and the bowel wall.

✧ *Small bowel follow through (SBFT)*: The patient drinks radiologic contrast. The path of the contrast through the stomach and small bowel is followed at regular intervals by repeated X-rays. It is easier to perform than small bowel enema (see below), but provides less detail of small bowel due to dilution of contrast, time taken to empty from the stomach, and overlapping bowel loops.

✧ *Small bowel enema (SBE)*: A contrast medium instilled through a tube passed directly into the upper jejunum. It has a high diagnostic yield for small bowel tumors, Crohn's, and occult GI bleeding and malabsorption. Malabsorption shows flocculation and segmentation of barium, thickening of mucosal folds and dilatation of intestinal loops. There may be difficulty swallowing the tube and passing tube through the pylorus.

✧ *Small bowel magnetic resonance imaging (MRI)*: MRI with small bowel contrast using water or locust bean gum. While currently not universally used, it has increasingly been shown to be very accurate at imaging the small bowel. Most of the work has been done in Crohn's disease. The ability of this technique to indicate areas of inflammation may allow differentiation between fibrostenotic and inflammatory strictures.

✧ *Selective splanchnic angiography*: An angiography catheter is passed using the Seldinger technique through the femoral artery, and the catheter manipulated through the aorta into the visceral arteries (celiac, super, and inferior mesenteric arteries). Radiologic contrast is injected. Certain appearances are characteristic of certain lesions, e.g. intraluminal bleeding, tumor, or stenoses/occlusions of the celiac or mesenteric arteries indicating mesenteric ischemia. The technique allows identification of obscure GI bleeding not identified by endoscopy and is diagnostic for angiodysplastic lesions during active bleeding. It may be useful for diagnosis of mesenteric ischemia. This is an invasive technique associated with complications to do with arterial puncture, e.g. hemorrhage, hematoma, false aneurysm, and the use of radiologic contrast, e.g. allergic reactions, renal failure.

✧ *Ultrasound*: An ultrasound probe is passed over the abdomen using aqueous gel as a coupling medium. Images of the underlying organs are formed from the differential amounts of ultrasound reflected from different organs. Using the Doppler effect and color-coding, blood flow can be imaged in major arterial and venous vessels. The technique is useful for detecting fluid-filled loops of small bowel, detecting peristalsis, estimating bowel wall thickness, detecting intra-abdominal fluid, and detecting blood flow in major vessels.

Visualization of the Small Bowel
✧ *Small bowel enteroscopy*: A long endoscope is inserted into the duodenum, a balloon is inflated and gut peristalsis carries the scope to the cecum; confirmed by X-ray screening. The bowel is inspected as the instrument is withdrawn. The technique may be useful to visualize obscure bleeding, but is not widely available.
✧ *Capsule endoscopy (CE)*: The PillCam videocapsule contains a miniaturized camera, a light source and a wireless circuit for acquisition and transmission of signals. The patient swallows a capsule and the device is passively propelled through the GI tract by peristalsis. Images are transmitted to a data recorder and then downloaded to be reviewed on a monitor. The capsule is passed in the patient's stool, usually within 24–48 hours. Currently, the best evidence for its use includes evaluation of patients with obscure bleeding, inflammatory bowel diseases, suspected small bowel tumors, hereditary polyposis syndromes, and complicated celiac disease. It cannot be used in patients with motility disorders or mechanical obstruction.

Radio-isotope Techniques
✧ *Isotope scintigraphy*: Intravenous administration of radiolabeled compound or autologous cells. It may be useful for occult GI bleeding, suspected intra-abdominal localized inflammation/abscess, inflamed Crohn's, intestinal transit time, and evaluation of biliary-enteric anastomoses, but requires use of radioactivity and poorly localizes bleeding points or abscesses in the abdomen.
✧ *Small bowel transit time*: External scintigraphy after administration of isotope-labeled meals or by breath tests. For meals, the detection of cecal radioactivity is used as the end-point for the estimation of small bowel transit time (includes gastric emptying time as well). Breath tests are a simpler way of obtaining similar information.
✧ *White cell scan*: Indium-111 labeled autologous leukocytes are injected intravenously and settle in areas of abscess/inflammation. Abdominal scintiscan is performed at 2, 6, 20, and 24 hours. The technique can be used to detect extent and severity of inflammatory bowel disease, but 99m-sulcralfate suspension drink selectively binds to areas of ulceration in both small and large bowel. It is increasingly used as a screening test.

Tests of Small Bowel Function
✧ *Breath tests*: Used for detection of bacterial overgrowth and demonstration of carbohydrate malabsorption, and in the assessment of small bowel transit time.
   ∝ *Bacterial overgrowth* – the ^{14}C-glycocholate breath test can detect bacterial overgrowth in the small intestine. Bacteria deconjugate the compound which is absorbed into the bloodstream and exhaled. This can also be positive in the presence of ileal disease, and in this circumstance ^{14}C-d-xylose is more reliable.
   ∝ *Carbohydrate malabsorption* – ingestion of ^{14}C-lactose is the conventional test for lactose intolerance, i.e. brush border lactase deficiency.
   ∝ *Hydrogen breath test* – for small bowel transit time and bacterial overgrowth. The hydrogen breath test is supplanting other tests for small bowel transit time. The technique involves repeated measurements of H_2 in end-expiratory air after intake of lactulose or a meal of mashed potato and beans. When the meal reaches the cecum, bacterial fermentation occurs and results in increased breath H_2. The test includes gastric emptying time, but if the meal is radiolabeled with

technetium-99m then both gastric emptying and small bowel transit times can be calculated from the one investigation.

✧ *Tests of intestinal permeability*: ^{51}Cr-labeled EDTA is given orally; this is not absorbed in healthy people. A urinary estimation is performed, and if EDTA is detected this indicates abnormal intestinal permeability. The test may be useful in the diagnosis of obscure cases of Crohn's, etc., but is not widely available.

✧ *Ileal malabsorption*: The Schilling test is performed to test the ability to absorb vitamin B12; and the SeHCAT (23-seleno-25-homo-tauro-cholate) test assesses bile turnover, and thus the ileal absorptive capacity for bile salts. Values less than 15% signify malabsorption.

Investigation of Specific Small Bowel Abnormalities
Investigation of Intestinal Bleeding

✧ *Causes* – Meckel's diverticulum, polyps, tumors, especially smooth muscle neoplasms and vascular malformations.

✧ *Investigations*:
  ∝ Upper and lower endoscopy are usually negative.
  ∝ Radionuclide methods include technetium-99m which shows a hot spot in 90% of Meckel's cases; 99m-sulfur colloid shows rapid bleeding; radiolabeled red cells are suitable for detecting intermittent bleeding not for active rapid bleeding.
  ∝ For rapid bleeding, perform angiography and embolization.

Investigation of Suspected Malabsorption

✧ *Causes* – malabsorption is either due to small bowel disease or bacterial overgrowth, or the result of pancreatic insufficiency.

✧ *First test* – abnormal fecal fat excretion (>6.0 g/day).

✧ *Second test* – small bowel enema. If normal, then perform mucosal biopsy, and if this is normal then perform pancreatic function tests. If small bowel enema is abnormal, then mucosal biopsy can be performed, or proceed directly to Schilling or SeHCAT test and follow with tests for bacterial overgrowth.

Syndromes Resulting from Disease or Surgery on the Gastrointestinal Tract

These include bacterial overgrowth (stagnant loop syndrome), short gut syndrome, and protein-losing enteropathy.

Bacterial Overgrowth

The causes of bacterial overgrowth include:

1. Excessive entry of bacteria into the small intestine. Causes include achlorhydria, gastrojejunostomy, partial/total gastrectomy, enterocolic fistulas, cholangitis, and loss of ileocecal valve following right hemicolectomy.
2. Intestinal stasis – due to Crohn's disease (stenosis), tuberculosis (stenosis), small bowel diverticulosis, afferent loop stasis, entero-enteric anastomosis, and other intestinal bypass procedures, subacute obstruction, blind loops, diabetes mellitus, radiation enteritis, scleroderma, and amyloidosis.

History

Weakness or malaise, nausea, and vomiting, excessive borborygmi, weight loss. Diarrhea is frequent and watery. Steatorrhea is less common.

Examination
Look for evidence of glossitis, stomatitis, anemia, hypoproteinemia with peripheral edema, tetany, osteomalacia, and rickets.

Investigation
^{14}C-glycocholate or ^{14}C-d-xylose breath tests.

Treatment
Treatment is of the underlying condition. Surgery is only indicated in treatment of anatomic causes related to previous operation.

Treat with intermittent courses of antibiotics (neomycin or metronidazole) for 10–14 days, which may give symptomatic improvement for several months. Fresh unpasteurized yogurt or *Lactobacillus* preparations should be given with and after antibiotics to inhibit re-colonization.

Follow-up
Follow-up is long-term at regular intervals, depending on the clinical condition.

Short Gut Syndrome
The causes of short gut syndrome include operations requiring extensive small bowel resection, Crohn's, mesenteric infarction, radiation enteritis, midgut volvulus, multiple fistulas, and small bowel tumors.

A small bowel less than 2 meters long has a diminished work capacity and those patients with less than 100 cm require parenteral nutrition for life. Those with borderline-length small bowel may benefit from enteral feeding and/or additional intravenous fluids.

Ileal resections are less tolerated than jejunal resections, largely because active transport sites for bile salts and vitamin B12 are localized in the ileum. Therefore, efforts should be made to try to retain a portion of terminal ileum and the ileocecal valve if possible.

Consequences of short gut syndrome include:

1. Malabsorption and malnutrition (also gastric hypersecretion – transient).
2. Gallstone formation, mainly cholesterol stones due to decreased bile salts.
3. Hepatic disease – fatty liver, onset of liver failure after jejunoileal bypass. Up to 6 months post-operatively, a history of flu-like illness, anorexia, nausea and vomiting, weight loss, decreased serum albumin is an indication to restore intestinal continuity.
4. Impaired renal function and stone formation – diarrhea and loss of electrolyte-rich fluid leading principally to hyponatremia. There may be metabolic acidosis and formation of urinary calculi. Increased aldosterone leads to chronic hypokalemia causing muscle weakness, anorexia, and cardiac arrhythmias.
5. Metabolic bone disease – hypocalcemia and hypomagnesium are common. Treat with 1-alpha-hydroxy-cholecalciferol.

History
Take a general small bowel history. Inquire about the causes of short bowel syndrome and the consequences of it (see above).

Examination
◇ Perform a general examination, looking for evidence of anemia and weight loss.
◇ Examine for evidence of the consequences of short gut syndrome.

Treatment

Support the patient until adaptation occurs; this may be up to 6 months post-operatively. Give transparenteral nutrition in the immediate stage. At 3–6 weeks, transition the patient to an oral diet. As long as 1 meter of small bowel remains, a normal diet may be achieved. However, these patients may require long-term enteral feeding with polymeric or elemental formula diets, and on occasions additional intravenous fluid. Supplements of calcium, magnesium, and vitamin C are needed; and in cases of ileal resection, vitamin B12 injections every 3 months for life.

Specialized intestinal lengthening procedures may provide benefits for some patients.

Follow-up
Follow-up is long-term at regular intervals determined by the clinical condition.
   Complications include:
1. *High output states* – sodium and water can be lost in significant amounts. Treat with a combination of oral fluid restriction, loperamide and on rare occasions infusion/subcutaneous injection of long-acting somatostatin.
2. *Steatorrhea* – the cause is excess fat in the diet. Treat by substituting fat with medium-chain triglycerides, which do not require the presence of bile salts for digestion.

Long-term treatments include combined hepatic and small bowel transplant or techniques such as reversed antiperistaltic small bowel segment to decrease diarrhea. If the patient is young and symptoms are not improving, then transplantation may be considered.

Protein-losing Enteropathy
The causes of protein-losing enteropathy include: celiac disease, Whipple's disease, bacterial overgrowth, and IBD.

History and Examination
The clinical picture is usually dominated by the underlying condition, but the loss of protein leads to hypoproteinemia with secondary hyperaldosteronism with water and salt retention. Albumin and immunoglobulin A (IgA) are depleted more than other, larger proteins.

Investigation
Albumin labeled with iodine-131 or chromium-52 is injected intravenously and levels monitored for 2 weeks. A plasma die-away curve is plotted and fecal radioactivity is measured. Daily enteric losses are calculated; excessive loss can be detected.

Treatment
Albumin infusions; surgery of the underlying condition. A high-calorie, high-protein diet is needed.

Follow-up
Follow-up is long-term at regular intervals determined by the clinical condition.

Vascular Anomalies, Hamartomatous Lesions, and Vasculitic or Connective Tissue Disorders of the Gastrointestinal Tract
Bleeding into the small intestine may be involved in systemic vasculitic and connective tissue disorders (CTDs). The conditions in which intestinal involvement is common are polyarteritis, Henoch–Schönlein purpura, pseudoxanthoma elasticum and Ehlers–Danlos syndrome.

Angiodysplasia

Angiodysplasia consists of clusters of arteriolar, venular, and capillary vessels in the mucosa and submucosa of the GI tract, which therefore are not visible or palpable from the outside. Rupture of the mucosal component causes bleeding. It commonly occurs in the right colon but also in the stomach and small intestine.

History
✧ There is an increased incidence in patients suffering from aortic valve disease and chronic lung disease.
✧ Colonic lesions are commonest between the ages of 50–55 years, and small bowel lesions between age 30 and 35 years.
✧ There may be episodic or chronic occult GI bleeding over years.
✧ May present as iron deficiency anemia, overt melena, or acute hemorrhage.

Examination
✧ Perform a general examination.
✧ Examine for signs of weight loss and anemia.
✧ Examine for general features of connective tissue disease.
✧ Abdominal examination may be normal, but rectal examination may reveal melena.

Investigation
✧ Upper endoscopy and colonoscopy to locate or exclude these sites as the source of bleeding. Colonic angiodysplasia is well visualized by colonoscopy – cherry-red lesions similar to a spider nevus.
✧ If the small bowel is suspected as the source, then options include radionuclide scan – ^{99m}Tc-, or Sc-labeled red cells.
✧ Selective mesenteric angiography is useful to demonstrate abnormal vessel patterns even in the absence of active bleeding.

Treatment
Conservative management of the patient, with blood transfusion only if clinically indicated.
✧ Endoscopic diathermy is especially useful in colonic lesions.
✧ Angiographic embolization can be useful, especially in the treatment of rapid bleeding.
✧ Laparotomy – pre-operative endoscopy can be used to transilluminate the bowel and localize the lesion for excision.

Follow-up
Intervals should be short, or the patient should be admitted for investigation until the source of bleeding is identified. Once this has been treated, follow-up at regular intervals (1–6 months) is indicated until further episodes are excluded.

Other Causes of Small Bowel Bleeding
✧ *Phlebectasia*: A meshwork of dilated veins in the submucosa frequently occurs in the esophagus, mid-small bowel and rectum, but these are a rare cause of bleeding.
✧ *Hemangiomas (vascular malformations)*: Occur in the small and large intestine. Treatment is by either surgical excision or selective embolization.
✧ *Hereditary hemorrhagic telangiectasia* – Peutz–Jeghers syndrome: Bleeding from polyps in the bowel. There is a risk of malignancy, so all polyps larger than 2 cm should be removed.

✧ *Polyarteritis*: Systemic necrotizing vasculitis with fibrinoid necrosis affecting the blood vessels of several organs, including the gut. Weakened vessels lead to aneurysm formation; these rupture, bleed, and thrombose.

Inflammatory Bowel Disease
Crohn's Disease
Crohn's disease most commonly affects the terminal ileum, colon and rectum, stomach and duodenum, and esophagus, in that order.

A chronic granulomatous disease, it is a segmental condition with areas of involvement strongly demarcated from contiguous normal bowel. Edema, sloughing and linear ulceration leads to the formation of pseudopolyps, mucosa bridges, etc. Ulcers are typically deep, penetrate into the muscle layers (fissuring), and account for the tendency to localized perforation, adhesions, and fistula formation.

History
Crohn's may present in a variety of ways, and this variable presentation often delays diagnosis. It is commonest in the third decade of life, with abdominal pain which varies from discomfort to severe and colicky. It is often associated with diarrhea and weight loss. Other signs and symptoms can include early satiety or sense of fullness, abdominal distension during bouts of abdominal pain, melena, or hematochezia.

✧ *Pseudoappendicitis syndrome*: Acute abdominal pain. Remove the appendix if the cecum appears normal. Only 1 in 8 cases of acute terminal ileitis are due to Crohn's. Always review the histology.
✧ *Small bowel obstruction*: Usually partial or subacute. It is more commonly due to adhesions or stricture. Early operation is advisable. Intermittent self-limiting episodes invariably have gross bacterial overgrowth, which may cause malabsorption.
✧ *Abscess*: Results from localized perforation or lymph node mass. It presents with local signs and increased catabolism, weight loss, fever, and anorexia. Abscess is commonest in the right iliac fossa. It may track through to the pelvis and under the inguinal ligament to the anterior compartment of the thigh. Free perforation causing peritonitis is rare.
✧ *Fistula*: A perianal fistula may present before intestinal disease. An enterocutaneous fistula is classified as high or low output. Spontaneous closure with parenteral nutrition is usually only possible with low-output fistulas.
✧ *Diarrhea*: Present in 70–80%. It is colonic, associated with mucus and blood. The small bowel is associated with protein-losing enteropathy and/or steatorrhea due to bacterial overgrowth or bile salt malabsorption.

Examination
✧ Perform a general examination.
✧ Examine for evidence of anemia and weight loss, and other systemic features of Crohn's such as clubbing, proximal myopathy, easy bruising, and in toxic cases raised temperature, tachycardia, and edema.
✧ Abdominal examination may be normal or there may be evidence of a mass, particularly in the right side of the abdomen.
✧ Examine anus for fissures, fleshy skin tags, sinuses, and abscesses.

Investigations
✧ Carry out a combination of luminal investigation (usually endoscopic) with appropriate histology, in association with raised inflammatory markers (CRP, ESR, and WBC).

◇ In addition, a number of serologic markers including anti-*Saccharomyces cerevisiae* antibody (ASCA) and antineutrophilic cytoplasmic antibody (ANCA)/pANCA, and outer membrane porin from *Escherichia coli* (OMP-C) may provide additional information.

◇ The Prometheus test panel is a commercially available serologic panel of antibodies (including pANCA/ANCA, ASCA IgA, ASCA IgG, and anti-OMP-C IgA) that has been proposed to help confirm the diagnosis of IBD, differentiate between Crohn's disease and ulcerative colitis, and possibly to assess disease severity.

◇ Diseased segments are demonstrated by conventional contrast radiology, conventional CT, CT enterography, and/or MRI. These studies can show narrowing of the lumen, a nodular mucosal pattern, irregularity, ulcers, strictures, and/or fistulas.

  ∝ The string sign refers to appearance of marked narrowing on a contrast study (the contrast resembles a frayed cotton string) that can occur with irritability and spasms associated with severe ulceration.

  ∝ Fistulas and sinuses can be defined by injection of contrast on fluoroscopic studies or CT scans.

Treatment

The management of Crohn's disease is dependent on the assessment of the disease location and its severity. The therapeutic goals are to induce a clinical remission, to maintain that remission, and to prevent post-operative relapse.

◇ *Mild to moderate disease* – the initial choice is 5-aminosalicylate (5-ASA), although there is little evidence to support its efficacy. Budesonide seems to be as effective as prednisolone, with a reduction in adverse effects. Metronidazole and ciprofloxacin regimens can give similar results to 5-ASA particularly in Crohn's ileocolitis and in perianal disease.

◇ *Moderate to severe disease* – steroids provide rapid remission but their use should be short and sharp to prevent side effects. There is no role for steroids in maintenance of remission. Introduction of immunosuppressives such as azathioprine or methotrexate will allow long-term control of the disease.

◇ *Severe disease* – patients are admitted to hospital. They require standard resuscitation and are then treated with intravenous medication. Options include steroids, cyclosporine, and biologic therapy such as infliximab.

Dietary Manipulations

Evidence exists to support the use of an exclusive enteral diet in the management of mild to moderate disease. This provides an equivalent, if slower, remission rate to that for oral steroids. Compliance may be a problem.

Surgery

Common indications for surgery include:

◇ Intestinal obstruction.
◇ Abscess formation.
◇ Fistula formation.
◇ Failure of medical treatment for limited disease.
◇ Need to raise an ileostomy to defunction diseased bowel.
◇ Nutritional failure.
◇ Small bowel perforation (rare).
◇ Acute severe hemorrhage (rare).

Procedures are small bowel resection, strictureplasty, and ileostomy.

Post-operative Follow-up
✧ Review with histology to confirm diagnosis and exclude other diagnoses, e.g. small bowel lymphoma.
✧ Examine for any post-operative complications including anastomotic leakage resulting in fistula formation or intra-abdominal abscess.
✧ Long-term follow-up is indicated to continue medical management in an attempt to reduce post-operative recurrence.

Complications of Surgical Treatment in Crohn's Disease
✧ The incidence of post-operative complications is 10–15%.
 ∝ *Acute* – anastomotic leakage, fistula formation, intra-abdominal abscess, and hemorrhage.
 ∝ *Late* – short bowel syndrome, urinary lithiasis, cholelithiasis, gastric hypersecretion, peptic ulcer disease.

Recurrence rates after small bowel resection are 30% at 5 years, 50% at 10 years. Medical treatment may influence the recurrence rate.

 Short bowel syndrome – treatment options include home parenteral nutrition, small bowel transplant, or small bowel and hepatic transplantation.

Ileostomy Care
✧ Ileostomy causes daily losses of 500–600 ml of fluid and 40–50 mmol Na^+. Patients thus require adequate water and salt intake.
✧ Local – complication of terminal ileostomies – stenosis, prolapse – may require revisional surgery.
✧ Peristomal irritation – occurs in 20–40% of cases but responds to regular cleaning and the use of skin barriers (Stomadhesive, Comfeel).
✧ Para-ileostomy hernia in 5% leads to ill-fitting appliances and leakage, and may cause internal strangulation. This may require surgical re-siting, but tends to recur so should be reserved for severe cases.
✧ Ileostomy diarrhea causes include proximal stoma, partial obstruction, internal abscess formation, and recurrence of Crohn's. Investigations include abdominal X-rays, small bowel enema (through the stoma), and endoscopic examination through the stoma.
✧ For treatment of high output ileostomy, see short bowel syndrome.

Tumors of the Small Intestine
These are rare – fewer than 10% of all GI neoplasms.

Benign Tumors
Historically, most have been detected as incidental findings on autopsy, but over time more are being found due to increased use of endoscopy and imaging. They include tubular and villous adenomas, lipomas, hemangiomas, and neurogenic tumors. Adenomas may also occur in association with familial polyposis coli, Gardener's syndrome (intestinal polyps and epidermoid cysts), and Turcot's syndrome (intestinal polyps and brain tumors).

 In addition to the known risk of colonic carcinoma, these patients are liable to develop carcinoma of the duodenum and biliary tract. In the non-familial group, villous adenomas are prone to malignant change.

History

May present acutely as intussusception or chronic bleeding causing iron-deficiency anemia, or occasionally overt hemorrhage. Most are asymptomatic.

Take a general small bowel history. Inquire regarding the symptoms of anemia, family history, or history relating to the rare causes outlined above.

Examination

♦ Perform a general examination.

♦ Depending on the mode of presentation, examination may be normal or there may be signs of anemia or, rarely, an abdominal mass.

♦ Rectal examination may reveal melena.

Investigations

♦ Fecal occult blood test (FOBT) may be positive for blood.

♦ Endoscopy is performed to exclude other causes of GI bleeding and to diagnose duodenal tumors.

♦ CT enterography or fluoroscopic contrast studies may be used to demonstrate other lesions in the small bowel.

♦ CT can be used to assess for metastatic disease.

Treatment

Surgical resection.

Follow-up

Follow-up is at short intervals until diagnosis is obtained and malignant tumors are excluded.

Post-operative Follow-up

Review the histology to confirm the benign nature of the tumor and ensure excision is complete. Detect complications related to laparotomy and small bowel resection. Discharge once asymptomatic. Follow-up is long-term for Gardner's and Turcot's syndromes.

Polyposis and Duodenal Tumors
Peutz–Jeghers Syndrome
Background

Peutz–Jeghers syndrome is an inherited autosomal dominant polyposis syndrome. Multiple hamartomatous polyps develop throughout the stomach, the small and the large bowel and patients usually have speckled pigmentation around the oral and buccal mucosa.

History

The polyps eventually produce symptoms such as obstruction or anemia secondary to chronic bleeding. Malignant change may occur in the polyps.

Investigations

Contrast radiology, endoscopy, and capsule endoscopy.

Treatment

Resection is indicated for small bowel polyps when symptomatic or when the size exceeds 1.0 cm in diameter. Endoscopic resection is the initial treatment, with surgery reserved for polyps not amenable to endoscopic resection.

Duodenal Tumors
Background
Duodenal neoplasms are rare and are most common in the first part of the duodenum. The risk of malignancy increases as they become more distal.

History
Presentation is most commonly with GI hemorrhage. Adenomas are the most common tumors. Presentation may be with obstructive symptoms or an abdominal mass.

Investigation
Endoscopy and cross-sectional imaging.

Treatment
Segmental duodenal resection or pancreatico-duodenectomy can be performed for resectable lesions. For unresectable or metastatic lesions, palliation can be achieved with stenting of the bile duct or duodenal obstruction or with surgical bypasses.

Duodenal Disease in Familial Adenomatous Polyposis
Background
Familial adenomatous polyposis (FAP) was previously known as familial polyposis coli, the change in name reflecting the recognition of extracolonic polyps and cancers. Adenomas tend to be noted in the duodenum approximately 15 years after colonic polyps occur.

Investigation
Regular endoscopy and biopsy. The severity of duodenal polyposis can be quantified using a staging system developed by Spigelman and colleagues, which relies on clinical and histologic assessment of the duodenum to provide a four-stage scoring system.

Natural History
Polyposis is associated with a high frequency of duodenal or periampullary cancer with estimates of the incidence of these cancers being between 1% and 12%. These cancers are the commonest cause of death for patients who undergo total proctocolectomy for prevention of colorectal cancer.

Treatment
Endoscopic surveillance with therapeutic options such as mucosal resection and argon-beam coagulation. Duodenectomy or pancreatico-duodenectomy is performed for more advanced polyps and/or cancer.

Malignant Small Bowel Tumors
These are rare and present late. They comprise adenocarcinoma (40%), carcinoid tumors (30%), lymphoma (25%), and smooth muscle tumors (5%).

Small Bowel Adenocarcinoma
Forty percent of these are duodenal, with 40% jejunal and 20% ileal. The majority of duodenal carcinomas are found in the periampullary region and in the third part of the duodenum. They typically spread to regional lymph nodes, the liver, and the peritoneal cavity.

Carcinoma in Crohn's disease has a particularly poor prognosis. It occurs in the 40- to 50-year age group, is more common in males (3 : 1), and affects the ileum in 75% of cases.

History
✧ Mainly occur in the over-60 age group.
✧ Present with epigastric or periumbilical discomfort or pain. Pain is usually postprandial and colicky.
✧ There may be nausea and vomiting, weight loss, GI bleeding, intestinal obstruction, or intussusception.
✧ Duodenal carcinoma can present with obstructive jaundice.

Examination
✧ Perform a general examination.
✧ Examine for evidence of anemia or jaundice.
✧ Abdominal examination may be normal, or there is a mass or evidence of small bowel obstruction.
✧ The liver may be enlarged due to metastases.

Investigations
Diagnosis is by endoscopy, capsule endoscopy, fluoroscopic contrast studies, or CT. Cross-sectional imaging is used to assess for metastasis. Carcinoembryonic antigen (CEA) can be used as a tumor marker.

Treatment
Surgical resection for local to regional disease. Tumors in the jejunum and ileum are often metastatic at diagnosis. Systemic chemotherapy is typically used for metastatic disease.

Follow-up
Follow-up intervals should be short (1–4 weeks) until diagnosis is obtained.

Post-operative Follow-up
Follow-up is long-term, looking for signs of recurrence. The five-year survival rate is 20–45%, but better for duodenal tumors.

Carcinoid Tumors
These tumors are classified into three groups:
1. *Foregut* – stomach, duodenum, pancreas, biliary tract, and bronchus.
2. *Midgut* – jejunum, ileum, and right colon.
3. *Hindgut* – left colon and rectum; these typically do not secret active peptides.

Foregut and midgut tumors may secrete almost any of the gut hormones and serotonin.

Size is a strong predictor of metastatic potential. Invasion occurs into the bowel wall, mesentery, parietal peritoneum, and adjacent organs. Carcinoid tumors are notable for local desmoplastic reaction. Most commonly, they spread to lymph nodes. The bronchus, small intestine, and rectum are the most common sites of origin.

History
✧ The commonest age group is 45–55 years.
✧ Duodenal carcinoids can present with vomiting or endocrine syndrome.
✧ Jejuno-ileal carcinoids can present with diarrhea, intestinal obstruction, and/or a palpable abdominal mass.
✧ Tumors of the appendix present usually as acute appendicitis.

✧ The presence of symptoms of the carcinoid syndrome indicates advanced disease with extensive hepatic involvement.

Examination
✧ Perform a general examination.
✧ Examine for presence of a tumor and metastases, e.g. enlarged liver.
✧ Examine for carcinoid syndrome (see below).

Investigations
✧ Endoscopy and biopsy can be used if the tumor is accessible.
✧ Cross-sectional imaging can be used to assess for liver metastasis (carcinoids tend to be vascular, so arterial phase imaging is important). Octreoscan can also be used to evaluate for metastatic disease.
✧ Chromogranin A can be used as a tumor marker.
✧ Measure urinary and/or serum levels of serotonin and its metabolite 5-hydroxyindoleacetic acid (5-HIAA) (see below).

Treatment
✧ Resection of tumor with wide margins of healthy tissue, regional lymph nodes and associated mesentery is standard.
✧ Somatostatin analogues (i.e. octreotide) can be used for treating unresectable or metastatic tumors.
✧ Chemotherapy is typically reserved for rapidly dividing tumors. Targeted agents are increasingly being used for some carcinoid tumors.
✧ Resectable hepatic deposits can be treated by surgical resection.
✧ Debulking of the tumor may help alleviate symptoms.

Follow-up
Intervals are short (1–4 weeks) until diagnosis is obtained.

Post-operative Follow-up
Follow-up is long-term to detect recurrence or onset of carcinoid syndrome. Many patients survive for long periods despite the presence of residual or metastatic disease. The five-year survival rate is 60%.

Carcinoid Syndrome
This is rare, affecting 10% of carcinoid tumors. It indicates advanced disease with extensive hepatic involvement. Inappropriate secretion of serotonin (5-hydroxytryptamine [5-HT]) and other vasoactive substances are responsible for symptoms.

History
✧ Patients may describe several types of flushing syndromes – cutaneous flushing affecting the upper part of the body accompanied by sweating, itching, edema, palpitations, and hypotension.
✧ Patients may also complain of intestinal colic and diarrhea, bronchospasm, hypoproteinemia, and edema.
✧ Other presentations include cardiac lesions (tricuspid insufficiency or pulmonary stenosis), photosensitive dermatitis, neurologic signs, peptic ulceration, and arthralgia.

Examination
◇ Perform a general examination.
◇ Examine for evidence of flushing and/or dermatitis and edema.
◇ Examine the chest for presence of cardiac lesions and bronchospasm.
◇ Examine the abdomen for evidence of a tumor and/or metastases (e.g. enlarged liver).
◇ Perform a neurologic examination.

Investigations
◇ Serum and urinary levels of serotonin and its metabolite 5-HIAA.
◇ Cross-sectional imaging can be used to assess for liver metastasis (carcinoids tend to be vascular, so arterial phase imaging is important). Octreoscan can also be used to evaluate for metastatic disease.
◇ Chromogranin A can be used as a tumor marker.

Treatment
◇ Complete surgical resection is performed when feasible. Debulking may help control symptoms and possibly prolong survival.
◇ Somatostatin analogues (i.e. octreotide) can be used for treating symptoms and can prolong survival.
◇ Chemotherapy is typically reserved for rapidly dividing tumors. Targeted agents are increasingly being used for some carcinoid tumors.

Follow-up
Follow-up is long-term at regular intervals determined by the clinical condition.

Primary Gut Lymphomas
Characteristically, primary gut lymphomas of the small bowel are seldom diagnosed pre-operatively and at operation may be confused with Crohn's disease. When gut lymphoma is diagnosed, one of the first tasks is to determine the type of lymphoma and whether this primarily affects the bowel or whether the bowel is involved as part of a systemic lymphoma.

Criteria for Diagnosis of Primary Gut Lymphomas
There is no uniform definition of primary small intestine lymphoma, but it typically refers to a lymphoma that predominantly involves the small intestine.

Primary gut lymphoma is rare – predisposing conditions include immunoprolifera-tive small intestine disease (IPSID), celiac disease, AIDS, and other immuno-deficiency states, and possibly IBD.
◇ *Site* – primary gut lymphoma arises in the following sites: duodenum 8%, jejunum 33%, ileum 59%, more than one site 32%.
◇ *Type of lymphoma*:
  ∝ Hodgkin's lymphoma accounts for less than 1% of gut lymphomas; non-Hodg-kin's lymphoma accounts for the vast majority.
  ∝ IPSID is thought to be a variant of extranodal marginal zone lymphoma of mucosa-associated lymphoid tissue (MALT).
  ∝ Celiac disease predisposes to enteropathy-associated T-cell lymphoma (EATL).
  ∝ Diffuse large B-cell lymphoma, mantle cell lymphoma, Burkitt lymphoma, and follicular lymphoma are other possible histologies.
◇ *Staging* – no uniform staging system exists for primary intestinal lymphomas. Tumors are staged by the involvement of lymph nodes and whether these lymph nodes are confined to the abdomen.

History
✧ Any age except infancy; incidence peaks in the sixth decade with a small peak in the first to third decades.
✧ Often presents as an emergency with intestinal obstruction, hemorrhage or perforation. Chronic symptoms are malaise, abdominal pain, weight loss, diarrhea/steatorrhea, anemia (patient may be normochromic).
✧ May be a previous history of celiac disease, previously controlled, with symptoms returning usually in the fifth to seventh decades.

Examination
✧ Perform a general examination. Examination may be normal or there may be evidence of weight-loss and anemia.
✧ Examine all lymph node sites and examine the abdomen for hepatosplenomegaly. An abdominal mass may be present.

Investigations
✧ ESR is increased and hypoproteinemia may be present. Perform complete blood count (CBC) to detect raised WBC.
✧ Most cases are diagnosed on imaging. Occasionally, laparoscopy and biopsy provides the diagnosis. Endoscopy can achieve a diagnosis when the lesion is accessible.
✧ Immunoproliferative small intestinal disease (IPSID) diagnosed by abnormal alpha chain on immunohistochemistry of tumor sections.
✧ Fluoroscopic contrast studies can be used to assess intestinal involvement. Capsule endoscopy may also assist with diagnosis and assessing intestinal involvement. CT can assess intestinal involvement and assess for extra-intestinal disease.

Treatment
The role of surgery has decreased over time. Surgery can be required for palliation or abdominal emergencies, and may be indicated for local to regional disease. Chemotherapy is usually the mainstay of treatment.

The histology is important in determining the optimal treatment approach.

Follow-up
Intervals are short (1–4 weeks) until diagnosis is obtained.

Post-operative Follow-up
Review with histology and consult with oncologists. Complete the grading and staging procedure. Detect early complications related to laparotomy and small bowel resection.

Gastrointestinal Stromal Tumors
Background
Gastrointestinal stromal tumor (GIST) was previously classified as leiomyoma and leiomyosarcoma.

History
Most common in the 60- to 70-year age group. They can present with bleeding, abdominal pain, anemia, or weight loss. Many are found incidentally. Sixty percent are gastric and 40% in the small bowel; rare elsewhere.

Examination
Most commonly, there is no detectable abnormality. Some patients may have a palpable mass.

Investigations
Cross-sectional imaging such as CT or MRI. Endoscopy with endoscopic ultrasound and fine needle aspiration can be considered if accessible.

Treatment
Segmental surgical excision for local disease. Unresectable or metastatic disease responds to tyrosine kinase inhibitors (imatinib). Adjuvant imatinib can be considered to increase disease-free survival in those at high risk of relapse.

Post-operative Follow-up
Review with histology to confirm diagnosis and adequate resection. Thereafter, follow-up is long-term to detect recurrence.

Chronic Infective/Inflammatory Conditions of the Small Bowel
Yersinia
Yersinia is one of the most common and clinically important infections. In the acute phase the differential diagnosis includes *Salmonella* and *Campylobacter*, which also may become chronic infections.

History and Examination
Acute infections are self-limiting. Chronic infections in children may simulate Crohn's disease. There is a swollen terminal ileum and colon exhibiting ulcerated, nodular, and cobblestone change.

Investigations
✧ Diagnosis is by recovery of organism from stool.
✧ *Yersinia* also causes a pseudoappendicitis syndrome in older children and adults.
✧ SBE may show typical Crohn's type changes.
✧ At operation, terminal ileum and lymph nodes are inflamed and edematous. Lymph nodes are sent for culture.

Treatment
The infection usually resolves and never progresses to Crohn's.

Intestinal Tuberculosis
Intestinal tuberculosis (TB) occurs in four macroscopic forms: hypertrophic, ulcerative, fibrotic and ulcerofibrotic.
✧ *Hypertrophic* – thickening of terminal ileum and colon. There is recent subacute obstruction, pain, vomiting.
✧ *Ulcerative* – terminal ileum has deep ulcers which may reach the serosa and perforate. There is subacute obstruction and pain, vomiting, and constipation.
✧ *Fibrotic* – terminal ileum, cecum, and ascending colon. Shortening and narrowing of segments.

History

✧ Take a general small bowel history.
✧ Mainly occurs in children and young adults.
✧ Twenty-five percent have coexisting pulmonary disease and give a history of chronic illness, malaise, anorexia, fever, night sweats, dyspepsia, weight loss.

Examination

✧ Perform a general examination. Examine for evidence of weight loss and general debility.
✧ Examine lymph node fields and the chest for evidence of systemic tuberculosis.
✧ Examine the abdomen for abdominal masses or intestinal obstruction (may be normal).

Investigations

✧ A Mantoux test may be negative. Try to culture TB from gastric washings, feces and peritoneal fluid and lymph node biopsy.
✧ Abdominal X-rays may show extensive calcification.
✧ Barium studies show the above changes according to the type of intestinal TB, but the changes may be indistinguishable from Crohn's. Laparoscopy and sampling of peritoneal fluid may be required for diagnosis.

Treatment

✧ In the absence of obstruction or perforation, give chemotherapy for 12 months.
✧ Surgery is performed for complications and failure of medical therapy, e.g. a right hemicolectomy.

Follow-up

Follow-up should be at regular intervals, e.g. every 3 months during the first 18 months, to detect obstruction or perforation, intra-abdominal abscess formation, etc. Discharge when chemotherapy has finished and the patient has remained asymptomatic.

Actinomycosis

This is rare; diagnosis usually follows perforated appendix.

History and Examination

The patient presents some weeks after appendectomy with abscess and sinus formation and a fixed indurated mass in the right iliac fossa. It may progress to abscesses in the liver.

Investigations

CBC, microbiology of pus. CT is typically used to evaluate abscesses.

Treatment

Penicillin and lincomycin – prolonged therapy.

Follow-up

Intervals are regular until patient is off all treatment and asymptomatic.

AIDS, Opportunistic Small Bowel Infection and HIV-1 Enteropathy

These are extremely common in AIDS, mostly due to opportunistic ulceration with protozoa, bacteria, viruses, and fungi. In some 30% of cases no pathogen is identified – this is AIDS enteropathy.

History and Examination
Diarrhea, weight loss, and abdominal pain.

Investigations
Sigmoidoscopy and stool cultures.

Treatment
Bacterial infection is treated with antibiotics. Otherwise, give symptomatic treatment with loperamide.

Follow-up
Follow-up is in conjunction with a specialist AIDS clinic. Regular stool cultures and sigmoidoscopy should be carried out until the patient is asymptomatic; then discharge to the specialist AIDS clinic.

Radiation-induced Bowel Disease
Symptoms are encountered in the majority of patients during the first few weeks of radio-therapy – anorexia, nausea and vomiting, and central nervous system (CNS) effects – and they should settle.

In true radiation-induced disease, the interval may be from 2 months to 2 years after radiotherapy.

History and Examination
Vague abdominal discomfort, diarrhea, mild rectal bleeding, and passage of mucus. Intestinal obstruction may be acute, subacute or recurrent.

Investigations
Evaluation of bowel with fluoroscopic contrast studies or CT enterography, malabsorption studies, flexible sigmoidoscopy, and colonoscopy.

Treatment
◇ Treatment is conservative whenever possible, and includes correction of nutritional deficiencies.
◇ Diphenoxylate/atropine (Lomotil), sulfasalazine and steroids are given. Give predni-solone enemas (Predsol) for radiation proctitis, antibiotics for bacterial overgrowth, and bile-salt-binding agents for ileal disease.
◇ Dietary management is through elemental diets. Extensive disease can require inter-mittent or indefinite parenteral nutrition.
◇ Surgical resection is performed in localized disease. Protect anastomoses with a stoma. For fistulas and extensive disease, carry out a complete bypass and exclusion of the diseased segment – these procedures can be safer than resection.

Follow-up
Follow-up is long-term at regular intervals until patient is asymptomatic or symptoms are well controlled.

Appendicitis Follow-up
Objectives
The main objectives of the follow-up visit after surgery are the detection of post-operative complications and the exclusion of underlying pathology such as IBD or tumors of the

appendix. Always ensure that you have read the histology report before you see the patient. Complications include:

✧ Chronic wound infection.
✧ Abscess/mass in right iliac fossa.
✧ Fecal fistula.
✧ Intraperitoneal abscess formation – solitary (pelvic/subphrenic) or multiple small loop abscesses.
✧ Recurrent intestinal obstruction – late complication secondary to adhesions.
✧ Pylephlebitis (infective suppurative thrombosis of the portal vein).

Specific Complications or Conditions
✧ *Superficial chronic wound infection* which has not responded to antibiotics, may indicate a stitch sinus, which can be treated by exploration of the wound either in the clinic or as a day-case local anesthetic procedure, with the residual stitch material removed.
✧ *Deeper chronic wound infection*, or the presence of a mass or fecal fistula may indicate the presence of an underlying condition such as Crohn's, a tumor, or chronic infective inflammatory conditions.
✧ *IBD* – the histology report may describe changes suggestive of Crohn's disease. In this situation, a full assessment for Crohn's is required including SBE (*see* Crohn's disease, p. 122).
✧ *Tumors of the appendix* – these include carcinoids, adenocarcinoma, mucinous neoplasm, and lymphoma. Assess according to the relevant section.
✧ *Carcinoid* usually occurs at the tip. There is invasion of the muscularis mucosa in 30% of cases, but nodal and distal metastases are rare. Appendectomy is often curative. Right hemicolectomy is indicated for tumors >2 cm in size or for vascular or neural invasion, involvement of the base of the appendix (or mesoappendix for tumors 1–2 cm), or atypical histologic appearance (i.e. goblet cell carcinoma).
✧ *Adenocarcinoma* – is rare, and may present as acute appendicitis or intestinal obstruction. The correct treatment is right hemicolectomy.
✧ *Mucinous neoplasm* – often this is a simple mucocele, which is definitively treated with appendectomy. Low-grade mucinous adenocarcinoma is treated with a right hemicolectomy unless pseudomyxoma peritonei is present.

Chronic Appendicitis
There is some controversy as to whether this condition exists, but removal of the appendix appears to be gaining in popularity when combined with a diagnostic laparoscopy and is successful in relieving the symptoms in a number of patients.

History
✧ Episodes of recurrent right iliac fossa pain which may be severe and debilitating. Pain is often colicky in nature but the patient appears otherwise well.
✧ Take a full GI and gynecologic history. In particular, enquire about bowel habits.
✧ Consider irritable bowel syndrome – ask questions regarding symptoms in other body systems which are suggestive of this, e.g. intermittent dysphagia.

Examination
✧ Perform a general examination; this is usually normal.
✧ Examine for abdominal masses and tenderness.
✧ Perform a rectal examination and arrange for a gynecologic examination.

Investigations
✧ Routine biochemistry and hematology, plus investigations to exclude IBD and gyneco-logic disease in females.
✧ The main finding in chronic appendicitis may be that a barium enema is normal but the appendix does not fill because it is often long, fibrotic, and contains fecaliths.
✧ Diagnostic laparoscopy combined with appendectomy is an alternative to invasive radiologic investigations.

Treatment
Conservative or laparoscopic appendectomy if other pathology has been excluded.

Follow-up
Follow-up is at regular intervals determined by the severity and impact of the symptoms until serious causes are excluded. Then, give treatment for the specific disorder, discharge with advice, or proceed to laparoscopic appendectomy.

Post-operative Follow-up
Review with histology. If normal, then discharge with advice and reassurance.

Meckel's Diverticulum
This arises from the antimesenteric border of the ileum within 90 cm of the ileocaecal valve. It is a true diverticulum, i.e. it contains all three layers of bowel wall. There is ectopic tissue (gastric, pancreatic, duodenal, colonic) in 50–70% of cases. Ulceration of ectopic gastric mucosa may cause copious rectal bleeding.

History
✧ Take a general small bowel history. The majority of patients are asymptomatic, but may complain of symptoms similar to peptic ulceration but in a different abdominal site, intestinal colic, or intermittent GI bleeding or melena.
✧ Unexplained anemia may be another presentation.
✧ May present acutely as acute appendicitis or perforation.

Examination
✧ Perform a general examination.
✧ Examine for evidence of anemia and abdominal tenderness.
✧ Occasionally there may be an inflammatory mass to palpate, but examination is often normal.

Investigations
Ectopic gastric mucosa can be identified by ^{99m}Tc scan.

Treatment
✧ If there is an uninflamed Meckel's at laparotomy with a wide base and normal to palpation, leave it.
✧ If there is a narrow neck, or it is nodular, chronically inflamed or fecaliths, excise it. Symptomatic Meckel's requires excision.

Follow-up
Intervals are short until diagnosis is obtained and other causes are excluded.

Post-operative Follow-up
Review with histology and ensure that all ectopic mucosa has been excised. Check for post-operative complications associated with laparotomy and small bowel resection. Discharge once patient has recovered and is asymptomatic.

Questions and Answers

Q1   Which of the following medications can be used as the initial treatment of mild Crohn's ileitis?

    A   Azathioprine
    B   Infliximab
    C   5-ASA
    D   Methotrexate
    E   Cyclosporine.

A1   C: Although there is little evidence to support its efficacy, 5-ASA is the initial treatment choice for mild Crohn's disease. Antibiotics and steroids are often added if there is no response. Immunosuppressive agents, such as azathioprine, methotrexate, and cyclosporine, and biologic therapies, such as infliximab (a monoclonal antibody against tumor necrosis factor alpha [TNFα]) are reserved for more severe or refractory disease.

Q2   Peutz–Jeghers syndrome predominantly results in the development of which type of polyps?

    A   Adenomatous
    B   Inflammatory
    C   Hyperplastic
    D   Pseudopolyps
    E   Hamartomatous.

A2   E: Peutz–Jeghers is a syndrome characterized by the development of multiple gastrointestinal hamartomas along with characteristic mucocutaneous pigmentation.

Q3   Which of the following is true regarding Meckel's diverticuli?

    A   All Meckel's diverticuli found at laparotomy need to be excised
    B   Meckel's diverticuli are actually false diverticuli
    C   The majority of Meckel's diverticuli are symptomatic
    D   Meckel's divericuli can present acutely as a lower GI bleed, an intestinal perforation, or as a mimic of acute appendicitis
    E   It is very uncommon for Meckel's diverticuli to have ectopic tissue from other gastrointestinal sites.

A3 D: Excision of the incidentally detected Meckel's diverticulum is generally reserved for the presence of a narrow neck, nodularity, chronic inflammation, or fecaliths. Meckel's diverticuli contain all three layers of bowel wall and thus are true diverticuli. The majority of Meckel's diverticuli are asymptomatic. The most common acute presentations for Meckel's diverticuli include lower GI bleeding, intestinal perforation, or as a mimic of acute appendicitis. Ectopic tissue (often gastric, pancreatic, duodenal, or colonic mucosa) occur in 50–70% of Meckel's diverticuli.

Q4 Carcinoid syndrome is caused in large part by the secretion of which substance?
  A Serotonin
  B Somatostatin
  C Norepinephrine
  D Epinephrine
  E Gherelin.

A4 A: Inappropriate secretion of serotonin (5-hydroxytryptamine [5-HT]) and other vasoactive substances are responsible for the symptoms of carcinoid syndrome. Somatostatin inhibits the release of numerous hormones, including serotonin. Synthetic analogues of somatostatin, such as octreotide, can be used in the treatment of carcinoid syndrome.

Q5 Which of the following is true regarding diagnostic modalities for the small intestine?
  A The Prometheus test is valuable in the work-up for carcinoid tumors
  B Capsule endoscopy is recommended for the work-up of motility disorders
  C The hydrogen breath test is useful in evaluating intestinal permeability
  D Selective splanchnic angiography may be useful for diagnosis of mesenteric ischemia
  E Compared with conventional CT scans, CT enterography has limited assessment of the mucosa and the bowel wall.

A5 D: The Prometheus test panel is a commercially available serologic panel of antibodies (including pANCA/ANCA, ASCA IgA, ASCA IgG, and anti-OMP-C IgA) that has been proposed to help confirm the diagnosis of IBD, differentiate between Crohn's disease and ulcerative colitis, and possibly to assess disease severity. Capsule endscopy is not recommended in the setting of motility disorders or mechanical obstruction, as this may result in the failure of the device to pass through the intestinal tract. The hydrogen breath test can be used for the work-up of small bowel transit time and bacterial overgrowth. This test functions by measuring hydrogen in the end-expiratory air after intake of lactulose or a meal of mashed potato and beans. When the meal reaches the cecum, bacterial fermentation occurs and results in increased breath hydrogen. Mesenteric angiography is the gold-standard diagnostic study for acute arterial ischemia but its use is limited by the invasive nature of the procedure. CT enterography is a specially protocoled CT scan that uses large volumes of ingested enteric contrast material to improve the assessment of the mucosa and the bowel wall.

The Spleen and Lymph Nodes

Clinton D. Protack and David T. Efron

SEVEN

The Spleen

The spleen has important hematologic and immunologic functions. However, the main involvement of the surgeon is to remove the spleen. One of the commonest indications for removal of the spleen is trauma, which seldom presents to the outpatient setting. However, patients return to the surgical clinic following splenectomy and it is important to have an appreciation of the implications of the long-term management of the asplenic patient.

In particular, many trauma patients are young, fit individuals who had an otherwise healthy spleen removed so no other clinical specialties (e.g. hematology) will have been involved. Splenectomy is also performed as an intentional part of resection for other pathologies, e.g. carcinoma of the stomach. In this instance, as well as managing the primary condition the effects of splenectomy must also be considered. The spleen may also be removed during operations on the pancreas or, less commonly, as part of the treatment of portal hypertension.

In other situations the patient will be referred from another specialty for consideration of splenectomy because the spleen itself is diseased or involved in a disease process, or is adversely affecting hematologic function.

In the commonest diseases to affect the spleen, enlargement occurs (splenomegaly) and a common result of this enlargement is that the spleen becomes overactive (hypersplenism). The commonest clinical features of a diseased spleen are splenomegaly and an abnormal blood film result. Key to understanding these disease processes and the effects of splenectomy is an understanding of the normal function of the spleen and the effect of an overactive or underactive spleen.

Hematologic Function

The spleen removes fragmented, damaged or senescent red blood cells (culling), and mature red blood cells (target cells have high membrane to intracellular hemoglobin [Hb] levels). It removes intra-erythrocytic inclusions (pitting), e.g. Howell–Jolly bodies (nuclear remnants), siderotic granules (hemosiderin), and Heinz bodies (aggregates of denatured Hb). It also removes irregular-shaped red blood cells (acanthocytes, irregular crenated cells, and target forms). All of these appear in the bloodstream after splenectomy. Within the spleen's volume is a large number of sequestered platelets.

Following splenectomy there is a transient thrombocytosis. There is no hematopoiesis after fetal life unless the bone marrow becomes diseased, e.g. myelofibrosis. There is storage of iron and factor VIII.

Immunologic Function

The spleen is involved in antibody production and cell-mediated responses. It is important in phagocytosis, maturation of lymphoid cells, and plays a significant role in lymphopoiesis.

Clinical Manifestations of Splenic Disorders

Most common disorders cause pathologic destruction or pooling of blood elements. Splenic enlargement, as occurs with venous thrombosis and congestion, causes entrapment and pooling resulting in destruction of normal cells.

Hypersplenism

Hypersplenism is splenomegaly plus decreased numbers of circulating blood elements (anemia, leukopenia, and/or thrombocytopenia). This is different from "work hypertrophy," where the spleen enlarges due to constant exposure of the spleen's phagocytic mechanism to abnormal cells. Hypersplenism leads to a decreased number of normal cells. If the bone marrow cannot compensate, the patient becomes anemic.

Splenomegaly

Causes of splenomegaly are as follows.
1. *Infections*:
    ∝ Acute (mononucleosis, septicemia)
    ∝ Subacute (bacterial endocarditis, tuberculosis [TB], brucellosis)
    ∝ Chronic (fungal diseases, syphilis, bacterial endocarditis).
2. *Congestive in a setting of portal hypertension* due to:
    ∝ Cirrhosis of all causes
    ∝ Prehepatic portal hypertension
    ∝ Posthepatic portal hypertension
    ∝ Segmental portal hypertension, usually due to splenic vein occlusion as a result of inflammation (post severe pancreatitis) or tumor.
3. *Hematologic*:
    ∝ Hemolytic disorders
    ∝ Myeloproliferative (myeloid metaplasia, polycythemia vera, essential thrombocythemia)
    ∝ Miscellaneous (megaloblastic anemia).
4. *Malignant*:
    ∝ Hematologic (acute or chronic leukemias, lymphomas, etc.)
    ∝ Intrinsic malignancies (primary – lymphosarcoma, plasmacytoma, fibrosarcoma; secondary – carcinoma, melanoma; benign – hamartoma).
5. *Inflammatory or granulomatous*: Felty's, systemic lupus erythematosus (SLE), rheumatoid arthritis.
6. *Storage*: Gaucher's, Wilson's.
7. *Miscellaneous*: Cysts – parasitic and non-parasitic. Other causes include amyloid, hyperthyroidism.

Hyposplenism

The causes of hyposplenism include:
1. Splenectomy.
2. Splenic agenesis.
3. Atrophy – celiac disease, dermatitis herpetiformis, sickle cell anemia, thrombocytopenia, SLE.

Assessment of Splenic Disorders

The main purpose of the assessment is to determine whether the spleen is enlarged because of a primary disorder or because it is involved in a generalized disease process. Therefore, assessment may also involve a hematologic investigation, investigation of hepatobiliary disease and portal hypertension (ultrasound and esophago-gastro-duodenoscopy [EGD]), and investigation of the causes of lymphadenopathy (lymph node biopsy).

Splenic History

The patient may be asymptomatic with regard to the spleen, or be referred from another specialty with the diagnosis already made, or be referred from the primary care physician (PCP) because of detection of an abdominal mass. Occasionally, if the spleen is very large the patient may complain of a heaviness in the left subcostal region, especially on exercise. The patient may complain of weakness, tiredness, or lethargy due to anemia, or complain of hemorrhage or the appearance of skin purpura or ecchymoses related to other hematologic abnormalities.

Further questioning is directed at differentiating the common causes of splenomegaly as outlined above. Remember to ask about other diseases, family history, drug history, and travel abroad.

Splenic Examination

✧ Perform a general examination, looking for any of the causes of splenic enlargement.
✧ Look for evidence of hematologic abnormalities, e.g. purpura, ecchymosis, lymphadenopathy, signs of liver disease, and portal hypertension.
✧ Examine the abdomen. Differentiate splenic from renal enlargement and other abdominal masses, e.g. stomach, colon. Features of an enlarged spleen are that the examiner's hand cannot get above it, it has a notched anterior border, enlarges toward the right iliac fossa and there is usually an absence of bowel gas in front of it (unlike kidney). With a renal mass the kidney moves downward on respiration and organ shapes are different.
✧ Examine for liver enlargement and the presence of ascites.
✧ Rarely, auscultation may reveal a rub when there is a splenic infarct.

Investigation of Splenic Disorders
Laboratory Investigations

✧ *Hematology*: Complete blood count (CBC) provides information on the number of blood cells circulating and the presence of abnormal cell types (as described above). Hypersplenism results in anemia, leukopenia and/or thrombocytopenia. Hyposplenism results in abnormal red blood cells (Burr cells, target cells, pitted cells), red-cell inclusions (Howell–Jolly bodies, siderotic granules), abnormal platelet morphology, thrombocytosis, leukocytosis (neutrophilia, lymphocytosis, monocytosis).
✧ *Tests of clotting, hemolysis, and bone marrow aspiration/biopsy* are part of the hematology work-up. Refer if initial blood results indicate a possible hematologic disorder.
✧ *Biochemistry*: Liver function tests (LFTs) – which include a clotting profile – may indicate underlying liver disease.
✧ *Immunology*: Autoantibodies – as a cause of hemolytic anemia. Investigation of rheumatoid arthritis, Felty's syndrome, and SLE.
✧ *Lymph node biopsy*: Investigation of lymphadenopathy associated with splenomegaly.

Imaging Techniques

✧ *Abdominal X-ray (AXR)*: May show an enlarged soft-tissue shadow or calcification in the spleen which may represent old infarcts, hydatid cyst, or TB.
✧ *Ultrasound*: First-line investigation to differentiate splenic from renal enlargement. Good for detecting all forms or splenic enlargement, e.g. splenic cysts. Also can detect other disease processes, e.g. portal hypertension, ascites, liver enlargement.
✧ *Computed tomography*: May give better visualization of the spleen than ultrasound, especially in the presence of ascites or obesity. Particularly useful for the detection of intra-abdominal lymphadenopathy. However, it is expensive and involves the use of radiation.

✧ *Magnetic resonance imaging (MRI)*: May give better visualization of the spleen and additional definition of tissues. It is expensive and time-consuming, and there is often limited availability.
✧ *Radio-isotopes*: Colloid labeled with technetium-99m colloid can be injected into the patient and scanned by a gamma camera to detect the position and size of the spleen, or to detect accessory spleens. A sample of the patient's own red blood cells are heat-damaged and then labeled with ^{51}chromium, or platelets are labeled with ^{111}indium, and re-injected. Scans with a gamma camera are performed after hours to days to provide information about the sequestration of these elements in the spleen. This provides quantifiable information on the activity of the spleen. It uses radioactivity, albeit in small doses, and is becoming less common.

Indications for Splenectomy
✧ *Definite*:
  ∝ Neoplasms of spleen (primary, lymphomas, benign)
  ∝ Splenic abscess (not small septic emboli)
  ∝ Echinococcal cysts
  ∝ Splenic vein thrombosis with segmental hypertension and resulting gastric varices
  ∝ Splenic artery aneurysm (asymptomatic splenic artery aneurysm <1.5 cm in diameter can be observed – rupture is common during pregnancy)
  ∝ En bloc resection of adjacent neoplasm
  ∝ Non-salvageable splenic injury.
✧ *Desirable*:
  ∝ Hereditary spherocytosis
  ∝ Idiopathic thrombocytopenia purpura
  ∝ Autoimune hemolytic anemia
  ∝ Genetic defects of red cells, e.g. pyruvate kinase deficiency
  ∝ Gastroesophageal devascularization procedures for esophageal varices (Sugiura operation).
✧ *Debatable*:
  ∝ Small splenic cyst – may be observed if less than 5 cm in diameter
  ∝ Small pseudocyst
  ∝ Thalassemia syndromes
  ∝ Lymphoma and specific cytopenia or pancytopenia
  ∝ Thrombotic thrombocytopenia purpura
  ∝ Myeloproliferative disorders.

Pre-operative Preparation
✧ Check CBC, clotting, and liver enzymes.

Platelet transfusion may be needed intra-operatively to correct thrombocytopenia (platelets are not usually given until the spleen has been devascularized, as otherwise they will simply disappear into the spleen and be ineffective – discuss with hematology).
✧ If thrombocytopenia is due to immune disease, do not give platelet infusion; instead, give human immunoglobulin G (IgG) to increase platelets.
✧ Correct coagulopathies with fresh frozen plasma or cryoprecipitate.

Post-operative Follow-up
Following splenectomy, patients are reviewed 6 weeks after leaving hospital. They are at specific risk of sepsis due to capsulated bacteria and require appropriate prophylaxis.

Ideally, *Haemophilus influenzae* type b (HIB), meningococcal (Meningovax), and pneumococcal (Pneumovax) vaccinations should be given prior to surgery, but if not given pre-operatively they may be given postsplenectomy once the patient is stable. Patients under the age of 2 years should also receive antibiotic prophylaxis (usually with penicillin/amoxycillin, or erythromycin in sensitive patients) until the age of 6 years. Additionally, patients should be advised to have annual flu vaccinations and take advice about additional prophylaxis if traveling to malarial areas. They should be advised to seek early medical advice should they become unwell. Most hospitals will now have a written protocol and patient advice sheet.

✧ *Early complications* – bleeding, left subphrenic collection. Immediately following splenectomy, thrombocytosis is common with an increased risk of thrombotic events. The platelet count should be monitored daily and will usually rise for a number of days before falling back to normal values. In addition to standard thrombo-embolic prophylaxis, if the platelet count increases to more than 10^6 platelets per microliter of blood, give an anti-platelet agent such as low-dose aspirin. Necrosis of the greater curve of the stomach due to poor surgical technique is a rare complication which may lead to subphrenic abscess and/or fistula. Trauma to the tail of the pancreas leads to subphrenic fluid collections, abscess, or pancreatic fistula. Diagnose by ultrasound or CT and treat by percutaneous drainage under imaging.

✧ *Late complications* – migrating thrombophlebitis or deep venous thrombosis (DVT) caused by thrombocytosis may occur and needs long-term anticoagulant therapy. There may be recurrence of presenting symptoms caused by retained accessory spleen – image with radiolabeled nuclear scan and plan curative surgical resection.

Remember to educate patients regarding overwhelming postsplenectomy infection (OPSI), and meningococcal, pneumococcal, and *H. influenzae* vaccination; make sure they have an advice sheet. Consider possible role of a "Medic Alert" bracelet.

Postsplenectomy Sepsis
Increased risk and incidence of postsplenectomy sepsis is related to the indication for splenectomy – trauma has a low risk with an incidence of 1–2%, while thalassemia has an incidence of 25%. *Streptococcus pneumoniae* is responsible for over half of all septic episodes; *Escherichia coli*, *H. influenzae* and *Neisseria meningitidis* for most of the rest. The mechanism responsible is thought to be impaired filtration, decreased phagocytosis, decreased IgM levels, and loss of opsonic tetrapeptide tuftsin.

Overwhelming Postsplenectomy Infection
This life-threatening disorder is a constant threat in patients who have had a splenectomy, and constant vigilance on the part of the patient and the surgeon is required if effective treatment is to be started in time.

History and Examination
This is an insidious, viral-like illness leading to high fevers, nausea and vomiting, dehydration, hypotension, and collapse.

Investigation
Gram stain of peripheral blood smears.

Treatment
Admit for intravenous antibiotics and fluids.

✧ *Prognosis* – mortality is 50–80%. Often a postmortem shows bilateral adrenal hemorrhage.
✧ *Prevention* – pneumococcal vaccine covers 90% of pneumococcal variants but leaves 10% uncovered. Vaccination should precede splenectomy by 10–14 days; not all patients convert, but those that do should have elevated pneumococcal antibodies for 42 months. However, no form of prophylaxis is completely effective – therefore close surveillance is necessary together with specific patient education to seek medical attention at the first signs of infection. The key to successful management is awareness of the risk of OPSI, and aggressive treatment.

Specific Disorders of the Spleen
Splenic Infarction
Apart from sickle cell anemia, this most commonly occurs with congestive disease, chronic myeloid leukemia (CML), and myelosclerosis, but can also occur as a result of arterial emboli (rare) or as a complication of severe acute pancreatitis.

History
Take a general splenic history. There may be sudden onset left-sided abdominal and loin pain. Infarction causes a capsular reaction irritating the left hemidiaphragm, leading to left basal pleurisy with or without rub and pain to the left shoulder. Pain may be worse on inspiration.

Examination
Perform a general examination. The patient may be in pain. Examine the chest for signs of a left basal rub or effusion. There may be tenderness in the left side of the abdomen and loin.

Investigations
Ultrasound may be useful to exclude other pathologies. CT with contrast is diagnostic.

Treatment
Appropriate analgesia; splenectomy is reserved for severe cases or diagnostic confusion.

Follow-up
Monitor for development of hyposplenism, but management of underlying condition will usually take precedence. Discharge if stable after follow-up and underlying condition resolves.

Post-operative Follow-up
As for splenectomy.

Splenic Abscess
A splenic abscess is a complication of severe sepsis, bacterial endocarditis, leukemia, diabetes, or prematurity. Multiple abscesses are often fatal.

History
Take a general splenic history. This may be non-specific – fever, pain with or without left upper quadrant (LUQ) tenderness.

Examination
Perform a general examination. Splenomegaly occurs in less than 50% of cases.

Investigations
Chest X-ray (CXR) shows left pleural effusion; ultrasound shows immobile diaphragm.

Treatment
Ultrasound-guided percutaneous drainage or splenectomy. A rupture is fatal.

Follow-up
If the patient recovers from the acute episode, monitor for development of hyposplenism. Discharge when stable.

Post-operative Follow-up
As for splenectomy.

Splenic Cysts
Most are post-traumatic – true cysts are rare and include hemangioma, lymphangioma, parasitic, epidermoid, and dermoid. They may occasionally rupture or become infected.

History
Symptoms are mostly size-related, but patients are usually asymptomatic.

Examination
Look for a mass in the LUQ.

Investigation
Ultrasound can identify cysts. Use CT with contrast if doubts exist.

Treatment
If small and asymptomatic, observe or perform laparoscopic deroofing. Splenectomy is performed for large or symptomatic cysts or any complications.

Follow-up
Monitor for development of complications or enlargement of cysts. Discharge when stable.

Post-operative Follow-up
As for splenectomy.

Splenic Vein Thrombosis
This follows acute pancreatitis or may arise in chronic pancreatitis or pancreatic tumor. Isolated splenic vein thrombosis (without portal vein thrombosis) results in splenomegaly and segmental portal hypertension (predominantly with gastric varices; esophageal varices are present but are less prominent). Portal venous pressure is normal. Varices are often missed on endoscopy.

History and Examination
Patients may present with massive gastrointestinal (GI) hemorrhage. Suspect in cases of GI bleeding with history of previous pancreatitis – look for splenic vein thrombosis.

Investigations
Endoscopy, duplex ultrasound, and selective visceral angiography. MRI is better.

Treatment
The condition is cured by splenectomy.

Post-operative Follow-up
As for splenectomy.

Splenosis
There is a need to differentiate splenosis and accessory spleens.
✧ Accessory spleens are found at the hilum of the spleen and omentum, number fewer than 10, and have hilar vessels with normal splenic architecture.
✧ Implantation splenosis tend to number greater than 20, there is a history of trauma, they are scattered over the peritoneum, and do not have a coordinated circulation.

Treatment
Neither condition needs therapy unless it is causing recurrent disease.

Gaucher Disease
This is a hereditary lipid storage disease. Clinical signs are hypersplenism and massive splenomegaly.
Treatment is splenectomy for symptoms and complications of hypersplenism.

Disorders Affecting the Spleen and Lymph Nodes
Disorders affecting both the spleen and the lymph nodes can be considered in three main groups:
1. *Immunologic reactivity* – non-specific, granulomatous (caseating, non-caseating).
2. *Neoplasia* (mainly non-Hodgkin's and Hodgkin's lymphoma).
3. *Primary hematologic disorders* – myeloid leukemia, myelosclerosis and polycythemia rubra vera.

History
✧ Take a general splenic history. Ask questions regarding each of the causes of splenomegaly. Ask about foreign travel.
✧ If there is a history of prior pancreatitis or abdominal pain, exclude a splenic vein thrombosis.
✧ If there is pruritus, exclude polycythemia vera and other myeloproliferative disorders.

Examination
✧ Perform a general examination.
✧ A LUQ mass may be present; a spleen auscultation may reveal a rub. With a renal mass, the kidney moves downward on respiration, organ shapes are different, and there is usually colonic resonance in front of kidney.
✧ Search for lymphadenopathy, including posterior pharynx.
✧ Look for purpura or bruising.

Investigation
✧ Peripheral blood film and bone marrow.
✧ CBC and serology for infective causes. Mononucleosis shows atypical lymphocytes on blood film, positive Paul Bunnell test, and raised Epstein–Barr virus titer.
✧ If there is a positive history for travel, then perform blood smears for malaria or bone marrow for Leishman–Donovan bodies.

✧ If exposure history is questionable, test for TB.
✧ Ultrasound scan or CT.
✧ Splenic vessels – duplex, dynamic CT or selective angiography.

Splenic function – injection of labeled platelets.

Disorders of the Lymph Nodes

Palpable lymph nodes should be considered diseased until proven otherwise. Always remember that in addition to hematologic disorders and infection, a lymph node may be the first sign of metastatic carcinoma at a yet undetermined site. This is particularly important in the neck, where node biopsy should not be performed without an appropriate ear, nose, and throat (ENT) examination – such a biopsy may preclude potentially curative ENT surgical excision and block dissection of diseased lymph nodes.

Localized Lymphadenopathy
✧ *Acute infections* – usually subside.
✧ *Chronic infections*:
    ∝ Lymphadenopathy without signs of inflammation, e.g. cat scratch fever
    ∝ Single tender node – primary bovine TB
    ∝ Chronically enlarged lymph nodes matted together – syphilis, leprosy, fungal, lymphogranuloma venereum.
✧ *Occipital* – chronic scalp infection.
✧ *Posterior auricular* – rubella.
✧ *Anterior auricular* – bacterial infection of eyelids or conjunctiva.
✧ *Axillary* – distal upper limb infection, occasionally lymphoma or Hodgkin's.
✧ *Neck* – most common site for lymphomas.
✧ *Painless epitrochlear* – childhood viral illnesses, secondary syphilis, or TB.
✧ *Mediastinal hilar* – not noticeably enlarged with bacterial pneumonia, mainly TB (unilateral hilar lymphadenopathy). Infectious mononucleosis may cause mediastinal lymphadenopathy for several months. The most common cause of persistent mediastinal lymphadenopathy is malignant disease and sarcoidosis.
✧ *Intra-abdominal or retro-peritoneal* – lymphadenopathy is uncommonly inflammatory.

Generalized Lymphadenopathy
Noticeable lymph-node enlargement in more than one drainage site is most commonly viral, e.g. mononucleosis, viral hepatitis, influenza, cytomegalovirus, rubella, and other causes such as syphilis, TB, salmonella, and toxoplasmosis. However, malignant causes should always be excluded.

Malignant Conditions of Lymph Nodes
Metastatic carcinomas rarely produce a generalized lymphadenopathy – they present more often as a group of nodes adjacent to the primary tumor site. Hodgkin's and non-Hodgkin's lymphomas commonly present with superficial lymph-node enlargement.

Hodgkin's Lymphoma
Found mostly in men, presenting with a group of painlessly enlarged anterior cervical lymph nodes. Axillary is the first site in 20% of cases; mediastinal or inguinal in 15%.

History
Fevers, pruritus, malaise, weight loss, anorexia, sweats. Asymptomatic is classed as A; symptomatic as B.

Examination
Painless enlarged lymph nodes. Hepatosplenomagaly appears late.

Investigation
Lymph node biopsy (excisional) and bone marrow aspirate. A team approach is essential. Staging laparotomy has now been replaced by high-quality cross-sectional imaging.

Staging
Hodgkin's is classified into Stages I–IV. Staging is based on history and examination findings, CXR and AXR, and CT of the chest and abdomen.
Stage I: single lymph node region or single extralymphatic site.
Stage II: Two or more lymph node regions on the same side of the diaphragm, or one lymph node region and a contiguous extralymphatic site.
Stage III: lymph node regions on both sides of the diaphragm.
Stage IV: disseminated involvement of extralymphatic organs.

Treatment
- ✧ Hodgkin's I and II – wide-field radiotherapy.
- ✧ IIIa – radiotherapy and/or chemotherapy.
- ✧ IIIb and IV – multi-agent chemotherapy.

Follow-up
Follow-up is under a hematologist/oncologist.

Non-Hodgkin's Lymphoma
Patients may present with painless enlargement of one or more superficial lymph nodes. Extranodal disease may be present. Biopsy should be assessed with multiple immuno-stains to accurately define cellular type and direct treatment.

Staging
Staging depends on results of node biopsy, bone marrow biopsy, and cross-sectional imaging.

Treatment
Localized disease is commonly managed with radiotherapy. More advanced disease is managed with various chemotherapy regimens, including monoclonal antilymphocyte preparations such as rituximab.

Tumors of the Peritoneum
These tumors are mainly secondary and include pseudomyxoma peritonei. Primary mesothelioma may occur, but is rare.

Pseudomyxoma Peritonei
The peritoneum is filled with yellow/browm mucoid substances caused by the presence of a well-differentiated pseudomucinous cystadenoma/carcinoma. The most common primary is the ovary, then the appendix, uterus, bowel, and urachus. The primary tumor is often slow-growing and rarely metastasizes or invades adjacent viscera.

History
Patients complain of increasing abdominal distension or present acutely with abdominal pain, peritonitis, or intestinal obstruction.

Examination
Perform a general examination. The main finding is abdominal distension.

Investigation
Diagnostic peritoneal tap and biopsy.

Treatment
Aggressive surgical evacuation, resection of primary tumor. This is followed by systemic chemotherapy including cisplatin. Radiotherapy is ineffective.

Prognosis is guarded, but long-term survival can occur. One useful prognostic factor appears to be the number of cells in the mucus. There is a poor correlation between histology of the primary and survival. Management following diagnosis is usually in a regional or supra-regional specialist center.

Follow-up
Follow-up is long-term to detect deterioration and provide symptomatic support.

Peritoneal Mesothelioma
This carries a poor prognosis of 8–12 months' survival. There are two main types – *diffuse malignant* (the majority) and *fibrotic benign* (rare; can be cured by surgical excision). Among malignant tumors, the only treatable lesions are stage I tumors confined to one hemithorax or peritoneum.

History
Patients present with anorexia, ascites, and intestinal obstruction. There is fever and weight loss.

Investigations
Paracentesis and laparoscopy and peritoneal biopsy.

Treatment
Stage I – surgical resection and radiotherapy and chemotherapy (systemic and intraperitoneal).

Follow-up
Follow-up is long term to detect deterioration and provide symptomatic support.

Desmoid Tumors (of the Abdominal Wall)
These are slow-growing, well-circumscribed hard tumors which involve fascial and muscle layers; they recur after local excision (10–20%). They may be associated with Gardner's syndrome.

Treatment
Treatment is surgical, wide local excision.

Follow-up
Follow-up is long-term to detect recurrence, or discharge with advice to PCP to continue follow-up.

Questions and Answers

Q1   Which of the following are not associated causes of splenomegaly?
   A   Portal hypertension.
   B   Bacterial endocarditis.
   C   Wilson's disease.
   D   KRAS mutation.
   E   Acute myelogenous leukemia.

A1   D: All of the above are associated with splenomegaly except for KRAS mutation, which is associated with gastric cancer.

Q2   All of the following are indications for splenectomy except:
   A   A 2 cm splenic cyst.
   B   Splenic abscess.
   C   Splenic vein thrombosis with resultant gastric varices.
   D   Echinococcal cysts.

A2   A: Splenic systs less than 5 cm may be observed and do not require splenectomy.

Q3   The risk of postsplenectomy sepsis for a patient undergoing splenectomy due to traumatic rupture is:
   A   100%.
   B   50–75%.
   C   25–40%.
   D   10–20%.
   E   1–2%.

A3   E: The rate of postsplenectomy sepsis after traumatic rupture is 1–2%.

Q4   Gaucher disease is associated with abnormal accumulation of:
   A   Protein.
   B   Nucleic acids.
   C   Lipids.
   D   Zymogens.

A4   C: Gaucher disease is a hereditary lipid storage disease.

Q5   The majority pathogen of postsplenectomy sepsis is:
   A   *Haemophilus influenzae.*
   B   *Streptococcus pneumoniae.*
   C   *Escherichia coli.*
   D   *Neisseria meningitides.*

A5   B: *S. pneumoniae* is responsible for over half of all postsplenectomy sepsis events.

Liver, Biliary System, and Pancreas

Kenneth R. Ziegler and Seth A. Spector

Potential Consultations
✧ Right upper quadrant (RUQ) pain.
✧ Jaundice.
✧ RUQ/epigastric mass/hepatomegaly.
✧ Liver tumors/metastases.
✧ Post-cholecystectomy.
✧ Post-pancreatitis.
✧ Pancreatic tumors.
✧ Rare hepatopancreaticobiliary disorders.

Introduction
Disorders of the liver, pancreas, biliary system, and spleen are considered separately in this chapter. However, it is important to appreciate that these systems are closely inter-related, and may present with similar clinical features. For example, a patient may be jaundiced due to a primary liver disorder such as cirrhosis, a biliary pathology such as choledocholithiasis, or obstruction of the extrahepatic bile duct by a pancreatic neoplasm. Conversely, each of these diagnoses can, in turn, cause secondary biliary cirrhosis if not corrected. When a patient presents with jaundice, one of the initial tasks is to elucidate the primary disorder, and then determine the effect this diagnostic entity has had on the function of the liver, the pancreas, and the biliary system.

Assessment of Liver Disorders
Liver Disease
The most common presenting clinical features of liver disease are jaundice and the stigmata of liver failure. As the assessment and management of liver disease is complex, it is useful to review an overview of the consultation objectives.

Objectives
Confirm that the signs and symptoms of liver disease are present.
1. *Determine the cause*: history, physical examination, urine and serum chemistries, serology, imaging, and histology.
2. *Detect the clinical consequences of liver disease*: history, physical examination, urine chemistry, serology, imaging, endoscopy, and Child–Pugh Score (detailed later in this chapter).
   ∝ Encephalopathy
   ∝ Ascites
   ∝ Portal hypertension
         i hypersplenism
         ii gastrointestinal bleeding – varices (esophageal, gastric, rectal)
         iii ascites
   ∝ Jaundice
   ∝ Clotting defects
   ∝ Hepatorenal failure.
3. *Treat the underlying cause* of the liver disease which may lead to improvement in the clinical consequences of liver disease.

4. *Treat the clinical consequences*:
   - ∝ Measures to reduce encephalopathy
   - ∝ Treat ascites
   - ∝ Portal hypertension – treat the consequences of portal hypertension
        i hypersplenism: splenectomy if surgery for portal shunt considered
        ii varices: injection sclerotherapy, fibrin glue, transjugular intrahepatic portosystemic shunt (TIPS), surgical shunt
        iii ascites: medical management, paracentesis, peritoneovenous shunt
   - ∝ Jaundice: symptomatic therapy, relieve obstruction if present
   - ∝ Clotting defect: correct with vitamin K, fresh frozen plasma
   - ∝ Hepatorenal failure: treat underlying liver condition and provide renal support.

Liver History

Begin by taking a general gastrointestinal (GI) history; when responses indicate a possible liver problem, focus on a more detailed liver history. This includes questions about general symptoms, etiologic factors, and symptoms related to the clinical consequences of liver disease.

General symptoms that may indicate liver disease include jaundice, fatigue, malaise, headache, myalgia, arthralgia, and fever. To determine the etiology of the liver disease, ask about excessive or chronic alcohol ingestion, drug use (therapeutic or recreational), occupation, pets, foreign travel, contact with jaundiced individuals, family history of jaundice or liver problems, recent anesthetic exposure, recent surgery or blood transfusions, ingestion of raw shellfish or wild mushrooms, and sexual contacts.

The clinical consequences of liver disease include:
- ✧ *Encephalopathy* – a range of reversible neuropsychiatric states ranging from confusion and forgetfulness to coma.
- ✧ *Ascites* – the presence of intra-abdominal fluid.
- ✧ *Portal hypertension (varices)* – which may be asymptomatic or present with end stage complications of hematemesis (vomiting of bright red blood) or melena.
- ✧ *Jaundice* – patients may simply report that they have turned yellow; one should inquire about pale stools, dark urine, and pruritus, and determine if the jaundice is painless or associated with RUQ or epigastric abdominal pain.
- ✧ *Clotting defects* – spontaneous bleeding, easy bruising.
- ✧ *Hepatorenal failure* – increasing lethargy, nausea, edema.

Liver Examination

Always perform a general physical examination, then, focus the examination on general signs of liver disease, etiologic signs, and signs associated with the clinical consequences of hepatic insufficiency.

Liver disease commonly presents with jaundice. However, other signs may also be present: palmar erythema, digital clubbing, leukonychia, bruising, asterixis, spider nevi, gynecomastia, muscle wasting, evidence of pruritis, ascites, caput medusa, hepatosplenomegaly, testicular atrophy, loss of axillary and pubic hair. Suspicion of hepatomegaly may arise due to extention of dullness past the costal margin; this sign may reflect actual enlargement or may reflect caudal displacement from an overinflated lung. Hepatic enlargement may be focal or generalized, smooth or irregular. Liver tenderness may be elicited by palpation or percussion through the rib cage. Etiology may be indicated by the smell of alcohol, the presence of tattoos, or evidence of intravenous drug use (e.g. track marks, puncture wounds in the antecubital fossa).

Signs of clinical consequences include:

✧ *Encephalopathy* – diminished performance on cognitive function tests, mental status exams, asterixis, overall decreased level of consciousness. *Peripheral neuropathy* may reflect the effect of liver failure on the peripheral nervous system.

✧ *Ascites* – abdominal distension; auscultation reveals flank dullness in supine position and shifting dullness, eversion of the umbilicus if umbilical hernia present.

✧ *Portal hypertension* – dilated periumbilical veins (caput medusa is a late sign), anemia, ascites, splenomegaly, hepatosplenomegaly, internal hemorrhoids.

✧ *Jaundice* – yellow skin, yellow conjunctiva, yellow oral mucosa, pale stool on rectal examination, dark urine.

✧ *Clotting dysfunction* – evidence of bruising.

✧ *Hepatorenal failure* – edema, decreased urine output, uremia.

Examination of Liver Disorders
Diagnostic Tests
Urinalysis

✧ *Technique* – dipstick urinalysis. Numerous dipsticks are available which can test for a variety of substances in a fresh specimen of urine, including conjugated bilirubin. Generally, the presence of conjugated bilirubin in the urine indicates obstructive jaundice, although this finding can also reflect the presence of some conditions associated with excess bilirubin production.

✧ *Results* – dipsticks are read and compared against a reference chart.

✧ *Advantages* – a quick and easy method that can be performed in the clinic.

✧ *Disadvantages* – limited information is derived from this test.

Blood Tests
Examination of the blood plays an integral role in the diagnosis of liver disorders. The most common tests to aid these pathologies are described below.

Serum Biochemistry
1. *Released integral membrane enzymes* – reflect hepatocellular damage.
   ∝ *Alanine transaminase (ALT or SGPT), aspartate aminotransferase (AST or SGOT):* Minor increases in level occur in cholestasis and chronic liver disease; major increases are associated with acute hepatitis or with liver cell necrosis of any cause.
   ∝ *Alkaline phosphatase (ALP):* immunoassay can differentiate between liver, biliary tract, bone, intestine, kidney, and placenta sources of ALP. Cholestasis and obstructive jaundice are associated with an increased alkaline phosphatase level.
   ∝ *Gamma-glutamyl-transpeptidase (GGT):* Elevation of GGT levels, especially isolated elevation or a disproportionate rise compared with liver transaminases, is particularly associated with alcoholic liver disease. Increased levels are also associated with obstructive jaundice from any cause. Secondary tumor deposits cause a rise in ALP and GGT, as well as a small rise in bilirubin; these can vary depending on the burden of underlying disease.
2. *Serum protein changes* – hypoalbuminemia often occurs in liver disease. Altered albumin : globulin ratio may occur in the presence of a normal albumin, e.g. increased immunoglobulin G (IgG) in cirrhosis and chronic active hepatitis. Primary biliary cirrhosis is associated with increased IgM and antimitochondrial antibody.
3. *Tumor markers*
   ∝ *Alpha-fetoprotein (AFP):* The most commonly used tumor marker for hepatocellular carcinoma (HCC). It may also be raised in pregnancy, germ cell tumors, and chronic liver disease. A normal AFP level does not rule out HCC.

∝ *Des-gamma carboxyprothrombin (DCP)*: Increased in 90% of primary hepato-cellular carcinoma (>300 ng/ml = primary HCC). Small increases in level with other disorders. Levels decrease or are eliminated after curative resection or chemotherapy. Interestingly, there is little correlation between DCP and AFP.

∝ *Human chorionic gonadotropin, beta subunit (beta-hCG)*.

∝ *Carcinoembryonic antigen (CEA)*.

4. *Electrolytes, blood urea nitrogen (BUN), creatinine* – may show generalized electro-lyte abnormalities, particularly hyponatremia and hypoglycemia. Evidence of raised urea and creatinine levels may indicate impaired renal function associated with liver disease (hepatorenal syndrome).

Hematology

✧ *Complete blood count (CBC)* – may reveal anemia of chronic disease or indicate blood loss from GI bleeding. Other abnormalities may be detected, such as hemolytic ane-mia, leukemia, and lymphoma. Thrombocytopenia can suggest hypersplenism in this setting.

✧ *Coagulation tests* – international normalized ratio (INR) may be abnormal in liver disease due to the defective production of clotting factors.

Immunology

Hepatitis serology is routine screening in liver disease for hepatitis A, B, and C. Also screen for autoimmune disease and primary biliary cirrhosis (antimitochondrial antibody).

Imaging
Ultrasound

✧ *Technique* – an acoustic water-based gel is applied to and an ultrasound probe manipu-lated over the abdomen by the sonographer. High-frequency sound waves enter tissues and are disparately reflected from structures of different composition. The reflected waves are detected and used to construct representative images of the underlying tissues.

✧ *Results* – written report compiled by radiologist or sonographer. May be accompanied by a selection of ultrasound photographs.

✧ *Advantages* – ultrasound is a very good non-invasive technique for visualizing the liver parenchyma and can detect small (1 cm) focal lesions. These lesions may include liver cysts and abscesses, as well as primary and secondary liver tumors. Liver cirrhosis is suggested by areas of increased and irregular attenuation. The intrahepatic and extra-hepatic bile ducts, in addition to the gall bladder, are well visualized; dilatation and stones can be detected. Using color duplex detection modes, blood flow in the portal vein can be identified and the diameter measured, giving an estimation of the presence of portal hypertension. Ultrasound-guided biopsy can be performed.

✧ *Disadvantages* – accuracy is operator-dependent. Ultrasound is less reliable in obese or gaseous patients. It is less reliable than computed tomography (CT) for defining vascular or cystic lesions such as hemangiomas, but can be used to follow these lesions once CT has established the diagnosis.

Computed Tomography

✧ *Technique* – X-rays are used to obtain multiple cross-sectional slices of the patient which are then reconstructed by a computer to produce the images. Intravenous con-trast can be given to outline the vessels and focal lesions within the liver and multiple scans can be performed to give non-contrast, arterial, venous, and delayed phases of scanning (triple phase liver scan). Oral contrast agents can be given to outline the stomach and duodenum. Modern multi-slice spiral CT scans can be performed within seconds using thin slices, yielding higher detail and allowing more sophisticated reconstructions. See also *CT angioportography* and *Lipiodol CT* below.

✧ *Results* – CT images with reconstructions, and written interpretation by radiologist. It may also be useful to review the images with the radiologist.

✧ *Advantages* – when used with intravenous (IV) contrast, CT is more sensitive than ultrasound at determining the nature of lesions within the liver. CT is especially useful in differentiating between small tumors, cysts, or abscesses. CT guided biopsies can be performed. CT is invaluable in planning liver resections.

✧ *Disadvantages* – uses ionizing radiation. IV contrast can be allergenic, and can induce acute kidney damage. Technique can be expensive and time-consuming. Certain lesions such as hepatic adenomas or focal nodular hyperplasia may be difficult to differentiate on CT.

Liver Scintiscan

✧ *Technique* – uses isotopes technetium-99m, gallium-67 citrate or indium-113. The isotopes are injected intravenously and concentrated in liver lesions. Excess uptake is detected by a gamma camera.

✧ *Results* – written report and selection of images.

✧ *Advantages* – technetium-99m is taken up by the reticuloendothelial system and can detect lesions larger than 2 cm in about 66% of cases. Gallium-67 citrate is concentrated in neoplastic lesions and abscesses. Indium-113 is concentrated in hemangiomas.

✧ *Disadvantages* – utilizes radioactivity. Other techniques usually provide the same information without associated risks.

Magnetic Resonance Imaging (MRI)

✧ *Technique* – the patient is placed into the MRI scanner, which detects minute quantities of energy released by hydrogen ions when forced to change direction by a strong magnetic field.

✧ *Advantages* – provides detailed information regarding liver parenchyma disease, especially for certain types of cirrhosis, e.g. hemochromatosis, Wilson's disease, and primary biliary cirrhosis. Magnetic resonance cholangiopancreatography (MRCP) is very useful for non-invasive imaging of the biliary tree. MRI is very useful as an adjunct to other imaging modalities to further characterize liver lesions. Recent advances include liver-specific MR contrast agents. MRI does not utilize ionizing radiation.

✧ *Disadvantages* – expensive, time-consuming. The experience is often described as unpleasant; the scanner tube is known to induce anxiety in claustrophobic patients, as the tube is narrow and noisy. Gadolium contrast dye is associated with nephrosclerosis.

Angiography/Venography, Hepatic Wedge Pressure and Venography, Portography

✧ *Technique* – these invasive techniques to visualize the hepatic vasculature are being less commonly used. Contacting a radiologist directly to discuss the indications is recommended.

   ∝ *Portography*: The spleen is punctured percutaneously through an intercostal space and contrast is injected to outline the splenic and portal veins and measure the portal venous pressure. A transhepatic route may also be used.

   ∝ *Hepatic Wedge Pressure and Venography*: A catheter is passed from the brachial vein or internal jugular vein through the superior vena cava into the hepatic veins until wedged, at which point the wedge pressure is measured;

under certain circumstances this is representative of the portal venous pressure. Injection of contrast can demonstrate the presence of thrombus or occlusion, e.g. Budd–Chiari.

∝ *Angiography/Venography*: The celiac and superior mesenteric arteries can be selectively catheterized. The arterial supply of the liver can be visualized and the venous phase can demonstrate the portal system. Selective angiography can be combined with CT scanning for the technique *CT angioportography* – contrast is delivered into the splenic artery or superior mesenteric artery (SMA) and enhances the liver via the portal venous blood. Liver tumors are supplied almost exclusively by hepatic artery blood and are therefore visualized as non-enhancing lesions. Another variation is *Lipiodol CT*: iodized poppy seed oil injected via angiography of the hepatic artery is retained for long periods by hepatocellular carcinoma, causing dense enhancement of these lesions on subsequent CT scan (usually two weeks later).

✧ *Results* – a written report by the radiologist and a selection of images.
✧ *Advantages* – provides direct measurements and images of the portal system. Selective arteriography is useful in planning resection of liver tumors.
✧ *Disadvantages* – invasive and associated with complications. Much of this information can be obtained by less invasive means, e.g. duplex ultrasound, MRI angiography, spiral CT.

Liver Needle Biopsy
✧ *Technique* – this biopsy can be performed on an inpatient basis, or it may be scheduled as an outpatient/same-day case in selected patients.
  ∝ Indications for liver biopsy include alcoholic liver disease, cholestatic jaundice without dilatation of the bile ducts on ultrasound, unexplained hepatomegaly, drug-induced liver disease, and unexplained focal lesions of the liver (after consultation with a liver surgeon). The procedure may require blood products to be given if the INR and platelet count are not normal.
  ∝ The patient is placed supine with the right arm abducted. A lateral intercostal approach is used; if a focal mass is apparent, it is approached directly, usually under ultrasound guidance. The liver is percussed, with the borders marked on the skin. Local anesthetic is infiltrated and a small incision is made in the skin. The patient is instructed to hold respiration at maximal expiration and the needle is inserted, the sample taken, and the needle removed. The patient can then resume respiration, and the sample is placed whole into fixation fluid.
✧ *Results* – written report from the histopathologist.
✧ *Advantages* – provides a tissue core for histologic diagnosis.
✧ *Disadvantages* – complications include hemorrhage, intrahepatic hematoma, pleurisy, arteriovenous fistula and biliary peritonitis. If there is any suspicion of a pnemothorax, an urgent plain film of the chest should be obtained and a chest tube placed if identified; if tension pneumothorax is suspected, do not wait for a chest film prior to intervention.

Exploratory Laparoscopy
✧ *Technique* – this procedure is a much more invasive method to visualize the liver and possibly obtain biopsies. A general anesthetic is required. The laparoscope is through an umbilical approach; additional ports may be created if necessary. The technique can be adapted to obtain an intra-operative liver biopsy, ultrasound, and/ or cholangiography.

✧ *Results* – direct visualization by the operating surgeon, operative note dictating the main intra-operative findings. Histology report if any biopsies were obtained.
✧ *Advantages* – hemostasis after biopsy. In experienced hands, ultrasound applied directly to the liver is another mechanism in detecting abnormalities.
✧ *Disadvantages* – invasive, requires a general anesthetic which can be very detrimental to these patients. Expensive and can be time-consuming. Risks and benefits must be carefully balanced. In patients with significant cirrhosis, ultrasound is not a very good method to assess the liver, even intra-operatively.

The Clinical Consequences of Liver Disease
Assessment of Hepatic Dysfunction
Clinical management options in liver disease depend on an objective assessment of the degree of end-organ impairment. One such assessment is Pugh's modification of Child's Scoring for hepatic dysfunction (Table 8.1). A worse prognosis is associated with a higher score.

Hepatic Encephalopathy
A spectrum of syndromes exists:
1. Acute (fulminant) liver failure.
2. Cirrhotic patients with a precipitant.
3. Chronic portal-systemic encephalopathy.

Grades are:
I – mild confusion.
II – drowsiness.
III – somnolent, but rousable.
IV – coma.

Causes are: acute liver failure from any cause, exacerbation of chronic disease by precipitants such as GI hemorrhage, infection, drugs, hypokalemic alkalosis, diuretic therapy, sedation, sepsis, and portosystemic surgical shunting.

History
✧ Presence of chronic liver disease.
✧ Symptoms of intellectual impairment.
✧ History of recent GI hemorrhage, diuretic therapy, or other causes of encephalopathy.

TABLE 8.1   Pugh's modification of Child's Score for hepatic dysfunction

	1	2	3
Encephalopathy	None	1-2	3-4
Ascites	Absent	Slight	Moderate
Albumin g/L	35	28-35	<28
Prothrombin time (sec prolonged)	<3	4-10	>10
Bilirubin (micromol/L)	<34	35-51	>51
Grade A (good) = 5-6, Grade B (moderate) = 7-9, Grade C (poor) = 10+			

Physical Examination

Decreased level of consciousness and abnormalities on cognitive testing. Apraxia. Asterixis. Hyperactive stretch reflexes.

Treatment

✧ Address underlying cause (e.g. cessation of sedatives), stop hemorrhage, give phosphate enema, and treat infection.
✧ The effect of GI hemorrhage is reduced by purgation with magnesium sulfate.
✧ Bacterial production of protein metabolites within the bowel is reduced using neomycin, metronidazole, and lactulose.
✧ Protein-restricted diet may be advised (questionable efficacy).
✧ Lactulose is often used as chronic therapy.

Chronic Treatment

Decreased protein diet but not less than 40 g/day. Severe encephalopathy after insertion of surgical shunts is treated by radiologic blocking of the shunt.

Follow-up

Follow-up is long-term at regular intervals (1–3 months) with frequent assessment for the presence of sub-clinical encephalopathy.

Portal Hypertension

Obstruction of portal venous flow results in increased pressure in the splanchnic venous circulation. Normal portal vein pressure is 5–10 mmHg, with a flow velocity around 1.5 L/min. Portal hypertension occurs when the pressure in the portal venous system exceeds 20 cmH$_2$O or 12 mmHg. Causes of obstruction, by level, include:

1. *Proximal to liver* – extrahepatic compression of the portal vein, or thrombosis of portal, mesenteric or splenic veins. Twenty-five percent of patients with portal hypertension will have an extrahepatic blockage, and a significant proportion of these patients will have underlying liver disease or polycythemia. Chronic pancreaticobiliary disease or a pancreatic neoplasm may precipitate portal vein thrombosis.
2. *Within the liver* – compression of portal venous radicles by disease. This obstruction is most commonly sinusoidal and results from cirrhosis of the liver. In cirrhosis, portal hypertension is due to both obstruction and increased splanchnic blood flow secondary to elevated levels of endogenous vasodilators, e.g. glucagon, and decreased sensitivity to vasoconstrictors. Pre-sinusoidal obstruction can develop in schistosomiasis.
3. *Distal to liver flow* – obstruction to venous outflow, usually due to thrombosis of the hepatic veins (Budd–Chiari syndrome). Causes of thrombosis include the use of oral contraceptive in women, ingestion of Bush teas, congenital diaphragm of the vena cava, or congestive right heart failure. These patients rarely present with bleeding, but have intractable ascites, painful hepatomegaly, and rapidly deteriorating liver function.

Obstruction of portal venous flow results in enlargement of portosystemic communications and increases the risk of bleeding from esophageal and gastric varices. Bleeding from varices usually occurs when portal hypertension exceeds 30 cm H$_2$O; however, only 50% of varices ever bleed, and only 15–40% of patients with chronic liver disease develop portal hypertension.

Clinical Features of Portal Hypertension
Three clinical disorders can be attributed to portal hypertension:
1. Hypersplenism.
2. Gastrointestinal bleeding.
3. Ascites.

Clinical Objectives
Detect portal hypertension, determine the cause of portal hypertension, detect the disorders associated with portal hypertension, treat portal hypertension, treat the effects of portal hypertension.

Hypersplenism
Increased pressure in the splenic vein due to portal hypertension causes the spleen to enlarge (splenomegaly). Enlargement of the spleen causes increased sequestration of blood elements, resulting in hemolytic anemia, leukopenia, and thrombocytopenia. These blood abnormalities seldom cause major symptoms, but may be debilitating. After portal decompression, hypersplenism may remain; therefore, pancytopenia in patients requiring portal decompression may be an indication for concurrent splenectomy.

Gastrointestinal Hemorrhage
The main causes of hemorrhage are esophageal varices and gastric fundus varices. Colonic and rectal varices are detectable, but seldom cause hemorrhage. After the initial diagnosis of varices, 30% of patients bleed within 2 years; a smaller proportion bleed each year after that.

Increased risk of bleeding is associated with the following endoscopic characteristics: size – graded from I (small) up to III, cherry red spots, overlying varices, red whale markings, blue varices (as opposed to white). Grade I varices may be reversible with improvement of the liver condition; other grades do not regress.

History
Presentation varies with severity of bleed, from signs and symptoms of anemia to massive hematemesis, or a herald bleed (e.g. a mouthful of bright red blood, melena).

Physical Examination
There may be stigmata of chronic liver disease.

Diagnostics and Imaging
The primary imaging modality is endoscopy performed by an operator experienced in dealing with variceal hemorrhage. CBC may reveal anemia; massive acute bleeding often is not reflected as abnormalities in an initial CBC. Coagulation testing may detect a raised INR. Liver function tests (LFTs) may be abnormal. Blood urea may be elevated.

Treatment
The initial management of acute variceal bleeding is resuscitation and the institution of measures to decrease encephalopathy. Mechanisms to control hemorrhage include drug therapy such as somatostatin, to lower transhepatic venous gradient, or other vasoactive drugs like terlipressin. Pentagastrin induces contraction of the lower esophageal sphincter, as does metaclopramide. Physical measures include balloon tamponade (Blakemore–Sengstaken tube), followed by endoscopy and sclerotherapy, banding, or fibrin glue. If these measures fail to arrest the bleeding, a transjugular intrahepatic portosystemic shunt

(TIPS) procedure should be considered. Surgical correction can be an option, but the procedure carries significant mortality in the acute setting.

After the bleeding has stopped, management is aimed at preventing recurrent bleeding by treating the underlying liver condition, treating the varices and reducing the portal hypertension.

✧ *Endoscopic sclerotherapy* – sclerotherapy (ethanolamine oleate, 3% tetradecyl sulphate or absolute alcohol) is repeated every 3 weeks until all the varices are obliterated.
  ∝ Complications of sclerotherapy: esophageal ulceration, perforation, stricture, acute respiratory distress syndrome (ARDS), mediastinitis, bacteremia (10%), anaphylaxis (especially with ethanolamine), pneumatosis intestinalis, pneumoperitoneum, and portal vein thrombosis (up to 36% of all patients; use with caution in good risk Child's A patients who may later require a shunt operation or liver transplant).
  ∝ Recurrence of esophageal varices after initial obliteration by sclerotherapy occurs in about 60% of patients. Failed sclerotherapy is managed by esophageal transection or shunt procedure.
✧ *Endoscopic banding* – rubber-band treatment to ensnare the varices produces results as effective as sclerotherapy.
✧ *TIPS* – a transjugular intrahepatic portosystemic shunt can be considered for suitable patients without extrahepatic venous thrombosis in persistent bleeding. Access is obtained by cannulating the internal jugular vein and advancing the catheter to the middle hepatic vein. A needle is then passed from the hepatic venous system to the portal venous system, which is replaced by an expanding metal stent placed over a wire.
  ∝ Complications of TIPS: Hemorrhage, stent dislodgement or occlusion, infection and shunt encephalopathy.
✧ *Surgical treatment* – indications include patients who continue to bleed (therapeutic failure) or those with recurrent bleeding. Bleeding often progresses a patient from Child's grade A/B to C. Portosystemic shunting in the emergency setting carries a prohibitive mortality; esophageal transection is generally performed instead. In the elective situation, two groups of patients are considered suitable for surgery:
  ∝ Bleeding arrested and good liver function (Child's grade A/B), with no effective method for prevention of further bleeding – portosystemic shunting is the first and best option, and esophageal transection with devascularization (the Sugiura procedure) can be considered if shunts are not successful.
  ∝ End-stage liver disease (Child's C), controlled by sclerotherapy. Consider for transplantation. In patients considered for hepatic transplantation, surgery should be avoided, but TIPS has been successfully employed to achieve portal decompression and avoid further bleeding.

Liver transplant should be considered in all patients with variceal bleeding and good liver function but whose quality of life is poor.

Follow-up
Review every 3 weeks until all varices are obliterated. Look for other signs of liver dysfunction and syndromes associated with portal hypertension. Detect complications of sclerotherapy.

Estimate the Child's Score and formulate a plan for definitive management. Follow-up endoscopy every 6–12 months is recommended. Beta-blockade should be considered. If rebleeding occurs after successful obliteration of varices, a shunt procedure or esophageal transection procedure should be considered. Consider liver transplantation for suitable candidates.

Ascites

Clinically detectable when volume exceeds one litre.

Causes of ascites include:

✧ *Infection*: Tuberculosis (TB), peritonitis.
✧ *Inflammation*: Crohn's, starch peritonitis.
✧ *Hypoproteinemia*: Nephrotic syndrome, liver disease, protein-losing enteropathy.
✧ *Lymphatic obstruction*: TB, filariasis, lymphoma, metastatic carcinoma, Milroy's disease, rupture/damage of abdominal lymphatics.
✧ *Increased lymph flow/pressure*: Cirrhosis, congestive heart failure, constrictive pericarditis, Budd–Chiari syndrome.
✧ *Neoplasms*: Primary and secondary tumors of the peritoneal cavity.
✧ *Chronic pancreatitis*: Pancreatic ascites (caused by disruption of the pancreatic duct).

Differential diagnosis – Large ovarian cysts, pancreatic pseudocysts, mesenteric cysts, hydramnios, and acute gastric dilatation.

Intractable ascites is seen in advanced chronic liver disease, Budd–Chiari syndrome, and in patients with peritoneal carcinomatosis. These patients cease to respond to diuretic therapy and develop pre-renal azotemia. Pericardial effusions occur in 60% of alcoholic cirrhotics.

Objectives

Determine etiology, treat underlying disorder, treat ascites.

History

Obtain general history, focusing on liver complaints. Patients may report increasing abdominal girth and fullness. They may also complain of leg swelling or difficulty breathing due to loss of excusion of the diaphragm. Ask about symptoms associated with each of the causes outlined above.

Physical Examination

✧ Perform a general examination.
✧ Early signs include dullness in the flanks in the supine position; shifting dullness and a fluid thrill may be elicited. Later, ascites may produce a tense, distended abdomen with grossly elevated intra-abdominal pressure, causing venous congestion and lower limb edema.
✧ Respiratory distress may occur due to splinting of the diaphragm.
✧ Umbilical hernias are not uncommon.
✧ Look for signs associated with each of the causes outlined above.

Diagnostics and Imaging

✧ Ultrasound to confirm presence of ascites.
✧ Diagnostic paracentesis: take off 20–50 mL and send samples of fluid for biochemistry, cytology, culture and sensitivity, and TB culture.
✧ Determine serum–ascitic fluid albumin ratio. Gradients less than 11 g/L are present in patients without portal hypertension. Gradients greater than 11 g/L are associated with portal hypertension. This ratio helps to distinguish high protein transudates in patients with portal hypertension from true exudates (e.g. TB and peritoneal carcinomatosis).

✧ Percutaneous peritoneal biopsy under CT guidance.
✧ Laparoscopy is useful for uncertain cases. It is often complicated by leaking ascites through the incisions and possibility of contamination of the ascites.

Ascitic fluid can be described as *serous, pseudochylous, bloodstained* (often malignant) and *myxomatous*. Chylous ascites fluid has a milky appearance and a high fat content on analysis. When chylous ascites arises spontaneously, it may indicate lymphatic obstruction by lymphoma or nodal deposits from carcinoma.

Treatment
Sodium restriction, spironolactone diuretic (note: loop diuretics increase the risk of encephalopathy, especially in the presence of subclinical renal impairment). The aim is for a gradual loss of fluid of about 3 kg/week.
   If this fails or patients become oliguric:
✧ Therapeutic paracentesis with intravenous 5% albumin infused over 2 hours with 50 mg of furosemide and 250 mL of 20% mannitol over 20–30 minutes. If diuresis is not established, peritoneovenous shunting is indicated.
✧ Peritoneovenous shunting – effective in decreasing hospital stay, increases muscle mass and provides adequate long-term control in patients with ascites and good liver function (Child's A and B). Ineffective and increases mortality in patients with advanced disease.

Contraindications to peritoneovenous shunting include encephalopathy, uncorrectable bleeding diathesis, renal failure due to primary renal disease, recent variceal hemorrhage, and cardiac failure. Risks of these types of shunts include disseminated intravenous coagulation (DIC). The standard shunt is a prosthetic shunt with a one-way valve. Patients are trained to use incentive spirometers throughout the day to maintain flow in the shunt.

Follow-up
Follow-up is long-term at regular intervals (1–3 months) to detect complications, which include blockage of the shunt and the development of DIC (most commonly occurs just after shunt insertion).

Renal Disease and Hepatorenal Failure
Hepatorenal syndrome is characterized by the development of renal failure in patients with severe liver disease without underlying renal disease. Diagnosis is dependent on a low glomerular filtration rate, absence of shock, ongoing sepsis, fluid loss, or hemorrhage; no improvement despite adequate plasma volume and diuretic withdrawal; proteinuria less than 500 mg/day and no evidence of renal tract obstruction. There are two types:
✧ Type 1 is rapidly progressive – less than 2 weeks in duration, with doubling of the initial creatinine, and is associated with a mortality of 80% at two weeks.
✧ Type 2 satisfies the criteria for diagnosis but is not rapidly progressive.

Hepatorenal syndrome does not usually respond to dialysis. Best treatment is to improve underlying liver function.

Jaundice
Jaundice is recognized when serum bilirubin exceeds 40 μmol/L. Underlying mechanisms include excess bilirubin production, impaired uptake by the hepatocytes, failure of conjugation, impaired secretion of conjugated bilirubin into bile canaliculi, impairment of bile

TABLE 8.2   Types of jaundice

Type	Mechanism
Hepatocellular	Defective secretion of conjugated bilirubin into the bile canaliculi
Cholestatic intrahepatic/extrahepatic	Impairment of bile flow subsequent to the secretion into the bile canaliculi
Hemolytic	Excess bilirubin production
Benign congenital hyperbilirubinemia	Defective bilirubin uptake, conjugation, or secretion defect

flow subsequent to the secretion by the hepatocytes (cholestatic or obstructive). Causes include hemolysis, liver disease, adverse drug reactions, and biliary tract obstruction (intrahepatic or extrahepatic). Types are shown in Table 8.2.

Hepatocellular Jaundice
✧ *Acute* – viral hepatitis, liver cell necrosis, acute alcoholic hepatitis.
✧ *Chronic* – chronic active hepatitis; cirrhosis – alcoholic, cryptogenic, primary biliary.

Characterized by increased transaminases on LFTs. If alcoholic, GGT is also elevated.

Cholestatic Jaundice
✧ *Intrahepatic* – functional (drugs, hepatitis), organic (obstruction of intrahepatic biliary tree).
✧ *Extrahepatic* – e.g. duct stones, pancreaticobiliary cancer.

Characterized by (1) conjugated hyperbilirubinemia; (2) increased alkaline phosphatase, GGT, and 5-nucleotidase – 5-nucleotidase is the most reliable indicator, as its levels are not influenced by bone disease and not induced by alcohol; (3) minor or no elevation of transaminases; (4) bilirubin in the urine (which is tea-colored); (5) elevation of serum cholesterol and bile acid levels.

Hemolytic Jaundice
Unconjugated hyperbilirubinemia results from hemolysis. Unconjugated bilirubin is not water-soluble, and is therefore carried in the blood bound to albumin. Increased unconjugated bilirubin leads to increased production of conjugated bilirubin, and this leads eventually to increased urobilinogen and urobilin in urine. Thus, prolonged and recurrent hemolysis may produce a cholestatic component.

Causes of hemolysis include structural abnormalities of red cells and increased red cell destruction.

Assessment of the Jaundiced Patient
Objectives
Diagnose jaundice, diagnose underlying cause, treat jaundice, treat complications of jaundice, treat the underlying cause.

History
Obtain a general history focused on liver and abdominal complaints. Inquire about drug intake (legal and illicit), injection with hypodermic needles (legal and illicit), alcohol abuse, recent anesthetics, transfusion of blood and blood products, contact with jaundiced individuals, family history, sexual contacts, travel to hepatitis-endemic areas, ingestion of raw shellfish and wild mushrooms. Ask about the color of urine, stools, pruritis, and previous surgical procedures.

Physical Examination

✧ Perform a general examination.

✧ Look for evidence of jaundice (e.g. yellow sclera) and evidence of parenchymal liver disease.

✧ Examine for palmar erythema, spider nevi, bruising, splenomegaly, hepatomegaly or decreased liver size, fluid retention (ascites and edema), muscle wasting, digital clubbing, leukonychia, enlargement of parotid gland, gynecomastia, and testicular atrophy.

✧ Scratch marks are commonly seen due to pruritis from bile acid deposits in the skin.

✧ Check for lack of coordination, neurologic signs: hyperreflexia, apraxia, altered sleep rhythm, confusion, asterixis, stupor, and fetor hepaticus.

✧ Examine the patient for evidence of malignancy: recent weight loss, enlarged left-sided supraclavicular lymph nodes, an enlarged nodular liver, palpable gall bladder (Courvoisier's sign), palpable intra-abdominal masses (epigastric, iliac fossa), new and rapid onset of ascites, rectal neoplasm on digital rectal exam (DRE).

Diagnostics and Imaging

✧ Cholestatic jaundice is characterized by dark and frothy urine (tea-colored) and pale stools (clay-colored). Bilirubin will be found in the urine. Serum alkaline phosphatase and GGT are elevated. Transaminases are slightly elevated, usually less than 400 iu/mL (400 iu/mL virtually excludes significant hepatocellular damage).

✧ Check hepatitis A, B and C status in all jaundiced patients.

✧ Ultrasound is good at locating bile duct dilatation, differentiating intrahepatic and extrahepatic etiology of jaundice, identifying stones, and demonstrating the level of obstruction. Further investigation into the nature of the obstruction involves cross-sectional imaging (CT or MRI) and a cholangiogram (MRCP, endoscopic retrograde cholangiopancreatography [ERCP] or percutaneous transhepatic cholangiography [PTC]). (For details of the ERCP and PTC techniques, see p. 181).

Intrahepatic cholestasis requires further investigation with liver biopsy for histology and serum auto-antibody screen (antimitochondrial, anti-smooth muscle and immunoglobulin titers). Liver biopsy can be performed (if clotting normal) percutaneously with ultrasound guidance, or during diagnostic laparoscopy. If liver biopsy suggests bile duct obstruction despite a non-dilated duct, visualization of the biliary tract is best achieved by ERCP.

Treatment

Treat the specific cause of the jaundice, treat the general effects of jaundice prior to any radiologic/surgical intervention.

General Management of Jaundice

Pre-operative management is aimed to minimize the incidence of complications associated with prolonged or severe cholestasis, including: infection (cholangitis, septicemia, wound infections), disorders of the coagulation, renal failure, liver failure, fluid and electrolyte abnormalities. Delayed wound healing is associated with malignancy rather than jaundice alone.

✧ *Correct disorders of nutrition*: Oral dietary supplements are preferred to intravenous supplements to control gut bacteria. Some centers advocate the oral administration of bile salts, and more recently lactulose, to reduce the intestinal absorption of endotoxin from intestinal microflora, thus minimizing the incidence of renal failure following surgical intervention. There are suggestions that probiotics may help modulate intestinal microflora. Hypokalemia is frequent and should be corrected.

✧ *Prevention of infective complications*: Prophylactic antibiotics to cover high-risk patients – all jaundiced patients, patients with rigors and pyrexia, patients undergoing emergency biliary procedures/operation, elderly patients, patients with common bile duct stones, patients requiring secondary biliary interventions.

✧ *Correct disorders of coagulation*: Prolonged prothrombin time is secondary to vitamin K deficiency (subcutaneous injection of 10 mg vitamin K until deficit corrected). Poor prognosis is associated with poor response, therefore give fresh frozen plasma (FFP) just prior to surgery. Severely jaundiced patients need careful monitoring of fibrinogen levels, D-dimer level, and platelet counts to rule out DIC. Stenting will relieve jaundice and may correct coagulopathy.

✧ *Stenting*: If jaundice is severe (serum bilirubin greater than 150 μmol/L), the patient is very distressed with pruritus, there are signs of cholangitis, there is going to be an undue delay in getting to surgery, or there are signs of impending liver failure, then a period of decompression is indicated by insertion of a biliary stent via ERCP. External percutaneous transhepatic drainage (PTC) can be performed if ERCP fails, and is more likely to be needed in obstruction at the hilum. This procedure will relieve the symptoms and allow better patient comfort and compliance. This may correct coagulopathy and relieve itching.

Hepatomegaly

A patient may be referred to the surgical clinic with an enlarged liver, or hepatomegaly may be discovered on routine abdominal examination. Generally, a liver that is palpable below the costal margin is thought to be enlarged, but this is not always the case. Determine the following features:

1. *Is the liver truly enlarged?* True enlargement is suggested by liver dullness extending from the fifth intercostal space to a point below the costal margin. Apparent enlargement may occur when a liver is displaced caudally by a hyperexpanded lung, as occurs in chronic obstructive pulmonary disease, and is suggested by lower level of liver dullness.

2. *Is the enlargement focal or generalized?* Localized swellings are caused by conditions such as Reidel's lobe, hydatid cyst, amoebic abscess and primary carcinoma.

3. *Is generalized enlargement smooth or irregular?* Causes of smooth enlargement include congestive cardiac failure, cirrhosis, reticuloses, Budd–Chiari syndrome, and storage diseases. Irregular enlargement is associated with metastatic liver tumors, macronodular cirrhosis, primary liver tumors, and polycystic disease (e.g. alpha-1-antitrypsin deficiency).

4. *Is jaundice present?* Smooth enlargement associated with jaundice includes viral hepatitis, biliary tract obstruction, and cholangitis. Irregular enlargement associated with jaundice occurs with macronodular cirrhosis and multiple metastases.

Objectives

Identify cause, identify treatable causes, treat cause.

History

✧ Take a general hepatobiliary history.
✧ If jaundice is present, take a general jaundice history (as above).
✧ Establish whether there has been previous treatment for malignancy. If not, are there symptoms in other systems to suggest malignancy?

Physical Examination
✧ Determine whether true liver enlargement exists. Determine whether this is localized or generalized, smooth or irregular.
✧ Determine whether jaundice is present.
✧ Perform a general examination looking for causes of liver enlargement and evidence of liver impairment.

Diagnostics and Imaging
✧ Urinalysis, LFTs, CBC, and clotting studies.
✧ Ultrasound is often diagnostic and answers the above questions in more detail, but CT or MRI will be more specific and allow better anatomic definition.
✧ Liver biopsy may be indicated in cirrhosis and tumors (after consultation with a liver surgeon).

Treatment
Treatment is according to the specific condition diagnosed.

Follow-up
Intervals should be short (1–2 weeks) until diagnosis is established and malignancy excluded.

Liver Cirrhosis
Cirrhosis is the end result of liver cell death by any cause. Three morphologic types are described:
1. Micronodular (alcoholic, malnutrition).
2. Macronodular.
3. Mixed.

Cirrhosis has two major clinical consequences: hepatocellular failure and portal hypertension.

Objectives
Diagnose cirrhosis, detect underlying cause, detect major consequences, treat cirrhosis, treat underlying cause, treat consequences.

History
✧ Take a general liver history.
✧ Uncomplicated cirrhosis is often asymptomatic.
✧ Ask about the complications of cirrhosis, e.g. gastrointestinal hemorrhage (varices), hepatocellular failure.
✧ Ask about possible underlying causes, e.g. alcohol, drugs, hepatitis, previous biliary disorders, metabolic disorders, autoimmune disorders.

Physical Examination
✧ Perform a general examination.
✧ Examine for palmar erythema or unexplained peripheral edema, muscle wasting, ascites, jaundice, or hepatic encephalopathy.
✧ Prior to any surgical procedure in the presence of liver disease, assess the risk using Child's Score.

Diagnostics and Imaging
✧ LFTs, ultrasound, and liver biopsy are usually diagnostic.
✧ Other useful investigations include CBC, coagulation tests, serology for hepatitis A, B, and C, autoimmune disease and primary biliary cirrhosis (antimitochondrial antibody).
✧ Esophago-gastro-duodenoscopy (EGD) to detect varices is performed if indicated.

Treatment
Treatment is primarily medical, but becomes important to the surgeon if a patient with cirrhosis is to undergo a surgical procedure or requires surgical intervention for the consequences of cirrhosis (e.g. bleeding varices).

Note that a cirrhotic liver does not regenerate as a normal liver does. There is no specific medical treatment for cirrhosis. Treatment is aimed at the underlying cause and detecting and treating the consequences of cirrhosis, such as hepatocellular failure and portal hypertension (see relevant sections).

Liver transplantation should be considered in patients heading toward end-stage liver failure, provided they meet the eligibility criteria.

Follow-up
Follow-up is long-term for detection of hepatocellular failure and portal hypertension. Periodic (every 6 months) estimations of AFP and liver ultrasound should be carried out to detect the development of primary liver tumors.

Alcoholic Liver Disease
Damage varies from fatty infiltration to alcoholic hepatitis, hepatic fibrosis, and cirrhosis.

Objectives
Diagnose alcoholic liver disease, assess the severity, treat alcoholic liver disease, treat underlying cause.

History
✧ Take a general liver history. There may be general symptoms of liver disease and a history of high and/or prolonged alcohol ingestion.
✧ Inquire about symptoms suggesting the development of liver failure or portal hypertension.
✧ There may be associated symptoms of alcohol damage to other organs, such as chronic pancreatitis, cardiomyopathy, myopathy, peripheral neuropathy, and neurologic effects (e.g. Wernicke–Korsakoff syndrome).

Physical Examination
✧ Perform a general examination. The most common and earliest sign of liver disease is hepatomegaly, which may progress to a tender liver, from fatty infiltration of the parenchyma, and jaundice.
✧ Examine for evidence of liver failure or portal hypertension.

Diagnostics and Imaging
✧ LFTs may show elevated transaminases.
✧ CBC may indicate anemia and there may be a leukocytosis indicating hepatitis.
✧ Pancytopenia may indicate alcoholic marrow suppression.

✧ An elevated mean corpuscular volume (MCV) may be present, but this can also be elevated in other conditions such as vitamin B12 and folate deficiency, which may be sequelae of nutritient deficiency associated with chronic alcoholism.

✧ Clotting abnormalities may be present.

✧ If liver biopsy is performed, early disease will be represented by fatty infiltration; later cases show the classic features of micronodular cirrhosis.

✧ Elevated GGT is suggestive of the diagnosis.

Treatment

✧ Abstinence from alcohol; assistance from psychiatry and addiction medicine may be necessary.

✧ Corticosteroids may be prescribed in alcoholic hepatitis.

✧ Liver transplant can be an option for synthetic failure or the complications of liver failure if the patient can demonstrate six months of abstinence.

✧ Otherwise, treatment is as for cirrhosis.

Follow-up

Follow-up is generally managed by a gastroenterologist with a liver interest, with the involvement of a surgeon if the patient is referred for treatment of coexisting disorders or being considered for transplant. If cirrhosis is present, follow-up is the same as for cirrhosis.

Cholestatic Liver Disease

This consists of impaired bile secretion/excretion leading to conjugated hyperbilirubinemia and raised ductular enzymes. Causes include excess alcohol ingestion, viral hepatitis, and obstructive lesions of biliary tract, both intra- and extrahepatic.

Primary Biliary Cirrhosis

Intrahepatic bile ducts are progressively destroyed by an immunologic process. Patients are often asymptomatic for long periods and diagnosed incidentally on abnormal liver function tests.

History

Take a general liver history. The patient may be asymptomatic or may complain of itching, weight loss, malaise, and icterus.

Physical Examination

✧ Perform a general examination. Examination may be normal in early disease, but in later stages, the liver becomes enlarged and the development of portal hypertension leads to splenomegaly.

✧ Deposition of cholesterol in the tissue around the orbits and extensor surface of the large joints may be detected.

✧ In advanced disease, intrapulmonary shunting leads to finger clubbing.

✧ Malabsorption of fat-soluble vitamins may lead to osteoporosis.

Diagnostics and Imaging

✧ Basic metabolic panel (BMP) to detect hyponatremia. LFTs are abnormal, alkaline phosphatase is elevated.

✧ Antimitochondrial antibodies are found in all patients with primary biliary cirrhosis.

✧ IgM and smooth muscle antibody also elevated.

✧ Clotting may be abnormal.
✧ Ultrasound may not be diagnostic but helps to exclude other causes such as extrahepatic biliary obstruction, and may even detect portal hypertension.

Treatment

There is no effective medical treatment. Treat symptoms – cholestyramine for itching, ursodeoxycholate for other symptoms; this may improve the LFTs. If there is no improvement, prednisolone may be effective in decreasing fatigue and itching, and may improve LFTs. Monthly injection of fat-soluble vitamins is given.

Surgical intervention is liver transplantation before onset of hyponatremia or significant osteoporosis. Indications for surgery include decreased quality of life or bilirubin >100 mmol/L and/or portal hypertension.

Follow-up

Follow-up is long-term, for life.

Metabolic Liver Disease

Metabolic liver disease can be classified into two categories:
1. Disorders of mineral deposition.
2. Disorders associated with defective enzyme production or release.

Objectives

Diagnose metabolic liver disease, diagnose underlying cause, treat cirrhosis, treat underlying cause, treat complications of cirrhosis.

Hemochromatosis

Hemochromatosis can be either *primary* (genetic, autosomal recessive) or *secondary* (acquired due to multiple blood transfusion and polycythemia) in etiology.

Primary hemochromatosis leads to progressive iron deposition in the liver, heart, pancreas, joints, and endocrine glands with sparing of spleen, lymph nodes, and bone marrow. Hepatic accumulation leads to cirrhosis, with an increased risk of hepatocellular carcinoma.

History

History of diabetes (75%) and increasing pigmentation (bronze diabetes).

Physical Examination

✧ Dusky brown pigmentation of skin, buccal mucosa, and conjunctiva.
✧ Sequelae of cirrhosis.
✧ Polyarthropathy, hypopituitarism, and hypogonadism.

Diagnostics and Imaging

✧ Liver biopsy demonstrates hemosiderin, excessive iron in the hepatocytes and Kupffer cells, with fibrosis or macronodular cirrhosis.
✧ Serum ferritin and transferrin saturation exceeds 55%.

Treatment

Phlebotomy, decrease dietary intake of iron, iron-chelating agents and long-term follow-up.

Follow-up
Follow-up is long-term. Monitor for development of hepatocellular carcinoma.

Wilson's Disease
In Wilson's disease there is copper deposition in liver, cornea, kidneys, and the central nervous system (CNS) (basal ganglia). Liver fibrosis and cirrhosis occurs at an early age.

History
Symptoms of Wilson's disease are similar to cirrhosis. Inquire about symptoms of liver failure and portal hypertension.

Physical Examination
✧ Ocular examination reveals a Kayser–Fleischer ring of pigment in the cornea.
✧ Examine for evidence of cirrhosis, liver failure, and portal hypertension.

Diagnostics and Imaging
✧ Start with routine liver investigations: CBC, coagulation parameters, LFTs, ultrasound, and liver biopsy.
✧ Carry out copper studies: These show abnormally low ceruloplasmin levels, but this may be normal in inflammation as ceruloplasmin is an acute-phase reactant. Serum copper and serum ceruloplasmin levels are reduced and urinary copper levels are elevated in all young patients with chronic liver disease.
✧ Aminoaciduria may be present.

Treatment
Chelation therapy with penicillamine or trientine, avoid copper and zinc supplements. Liver transplant can be considered for end-stage liver disease.

Follow-up
Follow-up is long-term for the treatment of copper storage and the consequences of cirrhosis.

Cystic Fibrosis
Twenty-five percent of patients with cystic fibrosis (CF) have clinical and biochemical evidence of liver disease, including fatty change, focal biliary cirrhosis, and portal fibrosis followed by multilobar biliary cirrhosis. They may progress toward developing intrahepatic and extrahepatic strictures.

Prognosis is determined by the extent of pulmonary disease rather than liver disease, although as CF patients are living longer with improved treatment, features of liver disease may become more common.

Treatment
Treatment is long-term for the development of cirrhosis. Ursodeoxycholic acid alters bile flow and composition, leading to an increase in less toxic hydrophilic bile acids.

Liver transplant, either alone or in combination with lung transplantation, can be considered for end-stage liver disease.

Alpha-1-antitrypsin Deficiency
Lack of inhibition of neutrophil elastase leads to pulmonary and liver damage.

Treatment
There is no effective medical treatment. Plasma-derived or synthetic alpha-1-antitrypsin has been used to treat pulmonary disease.

Surgical treatment is liver transplantation and is the second most common indication for liver transplant in childhood.

Hereditary Tyrosinemia Type 1
An autosomal recessive disorder resulting in the lack of the enzyme fumaryl acetoacetate hydrolase, leading to the accumulation of the toxic products of amino acid degradation in the kidney, liver, and nervous tissues. The acute form leads to liver failure in infancy and death in the first year of life. The chronic disease manifests as renal tubular dysfunction, rickets, progressive liver disease, and the development of hepatocellular carcinoma (40%).

Treatment
Hepatic transplantation.

Hepatic Abscess
There are two primary etiologies of hepatic abscesses: (1) *pyogenic* and (2) *amoebic*.

All abscesses are more common in the right lobe, and both forms have a high incidence of right lower lung abnormalities (50%). Mortality is increased by multiple abscesses, hyperbilirubinemia, and comorbid disease.

Objectives
Diagnose abscess, diagnose cause, treat abscess.

Pyogenic Abscess
The main source of the inciting infection is the biliary system (ascending cholangitis), caused by *Escherichia coli* and anaerobic organisms. Other causes generally stem from intra-abdominal infections, including portal pyemia (e.g. from complicated diverticular disease), septicemia, direct extension from suppurating cholecystitis, penetrating peptic ulcer disease, or devitalized liver from trauma. In the frail geriatric population, liver abscesses may be insidious, presenting with non-specific systems, and may be caused by *Streptococcus milleri*.

Pyogenic abscesses can be formed from either a pocket of pus surrounded by a fibrous capsule or, if antibiotics are used early in the course, a solid woody abscess containing inflammatory cells, dying liver cells, and fibrotic tissue mimicking a neoplastic lesion.

Amoebic Abscess
This is commonly caused by *Entamoeba histolytica*. The organism, also responsible for amoebic dysentery, spreads to the liver via the portal vein after invasion from the bowel. It tends to affect younger patients.

Hepatic Candidiasis
This occurs in immunocompromized patients and complicates systemic candidiasis. It often presents with combined hepatic and splenic involvement. The organism forms target lesions (i.e. a central mass of fungus surrounded by necrotic liver cells), as visualized by CT or ultrasound. Needle biopsy is *not* performed in these cases; these lesions need an open or laparoscopic wedge excision for diagnosis and treatment.

History
✧ Pyogenic abscesses tend to present with fever, rigors, profuse sweating, anorexia, and vomiting; pain is a late symptom.
✧ Amoebic abscesses present with a low-grade fever but with more pain, which is aggravated by movement and coughing.

Physical Examination
Hepatomegaly may be a feature, and half of all patients will have diarrhea. In right lobe disease, the patient may exhibit bulging and pitting of the intercostal spaces.

Diagnostics and Imaging
✧ CBC may demonstrate anemia and leukocytosis. LFTs usually show an abnormal alkaline phosphatase; alanine transaminase may also be elevated. The ESR is raised.
✧ Amoebic abscess is diagnosed by positive serologic tests (serum complement fixation test), amoebic trophozoites in abscess fluid, and a rapid response to anti-amoebics.
✧ Ultrasound and CT scan are performed, and diagnostic aspiration under imaging control is performed if indicated. Chest X-ray (CXR) may detect lung involvement.
✧ In pyogenic abscesses with no obvious source of sepsis in the gut or biliary tree, look for an occult focus of infection elsewhere (e.g. endocarditis, dental sepsis).
✧ As with any systemic infection, obtain blood cultures before starting antibiotic therapy.

Treatment
✧ *Pyogenic abscess* – aspiration or drainage under radiologic control and appropriate antibiotics based on microbiologic samples.
✧ *Amoebic abscess* – metronidazole. If there is no improvement and the cyst is single and unilocular, percutaneous drainage may be utilized. Otherwise, surgical drainage is indicated.

Follow-up
Treatment is mainly on an inpatient basis. After percutaneous or surgical drainage, monitor by frequent ultrasound until evidence of resolution, then discharge to appropriate location with advice to return if symptoms recur. Very occasionally, a neoplasm may mimic an abscess.

Liver Cysts
Liver cysts are best thought of in two etiologic categories: *non-parasitic* or *parasitic*.

Non-parasitic Liver Cysts
These may be developmental, traumatic, dermoid, or associated with other disorders such as congenital hepatic fibrosis, hamartoma, choledochal cyst – including Caroli's disease (Type V choledochal cyst) – or polycystic disease (liver, kidneys). Non-parasitic cysts are usually detected in middle-aged women.

Objectives
Diagnose cause, treat cause.

History
Most cysts are asymptomatic until they are large enough to exert a mass effect on other structures or distended the liver capsule. Those on the superior part of the liver may be irritated by contact with the diaphragm with respiration. They often present with

non-specific symptoms of vomiting, upper abdominal pain, and occasionally diarrhea. Torsion, rupture, or hemorrhage into a cyst can produce the sudden onset pain.

Physical Examination
Most affected patients have non-tender liver swelling. Jaundice is rare.

Diagnostics and Imaging
✧ LFTs are usually normal.
✧ Ultrasound is usually diagnostic, although CT can also be used. It is important to identify cystic neoplasms (e.g. biliary cystadenoma). If in doubt, do fine needle aspiration
(FNA) of the cyst fluid under ultrasound guidance and send the fluid for cytology and
CEA level (high levels suggest a mucinous neoplasm). Ultrasound is useful in detecting
cysts in the kidneys which develop before liver cysts in polycystic disease. Occasionally
multiple cysts can be confused for metastases. If the aspirated fluid is yellow, send
for bilirubin. This is confirmation that the cyst is in continuity with the biliary tree.

Treatment
Small, asymptomatic simple cysts do not require treatment unless complications occur.
Treatment is confined to single large cysts which are treated by laparoscopic surgical
unroofing. In polycystic liver disease, treatment is confined to those patients who develop
local symptoms or portal hypertension due to compression of the portal vein. Aspiration
of cysts with instillation of fibrosing agents is almost never effective. Laparoscopic unroofing and liver resection have been advocated in specialized centers.

Follow-up
Intervals should be short until a diagnosis is achieved and neoplastic lesions are excluded.
Thereafter, small asymptomatic cysts can be followed up yearly with an ultrasound to
detect enlargement.

Post-operative Follow-up
✧ Review histology. Detect general complications of surgery, such as wound healing.
✧ Regular ultrasound can be used to detect recurrence, or can be reserved until symp-
toms recur.

Parasitic Cysts (Hydatid Cysts)
Hydatid cysts are caused by ingestion of vegetables and water contaminated (usually by
canines) with the eggs of the parasite *Echinococcus granulosus* (unilocular cyst, good
prognosis) or *Echinococcus multilocularis* (multiple cysts, poor prognosis).

History
✧ Patients are usually in otherwise good health. In patients of all ages, pain, jaundice,
and ascites are uncommon.
✧ Presentation is often a painless liver mass or the sequelae of rupture complications,
though there may be complaints of RUQ pain with capsular distention.
✧ A history of contact with dogs or sheep is common.

Physical Examination
There is a smooth, round, tense liver mass. If there is a secondary infection, there may
be hepatomegaly, rigors, and pyrexia, and deep rooted continuous pain. Jaundice is
infrequent.

Complications

✧ Intrabiliary rupture of the cyst produces biliary colic, jaundice, and fever (Raynaud's triad). Vomitus may contain hydatid cysts and membranes.

✧ Intraperitoneal rupture results in severe pain and hemodynamic instability, with urticaria and pruritus.

✧ Intrathoracic rupture is characterized by bile-stained sputum.

Diagnostics and Imaging

An abdominal plain film will reveal a calcified reticular shadow. Following intrabiliary rupture, there may be gas in the cyst. Ultrasound shows an echogenic cyst.

CBC will demonstrate eosinophilia in 25% of cases. The complement fixation test for hydatids is positive in 93% of patients. Enzyme-linked immunosorbent assay (ELISA) yields positive results in 90% of cases (i.e. 10% of patients can be false-negative). Casoni's test has been largely abandoned. LFTs are usually abnormal and may demonstrate an obstructive picture.

Treatment

✧ Cysts with extensive calcification are usually sterile and best left alone.

✧ Medical treatment consists of albendazole; 30% of cysts disappear, 30–50% show reduction, and 20–40% remain unchanged.

✧ Interventional treatment is the PAIR routine: Percutaneous fine-needle puncture, Aspiration, Injection of hypertonic saline, and Re-aspiration. This procedure is associated with a small but real risk of anaphylaxis, and a theoretical risk of peritoneal seeding.

✧ Surgical treatment consists of removing the cyst entirely (cystectomy) with removal of the germinal and laminated layers and preservation of the host-derived ectocyst. Alternately, it may be possible to enucleate the cyst, but this is not recommended due to the risk of recurrence. Cysts complicated by secondary infection require surgical drainage. Treatment by partial liver resection may be required, especially if the cysts are large and/or multiple.

✧ Remember to administer a full course of albendazole before PAIR or surgery.

Follow-up

Follow-up is at short intervals until diagnosis is achieved, then treatment is arranged.

Post-operative Follow-up

✧ Check pathology results. Detect general complications of surgery.

✧ Ascites may complicate this surgery and may indicate disseminated disease.

✧ Repeat ultrasound scans until resolution of the cyst is confirmed, then defer routine follow-up to primary care with re-referral as warranted.

Benign Solid Tumors
Hemangioma

Hemangiomas are blood-filled congenital vascular malformations comprised of endothelial cells and fibrous tissue. Symptoms are often associated with a mass effect: large hemangiomas produce capsular distention and pain, vomiting, elevation of the diaphragm, and may produce heart failure in children due to arteriovenous (AV) shunting. There may be a palpable abdominal mass which may be associated with skin lesions in 85% of cases; a bruit is audible in 15%. Rupture is rare.

Lesions are hyperechoic on ultrasound. CT with intravenous contrast is usually diagnostic; if doubt still exists, a labeled red-cell scan can be performed. MRI can be useful in confirming the disease when equivocal on other imaging modalities.

Where the diagnosis is certain and the risk of bleeding is minimal, lesions can be observed. If the lesion is large and peripherally placed, it may be suitable for surgical resection. If the lesion is difficult to differentiate from neoplastic lesions, surgical resection is indicated.

Hamartoma
These are congenital lesions comprised of normal tissues in a disorderly arrangement. They present as large liver masses in children that produce pressure effects (pain, vomiting). Complaints include an expanding abdomen with a mass.

CT is diagnostic. Treatment is by surgical excision if the diagnosis is clear. Occasionally, these lesions are sarcomatous.

Adenomas and Focal Nodular Hyperplasia
✧ *Adenomas* are variable in size (4–30 cm); 90% occur in women between the ages of 30 and 60 years. There is an association with long-term use of estrogen contraceptive pills. Thirty percent of cases progress to rupture and hemorrhage, and can be difficult to distinguish from low-grade hepatoma. There is an increased risk of rupture in pregnancy. Adenomas are premalignant.
✧ *Focal Nodular Hyperplasia (FNH)* tends to occur in the same demographic as adenoma, but is not premalignant and may be observed without serious risk. If hemorrhage occurs, successful management can be achieved through resection.

History
✧ Obtain a general liver history.
✧ The majority of patients will be women aged 30–60 years, often with a history of oral contraceptive pill (OCP) use.
✧ One third of patients will present with an abdominal mass, another third with rupture, and the last third will be referred for an incidental finding.
✧ Symptoms are commonly vague, such as upper abdominal pain and discomfort.

Physical Examination
Perform a general examination. Evidence of jaundice and anemia are rare. The liver may be focally enlarged.

Diagnostics and Imaging
✧ LFTs are usually normal.
✧ Adenomas appear solid on ultrasound and have a characteristic arteriographic appearance. FNH also has a characteristic CT appearance with the presence of a central stellate scar.
✧ Percutaneous liver biopsy for histology can be performed when the diagnosis is unclear, but adenomas can be difficult to distinguish from well-differentiated hepatocellular carcinoma.

Treatment
✧ Ruptured and bleeding lesions are considered emergencies and require excision. Hepatic arterial embolization can be useful in controlling hemorrhage. Intracapsular hemorrhage presents as an expanding mass and requires partial liver resection.

✧ FNH does not need invasive treatment once confirmed on imaging, whereas adenomas should be excised as they are premalignant.

Follow-up
✧ Patients with multiple adenomas need prolonged follow-up with repeated imaging. Female patients should be cautioned to discontinue OCPs.
✧ If diagnosis is certain, then it is acceptable to monitor lesions every 6–12 months with ultrasound. If static or diminishing in size, then operative resection may be deferred.

Post-operative Follow-up
Enlargement of residual adenomas requires elective excision.

Adenomatous Hyperplasia
These are sizeable nodules which develop in chronic liver disease. They may have premalignant potential and require long-term follow-up.

Other
Cholangioma and biliary cystadenoma are rare lesions.

Primary Malignant Tumors of the Liver
The most common primary malignant tumor of the liver is hepatocellular carcinoma (HCC); the incidence and geographical distribution of HCC parallels that of hepatitis B infection. HCC usually develops in a background of cirrhosis, but can develop in a normal liver.

Rare primary tumors include hepatocellular cholangiocarcinoma, cystadenocarcinoma, sarcoma, and angiosarcoma. Hepatocellular cholangiocarcinoma shows features of both HCC and cholangiocarcinoma, and is thought to represent a coincidental occurrence of both. Cystadenocarcinoma tends to present as a large cystic tumor in adults. Sarcoma arises from the connective tissue elements of the liver and presents as a rapidly enlarging lesion associated with hypoglycemia. Angiosarcoma is an aggressive neoplasm associated with vinyl chloride exposure or ingestion of arsenic or anabolic steroids.

In children, the most common tumors are hepatocellular carcinoma and hepatoblastoma. Hepatoblastomas tend to occur by the third year of life and produce increased levels of alpha-fetoprotein and gonadotropins, occasionally causing precocious puberty. Liver resection produces long-term survival in 30% of cases.

Hepatocellular Carcinoma
Objectives
Diagnose hepatocellular carcinoma, differentiate from other causes of liver tumors, localize and stage the tumor, determine resectability, treat tumor.

History
✧ Obtain a general history, focused on liver issues.
✧ In areas of the world that screen for hepatocellular cancer, the tumor may be detected while it is still asymptomatic. The majority of HCC are asymptomatic.
✧ These tumors can grow to be very large and cause associated symptoms such as anorexia, weight loss, abdominal or chest pain, vomiting, fever, and weakness.

Physical Examination
✧ The diagnosis must be suspected in the presence of abdominal distension and a liver mass.
✧ Ascites is a common clinical feature in those patients with advanced cirrhosis.

✧ Additional infrequent clinical features include hypoglycemia, hypercalcemia, hyper-lipidemia and hyperthyroidism.

✧ Look for features of liver failure and portal hypertension during the exam.

Diagnostics and Imaging

LFTs are frequently abnormal due to underlying cirrhosis rather than the HCC. CBC may show either anemia due to bleeding or polycythemia from anomalous erythropoietin production. AFP is raised in one third of cases; it is often high in undifferentiated disease, and is useful as a marker for recurrence after resection. Hepatitis B and C serology needs to be done in all patients. Clotting may be abnormal.

✧ *Tumor markers*: AFP and abnormal prothrombin antigen (APT) serve as tumor markers for HCC. Very high levels are associated with undifferentiated disease and a poor prognosis. It is a variable predictor for detection of hepatocellular carcinoma, but any patient with chronic active hepatitis or cirrhosis who develops a rising level of AFP or a level exceeding 500 ng/mL should be worked up for hepatocellular carcinoma (e.g. ultrasound). One should also measure CEA and CA 19-9 (markers for biliary tract malignancies) during the workup of HCC.

✧ *Tumor localization*: Ultrasound or CT scan to demonstrate size and position, multiple deposits, and extrahepatic spread (e.g. porta hepatis). CXR may show pulmonary metastases. Occasionally, neither CT nor ultrasound will reveal a lesion in a cirrhotic patient who has a rising level of AFP. In these cases, MRI may be useful, or alternately, Lipiodol-CT scan. FNA cytology or core biopsy under ultrasound or CT guidance has been advocated to differentiate HCC from other benign lesions in both cirrhotic and non-cirrhotic livers; however, there is a proven risk of seeding tumor along the needle track and this procedure is only necessary if the diagnosis is in doubt. A classic radiographic finding of early enhancement on the arterial phase of the CT and washout on the venous phase and an AFP >100 is diagnostic.

✧ Multi-slice helical CT scanners have reduced the need for arterioportography. MRI scans carry a high diagnostic yield and can distinguish between benign and malignant lesions.

Pre-operative Preparation

Correct fluid, electrolyte, and clotting abnormalities. Determine the operative risk. Important considerations include that patients who are Child's grade B and C have already lost 50–60% of functional liver parenchyma, and that patients with cirrhosis may not be able to regenerate liver tissue.

Treatment

Surgical resection is the optimal treatment, and small tumors (<5 cm) carry the best prognosis. Favorable results have also been obtained with the use of local ablative techniques such as alcohol injection and radiofrequency ablation (RFA). Recently investigated modalities (e.g. radiolabeled ablation, laser photocoagulation, electrolysis) may become important.

Liver transplantation is a recognized treatment of HCC arising in a cirrhotic liver. Consideration is based on the Milan criteria: a single lesion less than 5 cm, no more than 3 lesions all less than 3 cm, no vascular invasion and no extrahepatic disease. The UCSF expanded criteria have included patients not meeting the Milan criteria. Radiofrequency ablation and transarterial chemoembolization are used as bridge therapies to transplantation.

Unresectable Lesions:

✧ *Chemotherapy* – both systemic and regional hepatic artery infusions give poor results, with response rates as low as 10–15%, but Sorafenib has recently been associated with a small survival benefit. Immunotherapy (e.g. interferon, cytokines) has not proved helpful.

✧ *Chemoembolization* – transarterial embolization of tumors with gelatin sponge and/or added transarterial chemotherapeutic agents may give symptomatic benefit, with slight improvement in overall survival in some studies. Microspheres containing cytotoxic drugs can be given by the hepatic artery.

✧ *Radiotherapy* – external beam radiation causes radiation-induced hepatitis and is rarely used. Microspheres containing radio-isotopes like yttrium-90 can be injected via the hepatic artery.

Follow-up
Intervals should be short (1–4 weeks) until the diagnosis and treatment plan have been decided. Many of these patients will have been followed for cirrhosis.

Post-operative Follow-up
✧ Check the histology for the pathology and adequate resection margins.
✧ Post-operative complications include intra-abdominal fluid collections and the development of liver failure; manage as indicated.
✧ The most common serious complication is tumor recurrence or new tumor. Monitor serum AFP levels and perform serial ultrasound of the liver every 4 months. Further resection, if recurrence is localized, can be performed and has been associated with extended survival. Median survival for these patients is about one year.

Metastatic Disease of the Liver
Metastatic disease from distant origins is the most common type of neoplasm of the liver. Direct invasion can occur from adjacent organs such as the stomach, pancreas, and hepatic flexure of colon.

Objectives
Diagnose metastatic lesions, differentiate suitable lesions for resection, stage the tumors, treat the tumors.

History
✧ Obtain a focused liver history.
✧ Many patients are asymptomatic.
✧ There may be a history of previous malignancy.
✧ Large lesions may cause capsular distention, and may be associated with abdominal and back pain.
✧ Flatulence and nausea may be clinical signs, with a subsequent decrease in appetite and weight loss. Eventually, malnutrition and cachexia will develop.
✧ Symptoms of cirrhosis may also be present.

Physical Examination
✧ Perform a general examination.
✧ There may be evidence of weight loss.
✧ Hepatomegaly may be present.
✧ Examine for underlying features of cirrhosis.

Diagnostics and Imaging

Ultrasound scan detects metastases larger than 1 cm in diameter; combination with CT reduces the false-negative rate. LFTs may be normal. Serial CEA detects 30% of metastatic livers with normal ultrasound scans (false-positive rate is 15%). Diagnosis can be obtained from percutaneous tumor biopsy. Positron emission tomography (PET) may be used to identify primary and metastatic disease. Laparoscopy can be performed, and should ideally be combined with intra-operative laparoscopic ultrasound.

Treatment

✧ Fewer than 5% of liver metastases are suitable for resection. Surgical resection of the liver is usually confined to metastatic colorectal, neuroendocrine, or congenital tumors. Rarely, other metastases may be considered for resection.

✧ Resection is contraindicated if less than 25% (fewer than two segments) of the liver can be retained. Likely residual volumes can be calculated from CT images.

✧ Liver resection for colorectal metastases carries a peri-operative mortality of less than 5% and a 5-year survival rate of 35–45%.

Unresectable Lesions

✧ *Chemotherapy* – regional hepatic artery infusion or systemic chemotherapy produces the same poor 2-year survival rate. Intraperitoneal infusion has also been studied.

✧ *Chemoembolization* – transarterial chemoembolization (TACE) using gelatin sponge + 5-fluorouracil (5-FU), doxorubicin, and cisplatin has been beneficial in ocular melanoma, advanced carcinoid syndrome, and islet cell tumors. Complications include post-embolization syndrome (nausea and vomiting, fever, abdominal pain, and ileus), infarction of the gall bladder, pancreatitis, and bleeding.

✧ *Other treatment modalities* – in-situ ablative techniques have received much interest in the surgical literature. These techniques of cryotherapy, radiofrequency, microwave and laser therapy, and electrolytic destruction, have yet to be tested in prospective randomized trials, but are now commonly used as adjuncts to surgical treatments or in patients deemed unresectable.

Follow-up

Follow-up is at short intervals until suitability for resection is determined. Arrange operative or non-operative treatment as appropriate.

Post-operative Follow-up

✧ Check the histology and adequacy of the resection margins. Post-operative complications include intra-abdominal fluid collections and the development of liver failure. Manage as indicated.

✧ Monitor for recurrences with regular CT scans at 3- to 6-month intervals with appropriate tumor marker levels. Occasionally, a "redo" resection is indicated.

The Biliary Tract

As stated in the introduction to this chapter, hepatic, pancreatic, and biliary disorders are closely related and should be considered as a group. For instance, a lesion in the head of the pancreas may cause obstruction of the biliary tract, which affects the function of the liver. One of the first objectives of the assessment is to determine which system contains the primary disorder, and then to determine what effect this has had on the function of the others.

Assessment of Biliary Tract Disorders
Biliary History

Obtaining a history in these referrals starts with a general gastrointestinal history; when responses indicate a possible biliary problem, a more detailed biliary history is required. This may also mean that a liver and pancreatic history is required.

The two main indicators of biliary disease are pain and jaundice, and the most common cause of these symptoms is gallstones.

✧ *Biliary colic* – pain originating with the gall bladder is colicky, severe, occurs in the RUQ, and may radiate around to the back. Biliary colic is caused by the gall bladder contracting to try to overcome an obstruction. Eventually, the contraction relaxes and the acute pain is relieved, leaving a dull ache until the next contraction starts. If the obstruction is caused by a gallstone, this obstruction can sometimes be overcome, and the stone is expelled; the bout of biliary colic resolves until the next stone produces another episode. If the stone becomes impacted, inflammation and infection of the biliary tract can ensue. When this occurs in the gall bladder, the result is cholecystitis and the pain becomes constant. If the bile ducts are affected, jaundice and cholangitis may be produced.

✧ *Jaundice* – obstructive jaundice typically causes pale stools, dark urine and often pruritus. An inquiry into possible liver and pancreatic disease is indicated. Usually, jaundice caused by gallstone disease is associated with episodes of biliary colic. The onset of painless jaundice should suggest a neoplastic rather than a benign cause.

✧ *Rigors* – a history of fever with rigors indicates infection of the biliary tree. When combined with pain and jaundice (Charcot's triad), this indicates an infected, obstructed biliary tree which requires urgent treatment to prevent septic shock.

Risk factors: Ask about previous biliary interventions or surgery. Recurrent biliary symptoms may be due to complications of these original treatments. There may be a family history of gallstones, or an inherited disorder that predisposes to the formation of gallstones (e.g. hemolytic anemia, hyperlipidemia, ileal disease or surgical resection, cirrhosis, cystic fibrosis).

Biliary Examination

✧ Perform a general and GI examination with particular attention to the signs of jaundice and liver disease.
✧ Between episodes of colicky pain, abdominal examination may be normal.
✧ An enlarged palpable gall bladder (Courvoisier's sign) in the presence of jaundice is suspicious of a neoplastic cause rather than gallstone disease. Severe inflammation of the gall bladder with adherent omentum may also produce a mass in the RUQ; however, all masses should be considered to be malignant until proven otherwise.
✧ Rectal examination revealing pale, clay-colored, toothpaste-consistency stools are typical of obstructive jaundice.

Examination of Biliary Disorders
Diagnostics
Urinalysis

✧ *Technique* – dipstick urinalysis. The presence of conjugated bilirubin indicates obstructive jaundice, although some conditions associated with excess bilirubin production will result in some bilirubin in the urine.
✧ *Results* – sticks are read and compared against a reference chart.
✧ *Advantages* – a quick and easy method that can be performed in the outpatient clinic.
✧ *Disadvantages* – limited information is available.

Blood Tests
Serum Biochemistry
1. *Release of integral membrane enzymes* – cholestasis and obstructive jaundice are associated with an increased level of alkaline phosphatase. GGT is especially elevated in alcoholic liver disease. Minor increases in ALT and AST occur in cholestasis and chronic liver disease. Significant increases are associated with acute hepatitis or with liver cell necrosis of any cause. Secondary tumor deposits cause a rise in alkaline phosphatase and GGT and a small rise in bilirubin.
2. *Electrolytes, BUN, creatinine* – electrolyte abnormalities may be present, particularly hyponatremia and hypoglycemia. Evidence of raised urea and creatinine levels may indicate impaired renal function associated with liver disease.

Hematology
✧ CBC may reveal anemia of chronic disease or indicate blood loss from the biliary system into the GI tract. Other abnormalities of the blood cells may be detected, such as hemolytic anemia, leukemia, and lymphoma.
✧ *Clotting tests* – coagulation, as reflected in the INR, may be abnormal in liver and biliary disease.

Immunology
Hepatitis serology: screen for hepatitis B and C. The patient should also be screened for autoimmune disease and primary biliary cirrhosis.

Imaging
Ultrasound
✧ *Technique, Results* – refer to liver section.
✧ *Advantages* – currently this is the first-line imaging modality for biliary disease, as ultrasound is an excellent non-invasive technique for visualizing the presence of stones, gall bladder disease, dilatation of the biliary tract and hepatic parenchymal disease. Ultrasound-guided biopsy of liver and pancreas can be undertaken. A common bile duct with a diameter over 10 mm is deemed dilated. A diameter above 15 mm indicates significant organic disease. However, there is a 5–10% incidence of ductal stones in a common bile duct (CBD) of 5 mm diameter. Other causes of duct dilatation include pancreaticobiliary cancer, chronic pancreatitis, congenital cystic disease, and parasitic infestation.
✧ *Disadvantages* – accuracy is dependent on the experience of the operator. Ultrasound may be unsatisfactory if the patient is obese, has undergone previous surgery, or if the exam is conducted in the presence of ascites or gaseous distension of upper abdominal viscera. In these cases, CT is indicated.

Computerized Tomography
✧ *Technique, Results* – refer to liver section.
✧ *Advantages* – intravenous contrast can be given to outline the vessels and focal lesions within the liver; multiple scans can be performed to give non-contrast, arterial, venous, and delayed phases of scanning. Modern multi-slice spiral CT scans can be performed quickly (15–30 seconds) using 5 mm cuts, giving more detail and allowing more sophisticated reconstruction. When used with contrast, CT is more sensitive than ultrasound at determining the nature of lesions within the liver, especially differentiating between small tumors, cysts, or abscesses. CT is better for detection of solid lesions in extrahepatic bile ducts (cholangiocarcinoma), pancreas, and liver. MRI is useful in

hilar carcinoma and primary carcinoma of the gall bladder, where it is superior to CT in assessing the presence and extent of extramural invasion.

✧ *Disadvantages* – though nearly ubiquitous, CT remains an expensive modality. In addition to exposing the patient to ionizing radiation, insignificant incidental findings on CT may necessitate further costly work-up.

Magnetic Resonance Imaging
✧ *Technique, Results* – refer to liver section.
✧ *Advantages* – MRI is useful in hilar cholangiocarcinoma and primary carcinoma of the gall bladder, where it is superior to CT in assessing the presence and extent of extramural invasion. Newer techniques include MRCP.
✧ *Disadvantages* – MRI is expensive and notoriously time-consuming. Many patients find the experience unpleasantly claustrophobic. The use of gadolinium dye has been associated with nephrosclerosis.

Percutaneous Transhepatic Cholangiography
✧ *Technique* – ultrasound is used to identify the dilated biliary system; under local anesthetic, a needle is inserted through the liver parenchyma into the dilated bile duct and contrast agent injected under fluoroscopy to visualize the biliary system. When an obstruction is detected, a percutaneous drain can be inserted to continue drainage after the procedure. Prior to the procedure, the patient should be covered with antibiotics and clotting abnormalities should be corrected.
✧ *Results* – written report and a selection of X-ray images.
✧ *Advantages* – while intended for the visualization of the biliary tract in the jaundiced patient, the procedure can be used to enable transhepatic drainage via the insertion of endoprosthesis. In practice, PTC is used when ERCP has failed, or for the insertion of stents for palliation of large bile duct obstructions due to inoperable/incurable malignancy. PTC can be a better modality than ERCP in hilar cholangiocarcinoma for enabling drainage and visualization of the biliary tree.
✧ *Disadvantages* – complications include septicemia, hemorrhage into peritoneal cavity and hemobilia, biliary peritonitis, intrahepatic arterioportal fistula, pneumothorax, and contrast reactions.

Endoscopic Retrograde Cholangiopancreatography
✧ *Technique* – ERCP is performed using a large-bore side-viewing endoscope. The scope is passed through the stomach into the second part of the duodenum. The duodenal papilla is cannulated and contrast injected under X-ray screening. The pancreatic and biliary duct systems are visualized.
✧ *Results* – written report and a selection of ERCP images.
✧ *Advantages* – ERCP can be performed in all patients with cholestatic jaundice irrespective of whether the ducts are dilated or not. By nature of the esophago-gastro-duodenoscopy (EGD) involved in the procedure, the stomach and duodenum are visualized and studied. A pancreaticogram can be performed. Certain lesions can be treated or palliated during the procedure: stone removal, endoscopic nasobiliary drainage, stent insertion for inoperable malignant bile duct obstruction. ERCP is good for diagnosis of ductal calculi, tumors of the bile duct and pancreas, and sclerosing cholangitis. In patients with complete biliary obstruction, the proximal biliary tree may not be visualized and PTC is then indicated.
✧ *Disadvantages* – the most common procedure-related complication is pancreatitis (1–2%). If sphincterotomy is performed, the complication rate rises to 6–10% and includes

hemorrhage, acute pancreatitis, cholangitis, retroperitoneal perforation, impacted dormia basket, acute cholecystitis, and gallstone ileus. Technical failure may occur in patients with duodenal stenosis, in those who have undergone a previous Billroth II resection, when duodenal diverticula are present, and when patients are uncooperative.

Endoscopic Ultrasound (EUS)

✧ *Technique* – EUS is performed using an upper endoscope with an ultrasound probe on the tip. The scope is passed through the esophagus, the stomach and into the second part of the duodenum. The upper GI, pancreatic and biliary duct systems are visualized. This procedure allows for assessment of lesions and determining depth of invasion. EUS can also be used to assess the biliary tree and the head of the pancreas. It can be used to obtain ultrasound-guided biopsies.
✧ *Results* – written report and a selection of EUS images.
✧ *Advantages* – EUS can be performed in all patients. By nature of the EGD involved in the procedure, the stomach and duodenum are visualized and studied. EUS is good for diagnosis of ductal calculi, tumors of bile duct and pancreas, and pancreatitis.
✧ *Disadvantages* – none.

Biliary Manometry

✧ *Technique* – performed during ERCP; the CBD is cannulated and the pressure in the bile duct is measured.
✧ *Results* – written report as for ERCP.
✧ *Advantages* – good for investigation of patients with biliary dyskinesia, including those with persistent pain after cholecystectomy, to characterize abnormalities of the sphincter (e.g. stenosis, dyskinesia). Measured parameters are basal sphincter pressure, rate and progression of sphincter contractions, and response to morphine and cholecystokinin. Dyskinesia is diagnosed by increased basal pressure, altered frequency and amplitude of phasic contractions, and reversal of normal peristaltic direction.
✧ *Disadvantages* – same as for ERCP. Results can be difficult to interpret.

Biliary Scintiscanning

✧ *Technique* – uses ^{99m}Tc-labeled compounds of iminodiacetic acid (HIDA, DISIDA, PIPIDA). HIDA is injected intravenously, taken up by hepatocytes, secreted into bile ducts, and then concentrated in a functioning gall bladder.
✧ *Results* – written report and a selection of images.
✧ *Advantages* – if HIDA scan demonstrates a lack of concentration in the gall bladder, the most likely diagnosis is cholecystitis; if the gall bladder is visualized, it is almost certain that the diagnosis is not cholecystitis (ambiguous results occur in chronic cholecystitis, gallstone pancreatitis, patients with alcoholic liver disease, and patients receiving parenteral nutrition). The technique is routinely used in the jaundiced neonate for the diagnosis of biliary atresia. HIDA scan is also useful for the functional evaluation of surgically constructed bioenteric anastomoses.
✧ *Disadvantages* – exposes patient to injected radioactivity. Not used routinely.

Laparoscopy

✧ *Technique* – a surgical procedure performed under general anesthesia. Laparoscopy can be used as an investigative technique alone, or can be combined with laparoscopic ultrasonography, cholangiography, biopsy or cytology, or modified to laparoscopic surgical intervention.
✧ *Results* – written operation note, sometimes with photographic images.

✧ *Advantages* – allows visualization of the liver, gall bladder, extrahepatic biliary system, pancreas, and peritoneal lining. Direct visualization enables diagnosis of hepatic disease, primary neoplasms, and secondary tumor deposits in liver and peritoneum, and enables biopsy of these lesions for histology. Staging of hepatobiliary and pancreatic tumors can also be undertaken due to visualization. Laparoscopy is also useful for liver biopsy in patients with chronic liver disease with a high risk of bleeding: hemostasis can be achieved and observed.

✧ *Disadvantages* – requires a general anesthetic and is thus associated with the attendant complications.

Intra-operative Cholangiography and Choledochoscopy
These are techniques used intra-operatively to assess the biliary system and to identify abnormal anatomy, the presence of stones, and confirm their absence or complete removal.

Disorders of the Biliary Tract
Cystic Disease of the Biliary Tract
Choledochal cysts include focal bile duct dilatation, choledochocele, bile duct diverticulae and/or liver cysts. There is an increased incidence of the disease in the Japanese. Sixty percent of cases occur in the first 10 years of life.

Complications of untreated cystic disease include cholangitis, pancreatitis, hepatic abscess formation, and cholangiocarcinoma.

History
Symptoms of increasing jaundice, RUQ pain, and symptoms indicating the presence of complications.

Physical Examination
Look for cholestatic jaundice, abdominal mass, and tenderness.

Diagnostics and Imaging
US and CT reveal the diagnosis; MRCP or ERCP define the anatomy.

Treatment
Surgical excision of the extrahepatic biliary tree and reconstruction in the form of a hepaticojejunostomy, with possible liver resection and drainage of simple liver cysts. Surgery is recommended even in asymptomatic patients to reduce the long-term risk of cholangiocarcinoma.

Gallstones
Cholelithiasis (gallstones) is very common, with a prevalence of up to 18.5% in autopsy studies. Three types of gallstones are recognized: (1) *cholesterol stones*, which are often radiolucent, multiple, or large and single; (2) *pigmented stones*, which are associated with infection or hemolytic disease; and (3) *mixed stones*.

✧ *Risk factors*: Gallstones are more common in females and are associated with obesity, fertility, increasing age (age >40 years), genetic and ethnic factors, a diet high in refined foods and animal fat, diabetes mellitus, ileal disease and resection, hemolytic states, infection of the biliary tract, parasitic infection, cirrhosis, and cystic fibrosis.

✧ *Differential diagnosis*: The majority of gallstones are clinically silent. Common coexisting causes of abdominal pain include colonic motility disorders and diverticular disease, gastritis and peptic ulceration, reflux esophagitis and hiatus hernia, pancreatitis, colonic cancer, renal disease, and ischemic heart disease. In addition to gall bladder imaging, an EGD (or barium upper series) and barium enema or colonoscopy may be necessary in patients undergoing elective cholecystectomy for chronic abdominal symptoms.

✧ *Silent gallstones*: The vast majority of gallstones will not cause symptoms or complications during a patient's lifetime. Therefore, there is no indication for cholecystectomy in the management of asymptomatic gallstones except in acromegalic patients on long-term somatostatin analogue, where gallstones can get very large, and in diabetic patients with gallstones.

Symptomatic Cholelithiasis

Cholecystectomy for gallstones is one of the most common operations performed in the Western world. This is partly because ultrasound is widely used during the work-up of abdominal pain and is very sensitive at detecting gallstones. Once detected, gallstones can be difficult to exclude as the cause of the pain until they are removed.

Objectives

Diagnose gallstones, rule out surgical emergencies, differentiate from other causes of abdominal pain, treat gallstones.

History

✧ Obtain a general history, focused on biliary complaints.

✧ Typically, patients report recurrent attacks of epigastric or RUQ pain, often radiating to the right side of back or scapula. The bouts of pain may last several minutes to hours, may subside or progress to acute cholecystitis. Nausea and vomiting may accompany each episode. Jaundice and dark urine may follow an acute attack and indicate a common bile duct stone.

✧ Intolerance to fatty foods, abdominal distension, and belching can occur with the same frequency in the general population as they do in patients with gallstones.

Physical Examination

✧ Perform a general examination. Look for jaundice and signs of liver disease.

✧ Examination may be normal or there may be tenderness in the RUQ.

✧ Occasionally, adherent omentum to a previously inflamed gall bladder may produce a RUQ mass.

Diagnostics and Imaging

LFTs may be normal or may demonstrate elevated transaminases and bilirubin. Ultrasound is diagnostic showing gallstones and maybe the presence of a dilated common bile duct, but there is no gall bladder wall thickening or pericholecystic fluid.

Treatment

The therapy of choice is surgery, and the current surgical standard is laparoscopic cholecystectomy. Advantages claimed for the laparoscopic approach include less pain, the potential for same-day or outpatient surgery, earlier return to work, fewer wound complications.

Patients should be informed that the operation may be converted to an open procedure if there are complications, severe inflammation, questions of anatomy, or bleeding. The conversion rate is widely reported as 5%.

Follow-up
Patients should be seen at 2 weeks for wound healing and to review pathology results. If there are atypical features to the history or examination, review sooner. After a second follow-up at 4–6 weeks after surgery, further follow-up should be deferred to primary care unless pathology results dictate otherwise.

Potential complications of surgery include wound infection, bile leak, abscess, bleeding, and wound pain; long-term complications include common bile duct injury (may present as progressive jaundice), damage to the duodenum, jejunum, and colon, and abscess formation around lost stones.

Persistence of the original symptoms may be due to residual stones or to alternative causes of abdominal pain, and is known as post-cholecystectomy syndrome (*see* page 191).

Alternate Treatments for Gallstones
Caveat: Cholecystectomy is the definitive treatment of choice.
✧ *Cholecystolithotomy* – this procedure is indicated in patients with a previous vagotomy for ulcer disease in the presence of a functioning gall bladder (demonstrated on biliary scintiscan). Post-vagotomy patients frequently develop symptomatic gallstones, but if a functioning gall bladder is removed, a high percentage will develop debilitating explosive diarrhea. Therefore, cholecystectomy is not performed and removal of the stones is the appropriate treatment, followed by oral bile salt therapy. However, cholecystectomy is the right treatment if the gall bladder is non-functioning.
✧ *Extracorporeal shock wave lithotripsy (ESWL)* – stone fragmentation is successful in 80% of patients with solitary small gallstones. ESWL will fail if the stones are larger than 3 cm, multiple, or calcified. Repeat treatments are frequently required. ESWL requires post-procedural maintenance therapy with bile salts. The recurrence rate is 50% at five years. The current role of ESWL is restricted to the fragmentation of occluding ductal calculi in jaundiced patients. ESWL is not performed routinely; 50% of patients require additional procedures to achieve stone removal.
✧ *Oral dissolution* – only applicable to patients with a functioning gall bladder on biliary scintiscan. Chenodeoxycholic and ursodeoxycholic oral bile salts result in dissolution after several weeks to months. Maintenance with ursodeoxycholate is then required. The recurrence rate is 12.5% after the first year, progressing to 61% by the eleventh year. The technique fails if the gallstone load is large (greater than 3 cm in size, or with multiple stones) and/or if the stones are calcified. Bile salt therapy is restricted to patients in whom cholecystectomy is contraindicated either as a primary treatment or after gallstone extraction, fragmentation or dissolution by MTBE.

Acute Cholecystitis
Whereas symptomatic cholelithiasis can be worked up, diagnosed, and treated on an outpatient basis, acute cholecystitis is best treated with surgery in the appropriate patient.

History
Patients often present to hospital for admission with acute abdominal pain and a progression of symptoms similar to symptomatic cholelithiasis. Acute cholecystitis may also occur in hospitalized patients, most frequently among critically ill patients who have been on parenteral nutrition.

Physical Examination

The hallmark findings of acute cholecystitis include RUQ pain and the arrest of inspiration with palpation of the gall bladder (Murphy's sign). In intubated and sedated patients, there may be no obvious signs of cholecystitis on physical examination.

Diagnostics and Imaging

CBC will reveal mild to moderate leukocytosis. LFTs may demonstrate mild elevation, highest in alkaline phosphatase.

US is the gold-standard examination modality, which will reveal gallstones, gall bladder wall thickening and pericholecystic fluid; additional findings may include common bile duct dilatation. Occasionally, gallstones may not be visualized despite the presence of other signs of acute cholecystitis. CT may be utilized when US is not immediately available.

Treatment

The definitive therapy for acute cholecystitis is cholecystectomy; the current standard of care is through a laparoscopic approach. The patient should always be consented for conversion to the open procedure.

IV antibiotics should be started after the diagnosis is made. In the event that emergency surgical intervention is not deemed safe (e.g. a debilitated cardiac patient who is not optimized for surgery, or a critically ill patient in the Surgical Intensive Care Unit [SICU]), a percutaneous transhepatic cholecystostomy tube should be placed by an interventionalist for drainage of the gall bladder, with definitive surgical correction to occur at a later date. The gall bladder should be sent for pathologic analysis.

Follow-up

Generally, patients should be seen at 2 and 4–6 weeks after discharge from hospital to check on wound healing and to review pathology results. Uncomplicated cases can be deferred to primary care follow-up after this time. Further surgical follow-up is dictated by the results of the gall bladder analysis.

Acalculous Chronic Gall Bladder Disease

Two etiologies of acalculous chronic gall bladder disease are known:
1. *Adenomyomatosis of the gall bladder*, characterized by diverticular formations of the epithelial lining.
2. *Cholesterolosis of the gall bladder*, in which the epithelial cells and macrophages in the gall bladder mucosa become laden with cholesterol, inducing chronic inflammation. This is seen as the "strawberry gall bladder."

Objectives

Diagnose the cause, differentiate from other causes of abdominal pain including gallstone disease, differentiate from cancer of the gall bladder, treat cause.

History and Examination

✧ Vague symptoms, similar to chronic cholecystitis.
✧ Examination may be normal, or possible tenderness in RUQ.

Diagnostics and Imaging

Ultrasound is normal or may show thickening of the gall bladder wall; by definition, gallstones will not be visualized on ultrasound.

Treatment
Cholecystectomy.

Follow-up
Patients should be seen for post-operative wound check at 2 and 4–6 weeks, during which time the pathology report can be reviewed. If there are atypical features to the history or examination, review sooner. If pathology confirms chronic cholecystic changes and the patient is symptom-free, further follow-up after 4–6 weeks can be deferred to primary care.

Mucocele of the Gall Bladder
This is a grossly distended gall bladder filled with mucoid material. Mucoceles are associated with cystic duct obstructions, usually, by gallstones that did not result in inflammation or infection.

Objectives
Diagnose mucocele, differentiate from other causes of abdominal pain and from cancer of the biliary tract, treat mucocele.

History
Obtain a general history, focusing on biliary complaints. The typical patient is usually elderly, presenting with a painless mass in the RUQ. There may be a history of acute pain in the RUQ, like in biliary colic or acute cholecystitis.

Physical Examination
Patients are usually not jaundiced. Often, there is a painless mass in the RUQ.

Diagnostics and Imaging
LFTs are usually normal. Ultrasound shows a distended gall bladder, but with a normal CBD diameter.

Treatment
Cholecystectomy.

Follow-up
The patient should be seen at short (2–4 week) intervals until malignant obstruction of the biliary system is excluded. Wounds should be followed up until 4–6 weeks after surgery. If pathology confirms chronic cholecystitis and the patient is symptom-free, further follow-up should be deferred to primary care.

Ductal Calculi
Ductal calculi are mostly found within the CBD; 5% are located in the intrahepatic ducts, more commonly in the left system of ducts. They arise as either secondary calculi from the migration of gallstones, or as primary calculi forming *de novo* within bile ducts. The predisposing factors to primary duct stones include stasis in the biliary tract caused by strictures, parasitic infestations, recurrent pyogenic cholangitis, and indwelling stents. Stone impaction may result in progressive jaundice, cholangitis, gallstone pancreatitis, secondary biliary cirrhosis, and portal hypertension.

Objectives
Diagnose cause, differentiate from other causes of pain/jaundice, treat cause.

History

Obtain a history focused on biliary complaints. Symptoms include recurrent bouts of biliary colic (with or without jaundice), episodic upper abdominal pain, and dyspepsia. Note that 15–20% of duct stones are asymptomatic.

Physical Examination

✧ Perform a general examination; the examination may be normal, as the patient may or may not be jaundiced.

✧ Examine for scars from previous biliary surgery, tenderness in the RUQ and evidence of liver disease.

Diagnostics and Imaging

LFTs reveal obstructive jaundice; ultrasound detects a dilated biliary system. MRCP defines the anatomy and the obstruction, whereas ERCP does the same but can be combined with sphincterotomy or endoscopic stent placement.

Treatment

✧ *Ductal calculi found incidentally during intra-operative cholangiography*: Stones less than 2 mm in diameter can be left alone, as more than 95% of them will pass spontaneously. If the stone becomes symptomatic, then remove during ERCP. Stones larger than 2 mm but smaller than 10 mm can be removed by intra-operative duct exploration (laparoscopic or open) or post-operative ERCP. Post-operative ERCP stone extraction is likely to fail for stones greater than 10 mm in diameter, and these are best removed surgically. Flushing of the duct or the administration of 1 ampoule of glucagon and flushing of the duct can be used in these cases.

✧ *Ductal calculi without previous cholecystectomy*: Cholecystectomy and CBD exploration. This can be performed either open or laparoscopically. In young patients with a small CBD, explore and clear the duct and insert a T-tube. If there are multiple ductal calculi and/or a grossly dilated duct, some form of drainage procedure may be required (e.g. Roux-en-Y hepaticojejunostomy). If the patient is elderly or a poor operative risk, then perform an ERCP and stone extraction and reserve cholecystectomy for those that develop symptoms.

✧ *Ductal calculi prior to laparoscopic cholecystectomy*: (1) Pre-operative ERCP and sphincterotomy. However, this carries the risk of a combined morbidity of two procedures and the unknown risk associated with sphincterotomy in the under-50-years age group; (2) Combined open or laparoscopic cholecystectomy and exploration of CBD.

✧ *Ductal calculi discovered after cholecystectomy and exploration of CBD with T-tube in place*: Missed stones are rare where intra-operative choledochoscopy is used, but increases to 8% for completion T-tube cholangiography. Treat by post-operative ERCP and sphincterotomy, utilizing flushing and drug-induced relaxation of the sphincter of Oddi. Other alternatives include dissolution with MTBE or percutaneous stone extraction via the T-tube tract; this is performed after 4–6 weeks of tract maturation. If stones are not detected during or soon after surgery (e.g. if the cholangiogram was not performed or a T-tube was not inserted at operation), recurrent symptoms from missed stones usually occur within 2 years of cholecystectomy. Ductal stones presenting beyond this period are generally considered to be primary.

✧ *Recurrent ductal calculi*: Often multiple and associated with gross dilatation of the bile duct with or without ductal stenosis. Duct stenosis may be primary (papillary stenosis) or secondary to previous bile duct exploration. Treat by either ERCP and sphincterotomy or surgically (e.g. Roux-en-Y hepaticojejunostomy).

✧ *Multiple intrahepatic calculi*: More common among Asian populations, associated with strictures of the hepatic ducts. Therapy is operative choledochotomy and stone extraction, transhepatic lithotomy, or resection of the involved lobe.

Follow-up
Schedule short-interval follow-up (1–4 weeks) until cancer is excluded and to prevent deterioration from jaundice. Consider inpatient admission and further investigation if the patient is frail or there is evidence of liver dysfunction.

Post-operative Follow-up
Follow up until symptom-free and LFTs return to normal. When stable, defer further care to primary care with notice for re-referral should bile duct strictures develop.

Cholangitis
This occurs as the infection of an obstructed biliary tract. Systemic symptoms result from bacteremia secondary to cholangiovenous reflux induced by biliary hypertension (greater than 20 cm H_2O). Most commonly, obstruction is due to gallstones, bile duct strictures, tumors of the bile duct, pancreatic head lesions, and periampullary lesions. Obstruction also occurs less commonly as a result of bilioenteric anastomoses, spontaneous bilioenteric fistulas, cystic disease of the biliary tract, and duodenal diverticula.

History
✧ Obtain a history with a focus on biliary complaints.
✧ The classical Charcot's triad of symptoms, indicative of cholangitis, are pain in RUQ, intermittent fever/rigors, and jaundice. Rigors are severe and nausea and vomiting are frequent.
✧ Reynold's pentad includes Charcot's triad with the addition of altered mental status and hemodynamic instability (hypotension/shock), and signifies the development of suppurative cholangitis and requires emergency intervention.

Physical Examination
Perform a general examination. Commonly, there is tenderness in the RUQ. Clinically apparent jaundice may not be present in the early stages.

Diagnostics and Imaging
Treatment should not wait for the results of investigations. LFTs and ultrasound confirm the diagnosis. Appropriate laboratory tests include blood cultures for specificity and sensitivity, CBC, coagulation screen, electrolytes, BUN, and creatinine to detect renal impairment.

Treatment
✧ Admission to hospital and resuscitation with IV fluids, supplemental oxygen as needed, and IV antibiotics (start with broad-spectrum antibiotics, ensuring coverage of anaerobic organisms; narrow as sensitivities return).
✧ Urgent biliary decompression is required (e.g. ERCP and sphincterotomy/stent or percutaneous transhepatic biliary drainage).
✧ Specific treatment is then directed at the underlying cause. Be highly suspicious of concomitant renal failure.

Follow-up
Follow-up depends on the underlying condition and the treatment performed.

Post-operative Follow-up

If a cholecystectomy and exploration of common bile duct was performed, follow up in the usual manner: review pathology, determine the presence of complications. When treatment regimen is complete and the patient is asymptomatic, further follow-up should be deferred to primary care, with notice for re-referral in the event of late bile duct stricture development.

Biliary Fistulas

Biliary fistulas are defined as abnormal connections between the biliary system and other viscera. They can be classified as either internal or external.

✧ *External fistulas* communicate with the skin and are caused by trauma or as a complication of surgery or therapeutic intervention (e.g. T-tube, stents, cholecystostomy).

✧ *Internal fistulas* occur between a variety of organs and are caused by differing etiologies (*see* Table 8.3).

Objectives

Diagnose fistula, determine underlying pathology, treat fistula, treat underlying cause.

History

Obtain a history from the patient, focused on biliary complaints. Symptoms of non-malignant internal fistulas involving the gall bladder are similar to symptomatic cholelithiasis, but jaundice and cholangitis are more common.

Physical Examination

✧ Perform a general examination.
✧ Examine for jaundice or evidence of underlying sepsis.
✧ Examine the chest.
✧ Examine for abdominal masses or tenderness.

Diagnostics and Imaging

LFTs show general derangement. Ultrasound and abdominal plain film may show gas in the biliary tree. CBC may reveal anemia and leukocytosis. Electrolytes, BUN, and creatinine may reveal renal impairment. Blood cultures should be taken prior to the infusion of antibiotics.

TABLE 8.3 Causes of internal biliary fistulas

Internal Biliary Fistula	Etiology
Bilioenteric	
Cholecystoduodenal	Gallstones
Cholecystocolic	Gallstones, carcinoma
Cholecystogastric	Gallstones, carcinoma, peptic ulceration
Choledochoduodenal	Ductal calculi, iatrogenic, duodenal ulcer, carcinoma
Biliobilial	
Cholecystocholedochal	Gallstones (Mirizzi's syndrome)
Other	
Bronchobilial, pleurobilial	Trauma, operative injuries, liver abscesses/hydatid, subphrenic abscess
Cholecystorenal	Gallstones

Treatment
✧ Treat the underlying gallstone disease via cholecystectomy; close the fistula.
✧ In cases of Mirizzi's syndrome, leave a cuff of gall bladder to close the fistulous opening.
✧ Explore the common bile duct through a choledochotomy.
✧ Management of bronchobiliary fistulas consists of adequate drainage of the hepatic/subphrenic abscess and decompression of the biliary tract.

Follow-up
Initially, the patient should be seen at short intervals (1–2 weeks) until the diagnosis is confirmed, for monitoring to prevent deterioration from the underlying condition, and to exclude neoplastic causes. Consider admission for investigation and treatment.

Post-operative Follow-up
Follow-up depends on the treatment and the procedure performed. Review with regard to the pathology and post-operative complications related to cholecystectomy and bile duct exploration. Monitor for the detection of bile duct stenoses with regular estimation of LFTs, ultrasound, and MRCP if necessary.

When the patient is symptom-free and the LFTs have returned to baseline, further follow-up should be deferred to primary care, with notice for re-referral if the patient develops symptoms of bile duct stricture.

Gallstone Ileus
This is a rare condition found primarily in the elderly. It is caused by intraluminal intestinal obstruction by a large gallstone, usually 10 cm proximal to the ileocecal valve, subsequent to the establishment of a cholecystoduodenal fistula.

History and Physical Examination
There may be a history of symptomatic cholelithiasis, though this is not always present. The primary presentation of this phenomenon is as a small bowel obstruction. Expect abdominal pain, constipation and/or obstruction, with abdominal distention and tympany. Nausea and vomiting may also be reported.

Diagnostics and Imaging
LFTs and ultrasound. Abdominal plain film will demonstrate pneumobilia due to the enteric fistula, and may also demonstrate an obstructing mass at the ileocecal valve. CT can be utilized for anatomic information.

Treatment
Begin treatment for small bowel obstruction, including gastric decompression and fluid resuscitation. Definitive treatment is surgical: enterolithotomy; check for other gallstones in the gut. The cholecystoduodenal fistula can be addressed at a later time if the patient is unstable or suboptimal for prolonged surgery; it is unclear whether there is an advantage of one-stage over interval biliary surgery in these patients.

Follow-up/Post-operative Follow-up
As for biliary fistula.

Post-cholecystectomy Syndrome
Post-cholecystectomy syndrome refers to the persistence of symptoms referable to the biliary tract after cholecystectomy (excluding diseases outside the biliary tract). A careful

history and investigation with laboratory tests, MRCP, and/or ERCP is advised in all patients. Common causes are:

1. Retained or recurrent calculi: Diagnose and treat by ERCP.
2. Gall bladder or cystic duct remnants: Diagnosed if operative note indicates leaving gall bladder remnants behind or cholecystotomy was performed. Ultrasound and ERCP are useful to confirm the diagnosis and exclude other causes. Treat by revision cholecystectomy.
3. Bile duct strictures and other unrecognized iatrogenic injuries (choledochoduodenal fistula).
4. Papillary stenosis, sphincter of Oddi dysfunction (SOD) syndrome, and biliary dyskinesia.

Papillary Stenosis
Fibrosis or fibromuscular hyperplasia of the sphincter of Oddi.

History
Pain similar to symptomatic cholelithiasis.

Physical Examination
Normal or slight tenderness in the RUQ.

Diagnostics and Imaging
LFTs show a slight derangement, including hyperbilirubinemia and elevated alkaline phosphatase. Ultrasound may demonstrate duct dilatation. ERCP shows that the trans-duodenal segment of the common bile duct is wider than the intrapancreatic segment. Biliary sludge and small calculi are often present. The resting sphincter pressure is raised and the normal phasic sphincter activity is lost.

Treatment
ERCP and sphincterotomy. Operative transduodenal sphincteroplasty is also an option.

Biliary Dyskinesia
There is persistent pain after cholecystectomy but no apparent abnormality on physical examination or routine laboratory tests. However, ERCP manometry demonstrates the following abnormalities:

1. Elevated resting pressure.
2. Tachyarrhythmia (increased phasic activity of the sphincter).
3. Retrograde contractions of the sphincter.
4. Paradoxical response to cholecystokinin.

Treatment
ERCP and sphincterotomy.

Benign Bile Duct Strictures
The most common cause of benign bile duct stricture is as a sequela of operative trauma. If left untreated, the late consequences are liver fibrosis, secondary biliary cirrhosis, and the development of portal hypertension. Strictures may develop many years after cholecystectomy. Alternately, damage to the CBD or common hepatic duct (CHD) may present in the immediate post-operative period with the development of an external biliary fistula associated with sepsis or the development of a subphrenic/subhepatic abscess.

Peritonitis may occur, and jaundice is often present but may not be severe or progressive. Other causes of bile duct strictures include penetrating and non-penetrating abdominal injuries, chronic duodenal ulcer, chronic pancreatitis, recurrent pyogenic cholecystitis, parasitic infestations, and sclerosing cholangitis.

Objectives
Diagnose stricture, detect underlying cause, differentiate from neoplastic causes, detect liver dysfunction, treat stricture, treat underlying cause, correct liver dysfunction.

History
✧ Take a general history focused on biliary complaints.
✧ Often, there is a history of previous biliary surgery; determine the details of the operation, ask about length of stay, and whether there were any complications at the time.
✧ The patient may complain of colicky RUQ pain similar to symptomatic cholelithiasis or present with mild painless jaundice.
✧ Ask about symptoms which would suggest any of the other causes.

Physical Examination
Perform a general examination. The patient may be normal or mildly jaundiced. Tenderness may be present in the RUQ.

Diagnostics and Imaging
✧ LFTs show elevated bilirubin and alkaline phosphatase.
✧ Ultrasound may show a dilated intrahepatic duct system and evidence of portal hypertension. In stable patients, MRCP is an excellent non-invasive method of visualizing the biliary tree. ERCP or PTC can be used to determine the relevant anatomy of the abnormality and provide information to assist reconstruction and treat the underlying condition.
✧ Liver biopsy may be indicated if cirrhosis is suspected.

Treatment
Therapy can be attempted using ERCP with balloon dilatation and indwelling stent for several months. However, the majority of injuries require surgical repair in a specialized center, as the correct treatment depends on accurate classification of the injury (e.g. Bismuth classification I–V). Numerous surgical procedures are possible depending on the exact injury, but most involve the use of a Roux-en-Y hepaticojejunostomy. Best results are obtained with the first surgical repair; thus the operation should be performed in a high-volume center.

Follow-up
After the initial visit, there should be short-interval follow-up (1–4 weeks) until the diagnosis is confirmed and malignant causes are excluded.

Following repair of bile duct injuries, there is a high incidence of further stricture formation and the development of biliary cirrhosis and portal hypertension. Therefore, these patients require long-term follow-up with ultrasound and LFTs at regular intervals.

Sclerosing Cholangitis
Sclerosing cholangitis is an obscure disorder of uncertain etiology which results in progressive fibrous obliteration of the biliary tract. It is currently considered an autoimmune disorder. Previously, it was considered to be two entities:

✧ *Primary* – no previous biliary surgery or biliary tract disease.
✧ *Secondary* – previous biliary surgery or tract disease.

However, both categories are often associated with inflammatory bowel disease (IBD) (usually ulcerative colitis, occasionally Crohn's). Classification is based on the extent of involvement of the biliary tree: total diffuse, localized hilar, diffuse intrahepatic, diffuse extrahepatic, and localized extrahepatic distal.

The disease progresses inevitably to cirrhosis and development of portal hypertension. Patients have a high risk of developing cholangiocarcinoma.

Objectives
Diagnose sclerosing cholangitis (especially in patients with ulcerative colitis or Crohn's), exclude cholangiocarcinoma, classify the disease, detect degree of liver impairment, treat sclerosing cholangitis, treat liver impairment.

History
Take a general history focused on biliary complaints. Symptoms may include vague ill-health, asthenia, RUC pain, jaundice, itching, pyrexia, and attacks of rigors.

Physical Examination
Perform a general examination. Look for jaundice, anemia, and signs of liver disease. Examination may be normal, but jaundice, a tender palpable liver, and an enlarged spleen is present in approximately 50% of patients.

Diagnostics and Imaging
LFTs show a cholestatic pattern, but the alkaline phosphatase is often elevated out of proportion to the bilirubin. The majority of patients are HBsAg negative. Antimitochondrial, anti-smooth muscle and antinuclear antibodies are found only in 20–50% of patients and are non-specific for this disease; if present, suspect primary biliary cirrhosis.

MRCP/ERCP/PTC show ducts are smaller in number and size with stricture formation. Saccular dilated areas between strictures are seen in diffuse disease. Differentiation from hilar and diffuse cholangiocarcinoma is difficult even with histology obtained from biopsies or cytology from brushings at ERCP.

Treatment
✧ Pruritus should be controlled by cholestyramine and ursodeoxycholate.
✧ Manage cholangitis episodes with intravenous antibiotics, with or without ERCP stenting.
✧ Progressive jaundice and recurrent cholangitis are indications for surgical intervention. The aim of surgical treatment is to reduce the dominant strictures. In the absence of cirrhosis, occasional good results in localized disease have been obtained by ERCP or percutaneous balloon dilatation and stent insertion. Surgical options include Roux-en-Y hepaticojejunostomy or intra-operative dilatation and external stent insertion. Stents are left in for 12 months, and progress is assessed by cholangiograms performed through the stent.
✧ Diffuse disease or the presence of cirrhosis require hepatic transplantation. Unexpected cholangiocarcinomas have been reported in 8% of livers removed at time of liver transplantation.

Follow-up
Arrange short-interval follow-ups until the diagnosis is confirmed and cholangiocarcinoma is excluded. Treat mild cases expectantly and monitor for the development of complications. These patients will require long-term follow-up.

Post-operative Follow-up
Follow-up depends on the operation and procedures performed. Review with pathology and examine the patient for complications of biliary surgery.

Long-term monitoring should look for the recurrence of symptoms or development of stenoses; LFTs, ultrasound, and ERCP may be useful in this goal. Perform a HIDA scan if stenoses or bilioenteric anastomoses are suspected.

Biliary Disorders in AIDS
AIDS patients are prone to develop acute acalculous cholecystitis, papillary stenosis, and abnormalities of the bile ducts similar to sclerosing cholangitis. Papillary stenosis and cholangiopathy produce symptoms of pain, develop elevated bilirubin and alkaline phosphatase levels, are diagnosed by ERCP, and should be treated appropriately. The treatment for acalculous cholecystitis is cholecystectomy.

Recurrent Pyogenic Cholangitis
The disease is most prevalent in South-east Asia, but is also known to occur among the immunocompromised. Recurrent bouts of bacterial cholangitis lead to formation of pigment stones and strictures. Recurrent pyogenic cholangitis affects intra- and extrahepatic ducts with a predilection for the left lobe of the liver.

History
Attacks of RUQ pain and rigors. The patient may also complain of the development of jaundice.

Physical Examination
May be normal, or patient may have tenderness in the RUQ. Mild jaundice may be present.

Diagnostics and Imaging
LFTs demonstrate bile duct obstruction. Ductal dilatation is seen on ultrasound. Diagnosis is made by ERCP.

Treatment
Surgical correction of strictures and stones.

Duodenal Diverticula
These diverticulae are present in 12.5% of patients who undergo ERCP. They are usually asymptomatic, but their clinical significance is that they are associated with an increased incidence of postprocedural bacterial infection and can make ERCP technically difficult to perform.

Hemobilia
Rare upper GI bleeding originating from the biliary system. Causes of hemobilia include iatrogenic percutaneous radiologic intervention, liver biopsy, blunt or penetrating trauma, and extrahepatic bile duct tumors. Diagnosis and treatment is by selective mesenteric angiography and embolization.

Tumors of the Gall Bladder
Benign Tumors
Benign neoplasms of the gall bladder include adenomas and papillomas. These are usually incidental findings on ultrasound during the investigation of RUQ pain. Treatment is by cholecystectomy to exclude carcinoma. At post-operative follow-up, determine that no malignant focus was detected and that excision was complete.

Carcinoma of the Gall Bladder
Carcinoma is often found incidentally on pathology analysis after cholecystectomy. The female-to-male ratio is 3 : 1, and is more common in the over-65-years age group. Gallstones are present in 75–90% of cases. The majority are adenocarcinomas. Rare types are neuroendocrine tumors and melanoma. If detected pre-operatively, these tumors can be difficult to differentiate from Klatskin tumors or Mirizzi syndrome.

History
This often presents with the same signs and symptoms as symptomatic cholelithiasis. Additional non-specific symptoms may be anorexia, nausea and vomiting, and weight loss.

Physical Examination
✧ Variable clinical presentation: The patient may have a normal examination, or have an inflammatory mass in the RUQ, or may present with acute cholecystitis.
✧ In advanced cases, there may be jaundice, an enlarged liver, and a palpable gall bladder (Courvoisier's sign). In very advanced cases there may be ascites.
✧ Anemia is present in 50% due to hemobilia.

Diagnostics and Imaging
LFTs may demonstrate elevated alkaline phosphatase despite a normal bilirubin level. CBC may show iron-deficiency anemia.

Ultrasound tends to identify only advanced cases. CT will reveal earlier-stage carcinomas. Abdominal plain films occasionally identify the intramural calcification of a "porcelain" gall bladder, a premalignant condition. ERCP/PTC is usually needed to define these lesions. Involvement of segment V bile duct by a gall bladder mass is indicative of cancer.

Staging
✧ *Stage 0 (Tis, N0, M0)*: Small cancer only in the epithelial layer of the gall bladder without external spread.
✧ *Stage IA (T1, N0, M0)*: Tumor extends into the lamina propria (T1a) or muscle layer (T1b), but does not extend outside of the gall bladder.
✧ *Stage IB (T2, N0, M0)*: The neoplasm grows into the perimuscular fibrous tissue without external spread.
✧ *Stage IIA (T3, N0, M0)*: The tumor grows through the serosal layer and/or directly grows into the liver or one other nearby structure. There is no lymph node spread or distant metastasis.
✧ *Stage IIB (T1–3, N1, M0)*: The tumor has spread to nearby lymph nodes in addition to local growth.
✧ *Stage III (T4, any N, M0)*: The cancer invades the main hepatic blood vessels or has reached more than one nearby organ, may or may not have spread into the lymph nodes.
✧ *Stage IV (Any T, any N, M1)*: Distant metastasis.

Treatment
Treatment is determined by stage:
- ◇ *Stage 0, IA*: Cholecystectomy. Usually, the carcinoma is found on pathology post-operatively, and requires no further immediate surgery.
- ◇ *Stage IB*: Radical resection. If found on post-operative pathology, patient should return to the operating room for a radical resection.
- ◇ *Stage II*: Controversial. May be amenable to radical resection and lymphadenectomy, albeit with high but acceptable morbidity and mortality.
- ◇ *Stages III and IV*: Unresectable disease. Treatment is chemotherapy with or without radiation. Surgical intervention is focused on palliation.

Follow-up
Follow-up is at short intervals until diagnosis is confirmed and treatment is instituted.

Post-operative Follow-up
Review within 2–4 weeks with pathology and complete the staging process. Detect any post-operative complications. Thereafter, follow-up is long-term and dictated by pathology and therapeutic goals.

Tumors of the Bile Ducts
Benign Tumors
Benign bile duct tumors include adenomas and papillomas. They are rarer than malignant tumors and have a tendency to recur after excision. The most common presentation is jaundice and hemobilia; CBC may reflect anemia.

Malignant: Cholangiocarcinoma
At least three staging systems exist for cholangiocarcinoma, but none has been shown to be useful in predicting survival. Rather, the potential for resectability dictates possible therapeutic success. Cholangiocarcinomas are best classified according to four positions:
1. *Intrahepatic*: Minor hepatic ducts.
2. *Proximal*: Right and left hepatic ducts, hilar confluence, and proximal common hepatic duct (Klatskin tumors).
3. *Middle*: Distal common hepatic duct, cystic duct, and confluence with common bile duct.
4. *Distal*: From common bile duct to the periampullary region.

Pathologically, cholangiocarcinoma can be divided into three forms:
1. *Stricture*: Difficult to differentiate from sclerosing cholangitis.
2. *Nodular*: Form extraductal nodules.
3. *Papillary*: Friable tumor in the distal duct tends to produce hemobilia.

Cholangiocarcinomas tend to grow slowly, infiltrate locally, and metastasize late. They have a special predilection for perineural spread and rarely metastasize beyond the liver.

Objectives
Diagnose tumor, differentiate from other lesions, classify tumor, determine resectability, treat tumor, follow up to detect recurrence.

History
- ◇ The primary presentation of cholangiocarcinoma is progressive obstructive jaundice accompanied by itching and anorexia (90% of all cases).

✧ The patient may also complain of a dull upper abdominal pain.
✧ Alternative presentations include cholangitis or acute cholecystitis.
✧ Duration of symptoms is usually short and measured in months.

Physical Examination
✧ Perform a general examination.
✧ Anemia may be present due to hemobilia, especially with periampullary lesions.
✧ Stools may have a silvery appearance due to steatorrhea and blood.
✧ Hepatomegaly may be present.
✧ There may be a palpable gall bladder in distal tumors.
✧ There may be a scar from previous cholecystectomy (an operative cholangiogram should never be regarded as normal unless there is adequate and complete filling of the intrahepatic biliary tree).

Diagnostics and Imaging
LFTs may show an obstructive pattern with elevated alkaline phosphatase and bilirubin levels and low albumin levels, indicating an impaired nutritional status. CBC may reveal an iron-deficiency anemia. Clotting may be abnormal. CEA and CA19-9 are often elevated.

Ultrasound identifies dilatation of the biliary tree. Triple-phase CT scan gives more detailed information about the anatomy and extent of arterial and venous involvement. CT-guided needle biopsy can be used to confirm the diagnosis. MRCP may be able to give a detailed pre-operative road map of the biliary system. ERCP/PTC are needed for decompression of the biliary tree; transbiliary biopsy can be performed with this procedure. Celiac axis angiography is sometimes performed to delineate vascular anatomy and tumor involvement at the hilum; color duplex Doppler ultrasound is a less invasive alternative.

Treatment
Surgical resection gives the best chance of cure, and also offers the best means of palliation. Hilar lesions are treated by an extended right or left hepatectomy with resection of the caudate lobe, resection of tumor and of extrahepatic biliary tree with hepaticojejunostomy. Mid-duct tumors can be treated by extrahepatic biliary tree excision alone, provided the proximal resection margins are negative. Periampullary tumors need a pancreatico-duodenectomy. Approximately 20% of lesions are resectable.

Unresectable lesions are treated by a surgical biliary bypass (Roux loop to segment III duct) or by percutaneous transhepatic or endoscopic stenting. Intracavity irradiation through stents is possible.

Photodynamic therapy can be used to treat unresectable tumors. This involves the administration of a photosensitizing drug that accumulates in cancer cells, followed by exposure of the tumor to the appropriate wavelength of light. This results in tumor destruction by the activation of the photosensitizer. These tumors have a poor response to chemotherapy.

Follow-up
Arrange follow-up at short intervals (2–4 weeks) until a diagnosis is established and treatment is instituted.

Post-operative Follow-up
Follow-up is long-term at regular 3–6 monthly intervals. Five-year survival is 30% for distal and periampullary tumors. With diffuse intrahepatic disease, most patients die

within 1 year. Five-year survival for proximal lesions is 5–15%.

Recurrence of jaundice may indicate anastomotic stenosis, which can be treated by stenting, or tumor recurrence.

Biliary Parasites

✧ *Ascaris lumbricoides* – patients present with biliary colic, pancreatitis, cholangitis, cholecystitis and eosinophilia. Abdominal plain film may reveal calcified worms and ultrasound can show linear filling defects that move. Treatment is by ERCP and removal of the worms, with laparotomy and removal of worms reserved for endoscopic failure. Antihelmintic therapy kills the worms, but physical removal is still required.

✧ *Clonorchis sinensis* – presentation is with cholangitis and septicemia. This infestation is associated with the development of bile duct carcinoma. Diagnosis is made by finding typical ova in the feces. It is treated by chloroquine 300 mg for 2–6 months, but relapse is common. The bile ducts must be cleared of worms and stones (surgically if endoscopic methods fail).

The Pancreas

Located in the retroperitoneum, the pancreas is a glandular organ that serves both endocrine and exocrine functions. While in close proximity to the stomach, duodenum, small bowel, large bowel, spleen, kidneys, portal vein, and vena cava, the pancreas shares an important anatomic feature with the hepatic and biliary systems, in that the common bile duct runs through the pancreatic head and meets the pancreatic duct at the ampulla of Vater. The organ is notoriously prone to inflammation and tumor formation.

Tumors in the head of the pancreas and lesions of the body and tail of the pancreas present with very different symptoms and signs. Lesions in the head of the pancreas tend to obstruct the common bile duct and present with obstructive jaundice, while lesions affecting the body and tail of the gland have a more insidious presentation with weight loss and pain as their primary symptoms.

Lesions of the exocrine pancreas produce symptoms and signs of malabsorption, while lesions of the endocrine pancreas produce a variety of endocrine syndromes (e.g. diabetes mellitus) and a wide range of syndromes associated with autonomous secretion of pancreatic and enteric hormones (e.g. insulinoma, gastrinoma, glugaconoma, pancreatic polypeptide-producing tumors [PPPoma]).

Inflammation of the gland is known as pancreatitis. Acute pancreatitis may be severe and life-threatening. Chronic pancreatitis can run a remitting and relapsing course with gradual destruction of the whole gland.

Assessment of Pancreatic Disorders

Pancreatic History

Start by taking a general GI history. When responses indicate a possible pancreatic problem, a more detailed pancreatic history is required.

✧ *Pain*: Site, severity, radiation, exacerbating and relieving factors.

✧ *Jaundice*: General questions regarding the etiology of jaundice (*see* page 161). Is the jaundice painless?

✧ *Endocrine function*: Symptoms attributable to diabetes mellitus or, if indicated, symptoms associated with rare disorders (e.g. insulinoma, Zollinger–Ellison).

✧ *Exocrine function*: Symptoms of weight loss and malabsorption, fat intolerance, frequent foul-smelling greasy stools that are difficult to flush away (floaters).

✧ *Etiologic factors for pancreatitis*: Gallstones, previous biliary surgery or interventions, alcohol intake, hyperlipidemia, hypercalcemia, medications.

✧ *Effect on other organs*: Symptoms attributable to liver failure, biliary obstruction, portal hypertension and hypersplenism, gastric outlet obstruction.

Pancreatic Examination
✧ Perform a general examination, with particular attention to signs of weight loss, anemia, jaundice, and evidence of liver disease.
✧ Patients may have an upper abdominal mass, liver and spleen enlargement, and/or portal hypertension.
✧ In some instances, the gall bladder may be palpable.

Examination of Pancreatic Disorders
The methods of investigation include imaging, assessments of endocrine and exocrine function, analysis of serum markers of pancreatic disease, and pancreatic biopsy for cytology/histology.

Diagnostics
Hematology
✧ *CBC* – the patient may have anemia due to hemobilia or chronic disease. Leukopenia and thrombocytopenia may indicate hypersplenism secondary to splenic vein thrombosis.
✧ *Coagulation* – the presence of liver disease may have concurrent increase in INR.

Serum Biochemistry
✧ *LFTs* – may reveal a cholestatic situation with an elevated alkaline phosphatase. Increased bilirubin levels may indicate bile duct obstruction while a raised GGT may indicate alcohol abuse.
✧ *Blood glucose* – high glucose levels may represent diabetes mellitus secondary to a glucagonoma or loss of islet cell function in chronic pancreatitis.
✧ *Serum amylase and lipase* – amylase levels are particularly useful in the acute setting for the diagnosis of acute pancreatitis; in late-stage chronic pancreatitis, it is unlikely to be elevated. A raised serum amylase level may be a marker of pancreatic trauma. Serum lipase is more sensitive and specific in the diagnosis of acute pancreatitis, but may not be routinely available.

Exocrine Function
✧ *Fecal fat excretion* – stool examination for fat is only useful for diagnosing malabsorption. However, 80% of pancreatic secreting capacity may be lost without detection by the test.
✧ *Direct measurement* – direct measurement of pancreatic, digestive, and secretory function is mainly used as a research tool, but is the best test for diagnosis of pancreatic exocrine insufficiency. The concentration of bicarbonate and pancreatic enzymes are measured in duodenal juice after stimulation by a meal (Lundh test) or injection of secretin/cholecystokinin (secretin-pancreozymin test).
✧ *Fecal elastase* – easy to perform. Absence of elastase in feces indicates exocrine insufficiency.
  ∝ *Results* – written report.
  ∝ *Advantages* – provides a direct measurement of pancreatic exocrine function.
  ∝ *Disadvantages* – invasive, expensive, and may not be universally available.

Endocrine Function
✧ *Fasting levels* – for the measurement of glucose and/or hormones secreted by islets: insulin, proinsulin, C-peptide, glucagon, somatostatin, and gastrin.
✧ *Provocative tests* – to measure hormone levels if fasting levels are not conclusive. For example, calcium perfusion of insulinomas and gastrinomas at angiography can cause a spurt of hormone release.
   ∝ *Results* – written report.
   ∝ *Advantages* – direct information regarding the level of hormones often provides the diagnosis.
   ∝ *Disadvantages* – specialized tests often not routinely available.
✧ *Tumor markers* – include CEA and CA 19-9.

Imaging Techniques
Indirect Imaging
✧ *CXR* – a plain film of the chest may occasionally demonstrate a pancreatic pseudocyst in the posterior mediastinum.
✧ *AXR* – an abdominal plain film may visualize the effect of the pancreas on the adjacent organs (e.g. the colon cut-off sign may indicate displacement, stricture, fistula of the transverse colon). Calcification usually indicates chronic pancreatitis, though occasionally radiating sunburst calcification may be seen in cystadenoma or cystadenocarcinoma.
✧ *Small bowel contrast series* – may show effacement or hypertrophy of folds in cases of malabsorption secondary to chronic pancreatitis. Enlargement of the pancreatic head may cause widening of the C-loop of the duodenum and/or displacement of the angle of Treitz (e.g. in cases of advanced pancreatic carcinoma). Contrast studies may also reveal post-bulbar duodenal ulceration which is characteristic of Zollinger–Ellison syndrome.

Direct Imaging
✧ Direct imaging of pancreatic parenchyma is provided by ultrasound, CT, and MRI.
✧ ERCP images the pancreatic duct system.
✧ Angiography visualizes the pancreatic and peripancreatic vasculature.
✧ MRCP and endoscopic ultrasound (EUS) are being increasingly used in the analysis of the pancreas.

Ultrasound
✧ *Technique* – acoustic water-based gel is applied to the abdomen and an ultrasound probe manipulated over the critical area by the sonographer.
✧ *Results* – written report compiled by radiologist. Occasionally, a selection of ultrasound photographs may be included.
✧ *Advantages* – ultrasound is a non-invasive technique that does not utilize ionizing radiation. Indicators of pancreatic disease include diffuse or localized atrophy, alteration of texture, dilated bile duct; abnormal dilatation of the pancreatic duct may be the result of cancer or chronic pancreatitis. EUS is an excellent modalitiy for studying chronic pancreatitis and endocrine tumors.
✧ *Disadvantages* – ultrasound quality is notoriously operator dependent. The non-visualization rate is 10–15%. Only 50% of changes caused by chronic pancreatitis are detected by traditional ultrasound. Due to the nature of the technique, visualization of internal organs is poor in obese individuals and when gaseous distension of the bowel is present.

Computerized Tomography

✧ *Technique* – X-rays are used to obtain multiple cross-sectional slices of the patient which are then reconstructed by a computer to produce the images. Intravenous contrast can be given to outline the vessels; oral contrast agents can be given to outline the GI tract. Modern multi-slice spiral CT scans can be performed within seconds using thin slices, yielding higher detail and allowing more sophisticated reconstructions.

✧ *Results* – written report by the radiologist and a selection of still CT images.

✧ *Advantages* – multi-slice helical CT scanners can now examine the pancreas with 5 mm slices and, when combined with contrast, arterial, and venous phase images, can give detailed pancreatic anatomy. CT produces better visualization of the gland than ultrasound, especially in the presence of ascites or abdominal obesity. CT is better at the detection of calcification, gas, dilatation, small intrapancreatic pseudocysts, and thick-walled pancreatic abscesses. The most valuable data accumulated is the presence of localized or diffuse enlargement of the pancreas.

✧ *Disadvantages* – uses ionizing radiation. IV contrast can be allergenic and can induce acute kidney damage. Can be expensive and time-consuming.

Endoscopic Retrograde Cholangiopancreatography (ERCP)

✧ *Technique* – a large-bore side-viewing endoscope is passed into the second part of the duodenum. The duodenal papilla is cannulated and contrast injected under fluoroscopy. The pancreatic and biliary system is visualized. Brushings or biopsies can be performed to provide a tissue diagnosis. Stents can also be placed during the procedure.

✧ *Results* – written report and a selection of ERCP images.

✧ *Advantages* – ERCP facilitates the diagnosis of a wide range of pancreatic conditions and allows for the collection of direct tissue samples and the placement of stents to treat obstructions. It is particularly useful in the diagnosis of ductal calculi, tumors of bile duct and pancreas, and sclerosing cholangitis.

✧ *Disadvantages* – a well-known complication of ERCP is pancreatitis (1%). If sphincterotomy is also performed, the complication rate rises to 6–10%. These include hemorrhage, acute pancreatitis, cholangitis, retroperitoneal perforation, impacted dormia baskets, acute cholecystitis, and gallstone ileus. Technical failure may occur in patients with duodenal stenosis, in those who have undergone a previous Billroth II resection, when duodenal diverticula are present, and when patients are uncooperative. In patients with complete biliary obstruction, the proximal biliary tree may not be visualized; PTC is then indicated.

Angiography

✧ *Technique* – generally, angiography may require admission to the hospital, although some centers do perform same-day or outpatient cases. Under local anesthesia, the femoral artery is cannulated and a catheter is manipulated into the celiac and superior mesenteric arteries. Contrast is injected and radiologic images are taken.

✧ *Results* – written report from the operator and a selection of angiography images.

✧ *Advantages* – angiography defines arterial variability for resection purposes. Other useful findings include arterial encasement, the narrowing or irregularity of a vessel caused by invasion of a tumor. Smooth encasement may be caused by chronic pancreatitis. Major venous involvement may indicate similar disease but is not as reliable a sign.

✧ *Disadvantages* – by its nature, angiography is a highly invasive technique. Common risks include hematoma formation at the puncture site and distal emboli. The technique is being phased out in favor of reconstruction of the vascular anatomy from CT or MR images, and by duplex ultrasound. Angiography still has a role in localizing pancreatic neuroendocrine tumors such as insulinomas using selective calcium stimulation.

Diagnostic Laparoscopy and Intra-operative Ultrasound
✧ *Technique* – laparoscopy enables direct visualization of the intra-abdominal structures. A special intra-operative ultrasound probe is inserted into the abdomen through a port, which enables ultrasound images of the pancreas to be obtained. Biopsy of lesions can be performed under direct vision.
✧ *Results* – direct surgical observations, operative dictation, and a selection of printed ultrasound images.
✧ *Advantages* – direct visualization of the liver may reveal multiple small metastases. Higher-quality ultrasound images of the pancreas can be obtained. Laparoscopy can give valuable information regarding resectability prior to a full laparotomy.
✧ *Disadvantages* – invasive operative procedure, risks associated with general anesthesia.

Disorders of the Pancreas
Congenital Anomalies of the Pancreas
✧ *Ectopic pancreas*: Presents with abdominal pain similar to peptic ulceration. Occasionally causes interference with gastric emptying.
✧ *Annular pancreas*: May present with vomiting with or without bile. Fifty percent of cases present in the newborn, where urgent operation is needed. The other 50% present between the ages of 20 and 70 years, when inflammation of the pancreas leads to symptoms of duodenal constriction.
✧ *Pancreas divisum*: Results from the non-union of the embryonic dorsal and ventral portions of the pancreas. Patients most commonly present with recurrent pancreatitis; occasionally, diagnosis is made after a single episode of pancreatitis which is initially thought to be idiopathic. Diagnosis is by MRCP, in which separation of the main and accessory pancreatic ducts is appreciated. ERCP can be both diagnostic and therapeutic via endoscopic accessory duct sphincteroplasty. Open accessory duct sphincteroplasty can be performed.

Pancreatitis
✧ Acute pancreatitis usually presents with typical epigastric abdominal pain and serum enzyme level elevations.

TABLE 8.4   Risk factors for pancreatitis

Alcoholism
Biliary tract disease (gallstones)
Congenital malformation (pancreas divisum)
Collagen vascular disease
Drugs (thiazides, steroids)
Iatrogenic (ERCP, surgery)
Infections (mumps, coxsackie B, mycoplasma pneumoniae,
   Epstein-Barr, sepsis)
Metabolic (hyperparathyroidism, hyperlipidemia)
Periampullary carcinoma
Trauma

✧ Although pain is a common feature of chronic pancreatitis, it can present with signs of pancreatic endocrine and exocrine insufficiency and little in the way of serum enzyme changes.
✧ Chronic relapsing pancreatitis describes a condition of repeated attacks of acute pancreatitis, usually resulting in gradual destruction of the gland.
✧ Risk factors for pancreatitis are listed in Table 8.4.

Acute Pancreatitis
Acute attacks are treated on an inpatient basis. After resolution and discharge from the hospital, patients are followed up in the outpatient office.

Objectives
The outpatient consultation has three main objectives:
1. Determine the underlying cause of the pancreatitis.
2. Arrange treatment of the underlying cause to prevent further attacks.
3. Detect any complications of pancreatitis (e.g. pseudocyst, pancreatic abscess).

Often, the underlying cause will have been identified during the inpatient hospitalization, but the outpatient visit gives an opportunity to review the history to identify any other significant factors; for example, gallstones and heavy alcohol consumption may coexist.
  Strategies for assessing and addressing the major causes of pancreatitis include:
1. *Alcoholism*: Get an estimate of the patient's weekly alcohol consumption (truthful or untruthful), detect the smell of alcohol on breath (or alternately, smell of strong mints), obtain GGT levels, and urine or serum ethanol levels. Some patients may respond to explanation, but there is often a need for referral to a psychiatrist with interest in alcohol addiction.
2. *Biliary tract disease*: Review ultrasound results if the patient received a scan during the inpatient treatment. Arrange intervention if indicated (e.g. laparoscopic cholecystectomy). In cases of previous pancreatitis, some assessment of the common bile duct is mandatory to exclude ductal stones even in the face of normal common bile duct diameter and LFTs; this may involve the use of MRCP, ERCP with or without sphincterotomy, or intra-operative cholangiography.
3. *Trauma*: Consider repeat imaging (ultrasound and/or CT) after the acute inflammation has subsided to determine whether trauma has resulted in distortion of the biliary system that can lead to long-term problems or will require long-term follow-up. LFTs should be monitored. MRCP with or without secretin will determine if there is duct disruption. ERCP may also give similar information; however, it is invasive and may have been the cause of the trauma in the first place.
4. *Drugs*: Review the history, physical examination and diagnostic findings to confirm that pancreatitis can be ascribed to this cause. Repeat tests if there is any doubt. Arrange for these drugs to be avoided or at least administered under close medical supervision in future.
5. *Metabolic disorders*: Assess serum calcium levels, serum parathyroid hormone levels, and fasting serum lipids. Treat as appropriate.
6. *Infections*: Review the history, examination and investigation findings. Viral titers often need to be repeated 4–6 weeks after the acute episode to provide a diagnosis.
7. ERCP can be utilized to assess for other major causes, such as pancreas divisum and periampullary carcinoma. At ERCP, biliary manometry can also be performed to exclude SOD and sample bile to exclude bile crystals (microlithiasis) as a cause of pancreatitis.

Diagnostics and Imaging

CT scan is the best modality for evaluation of a patient with pancreatitis. Acute elevations in amylase and lipase are diagnostic; treatment is determined not on the level of these enzymes but rather on symptoms of pain and infection. The most sensitive method is a lipase greater than three times normal values.

Treatment

Management is generally expectant, with inpatient admission, IV fluid administration, nil per mouth and bowel rest. Antibiotic usage is only appropriate in those cases with documented or suspected infection. The etiology must be determined and treatment of it provided.

If surgery is needed, such as in gallstone disease, it should be performed once the pain has resolved and the bile duct has been shown to be free of stones either by resolution in lab abnormality or by MRCP/ERCP.

Complications of Acute Pancreatitis

Any patient who has a persistence or reappearance of the inflammatory manifestations of acute pancreatitis must be suspected of having developed a pancreatic pseudocyst or a pancreatic abscess. Other local complications of pancreatitis include hemorrhage, peptic ulceration and erosions, left-sided portal hypertension and variceal hemorrhage, and vascular complications. These complications generally occur at the time of an episode of acute pancreatitis and must be treated at the time of the acute illness. Pseudocysts may exist for longer periods of time.

Pancreatic Pseudocyst

Pseudocysts are thought to arise secondary to pancreatic duct disruption and leakage. These are not considered true cysts, in that they lack an endothelial lining.

Objectives

Diagnose pseudocyst, differentiate those suitable for conservative therapy from those that require urgent treatment, monitor for the development of complications, treat pseudocyst.

History and Physical Examination

✧ Recurrence of pain, nausea and vomiting, anorexia, weight loss.
✧ Patients may manifest with a tender upper abdomen or a tender mass. Many are asymptomatic.

Diagnostics and Imaging

Leukocytosis and hyperamylasemia may be present.

Ultrasound or CT scan is diagnostic. Air within a pseudocyst suggests an abscess. Ultrasound may also detect splenic artery aneurysm and portal hypertension. In chronic or recurrent pseudocysts, an ERCP will exclude pancreatic duct stenosis as an etiologic factor.

Treatment

✧ *Acute pseudocyst*: Manage expectantly for 4–6 weeks. Spontaneous resolution is known to occur commonly; surgical therapy is also more effective if the cyst wall has been given time to mature.
✧ *Chronic pseudocysts*: Usually asymptomatic; no recent attack of pancreatitis can be identified on interview, but there may be a history of blunt abdominal trauma.

Spontaneous resolution is rare and there is a high risk of complications if treatment is delayed (e.g. hemorrhage due to erosion of major vessels, rupture, infection, and local mass effects).

Other factors for consideration in the treatment of pseudocysts are:
1. Size: Spontaneous resolution is more likely to occur with smaller pseudocysts compared with larger ones. Generally, pseudocysts smaller than 4 cm may be observed, whereas those larger than 4 cm may require endoscopic or surgical drainage.
2. Development of symptoms suggesting compression of adjacent organs or indicative of an impending complication such as rupture, hemorrhage, or infection.
3. Maturity: Pancreatic pseudocysts generally take 4–6 weeks to stabilize an adequately thick cyst wall.
4. Vascular complications: CT angiography or intra-arterial angiography have identified a subgroup of patients that develop vascular complications associated with acute pancreatitis, including pseudoaneurysms and left-sided portal hypertension from splenic vein thrombosis. Presence of a pseudoaneurysm is rare and treatment is usually angiography and embolization; if this fails, open exploration and exclusion of the aneurysm or pancreatic resection should be performed, rather than internal drainage of a pseudocyst. Presence of portal hypertension may be an indication for splenectomy with or without gastric devascularization if there have been repeated gastric fundal variceal bleeds which have failed endoscopic treatment.
5. Location: Pseudocysts located anteriorly that communicate with the primary duct respond to posterior cystgastrostomy, whereas those found in the head of pancreas close to the duodenum can be drained by cystojejunostomy or possibly cystoduodenostomy. Large pseudocysts bulging into the transverse mesocolon can be addressed using a Roux-en-Y loop to create a cystojejunostomy. Those in the tail or body of the pancreas may require a distal pancreatectomy or longitudinal pancreaticojejunostomy.

Infected or ruptured pseudocysts or acute pseudocysts with thin friable walls are best drained externally with wide-bore drains. In many instances, the resulting pancreatic fistula will spontaneously close, albeit gradually. Occasionally, a second procedure is needed to implant the fistulous tract into a Roux-en-Y loop of jejunum.

Percutaneous Drainage of a Pseudocyst
Percutaneous drainage is the optimal treatment for infected pseudocysts or cysts that are very large in the setting of an acute episode of pancreatitis. If a patient has pseudocysts on CT scan, they should be left alone. If there is concern for infection, as depicted by recurrent fevers, FNA may be performed and if the culture or the Gram stain are positive, then percutaneous drainage is indicated. Open surgical drainage is a last resort.

Prior to drainage, an MRCP or ERCP is required to delineate pancreatic duct anatomy. If the pseudocyst does not connect with the pancreatic duct, then external drainage can be considered. If the pseudocyst connects with the pancreatic duct, then drainage must be internal. Pseudocysts can also be drained by percutaneous cystogastrotomy or via EUS-guided stenting of the pseudocyst into the stomach or duodenum.

Surgical Drainage of a Pseudocyst
Lesser sac pseudocysts can be drained via a posterior cystogastrostomy. Pancreatic head or uncinate process pseudocysts should be drained into the duodenum. Pseudocysts bulging through the transverse mesocolon can be drained by a cystojejunostomy.

Surgical intervention should also address the gall bladder if it has been identified as the original cause of the patient's pancreatitis.

Follow-up
Review with ultrasound scans to ensure that pseudocysts being managed conservatively are resolving. If there is no resolution after 6 weeks, consider surgical or radiologic intervention if the pseudocysts are large or symptomatic.

Post-operative Follow-up
Review within 4 weeks after surgery and at regular intervals (3–6 monthly) thereafter. Determine the success of the operation and detect any complications. Review histology of the pseudocyst wall to exclude a neoplastic cyst. If symptoms are persistent, repeat abdominal ultrasound to confirm that the pseudocyst is resolving (cysts can still re-occur despite surgery).

Complications include those of laparotomy and general anesthesia. More specific complications depend on the procedure performed. Persistent leakage of fluid from a wound or drain site may indicate a pancreatic fistula; send fluid for amylase concentration, which is expected to be very high if derived from a pancreatic fistula. Pancreatic fistulas require admission for further assessment and treatment. Other complications include gastric outlet or small bowel obstruction related to the surgical procedure.

Pancreatic Abscess
Pancreatic abscesses are caused by extensive pancreatic and peripancreatic necrosis followed by the formation of a peripancreatic fluid collection that gets secondarily infected, usually by *E. coli*, enterococci, or fungi. Abscesses usually develop after the second week of acute pancreatitis; they carry a high morbidity and mortality. Occasionally, an infected pseudocyst may lead to an abscess.

Objectives
Diagnose pancreatic abscess, differentiate from pseudocyst, treat abscess.

History
Pancreatic abscesses usually become apparent 2–5 weeks after an attack of pancreatitis as the attack appears to be resolving. The patient often complains of increasing fever, abdominal pain, and tenderness.

Physical Examination
✧ Perform a general examination.
✧ Patients with a pancreatic abscess will look unwell with evidence of sepsis.
✧ An abdominal mass may be palpable.

Diagnostics and Imaging
CBC will reflect leukocytosis. Serum biochemistry will reveal hyperamylasemia. Blood cultures are usually negative in the early stages.

Abdominal plain film shows the "soap bubble" appearance of a retroperitoneal abscess in fewer than 20% of cases. Ultrasound or CT is usually diagnostic; CT may show air in the pancreas or may detect areas of low attenuation with contrast, suggesting necrosis.

Treatment

✧ *Surgical*: Retroperitoneal debridement and drainage. This may result in an open abdomen for daily packing.

✧ *Interventional*: Percutaneous drainage with wide-bore drains. Two drains can be placed side-by-side for irrigation and drainage. A sample of aspirate should be sent for amylase and microbiology, and appropriated antibiotics should be started. The interventional approach requires follow-up scans and drain adjustments with or without further drainage.

Follow-up

Affected patients are usually hospitalized for long periods until they recover from the acute episode. Possible long-term consequences of pancreatic debridement are endocrine and exocrine deficiency, for which insulin and pancreatic enzyme supplements may be necessary, and pancreatic fistulae.

Recurrent Pancreatitis

In patients who have experienced more than one attack of acute pancreatitis, further investigation is needed to determine the etiology. If the cause is unclear, consider rarer causes of recurrent pancreatitis, such as:

✧ *Stenosis of the sphincter of Oddi*: This phenomenon may occur due to fibrosis after passage of a stone. Diagnosis is made by ERCP and it is treated by sphincterotomy. If this fails or recurs, operative sphincteroplasty can be performed.

✧ *Pancreas divisum*: Due to failure of the pancreas to form properly during development, the duct of Wirsung is very small; thus, the duct of Santorini becomes the major ductal system but retains a small papilla, creating a relative stenosis predisposing to pancreatitis. Divisum is found in 3–4% of the population but in approximately 12% of patients with idiopathic pancreatitis. The relationship between pancreas divisum and pancreatitis is unclear and surgical treatment carries a poor prognosis. Diagnosis is made at ERCP, when pancreatic stenting may alleviate symptoms. Accessory duct sphincteroplasty can be performed at ERCP or during surgery if relief has been obtained after a trial of pancreatic stenting.

✧ *Biliary microlithiasis*: Biliary crystals can be seen at EUS or on microscopy of bile samples taken at ERCP. Treatment involves cholecystectomy and/or endoscopic sphincterotomy.

Chronic Pancreatitis and Chronic Relapsing Pancreatitis

These conditions may present with frequent attacks of pancreatitis requiring admission to hospital, or may be insidious in onset with increasing pancreatic insufficiency. Unlike acute pancreatitis, gallstones are thought to be an uncommon etiologic factor. Rather, alcohol is the primary causative factor in 60–70% cases, with no cause found in 30–40%. Rare causes such as pancreas divisum, neoplasia, trauma, cystic fibrosis, and radiotherapy are responsible for the rest. Family history is very important; in younger patients with a strong family history, suspect familial pancreatitis.

Objectives

Diagnose chronic pancreatitis, exclude pancreatic cancer, identify underlying etiologic factor, detect pancreatic insufficiency, treat pancreatitis, treat etiologic factor, treat pancreatic insufficiency.

History

Patients may complain of repeated bouts of upper abdominal pain, which may or may not be related to alcohol ingestion. The pain may radiate to the back or tip of the scapula and is constant and dull. Patients will report avoiding lying on their back as this makes the pain worse. Initially, pain is intermittent and episodic, but then progresses to constant pain.

On interview, the patient may admit to stools which are pale, bulky, oily, or difficult to flush away. Symptoms due to the onset of diabetes mellitus are unusual in the early stages. Patients may give a history of weight loss due to exocrine insufficiency and/or anorexia and nausea. Jaundice may be caused by biliary duct obstruction or inflammation and fibrosis in the head of the pancreas. Similarly, signs and symptoms of gastric outlet obstruction may result from an inflammatory mass in the head of pancreas. Hematemesis may be reported due to esophageal varices.

Physical Examination

✧ Perform a general examination. Look for evidence of weight loss, malnutrition, jaundice, and/or the stigmata of liver disease. Erythema ab igne from frequent application of a hot water bottle is often seen.
✧ Examination may be normal, but make sure to check for a palpable epigastric mass representing an inflamed, fibrosed pancreas or a pseudocyst.
✧ Rupture of a pseudocyst may produce ascites.
✧ Splenomegaly usually indicates splenic vein thrombosis.

Diagnostics and Imaging

Due to long-term damage to the pancreas, serum amylase may be normal. LFTs may indicate cholestasis. Blood glucose may be abnormal due to loss of islet cells in the pancreas, as may clotting. CBC may reveal leukopenia and thrombocytopenia secondary to hypersplenism. Fecal elastase will identify exocrine insufficiency.

Ultrasound and CT can identify features suggestive of chronic pancreatitis and detect complications such as a dilated biliary tract and splenic vein thrombosis. MRCP can delineate biliary and pancreatic duct anatomy. EUS can be used to obtain tissue for histology and to exclude a neoplasm.

Treatment

✧ *Medical*: Control pain and treat endocrine and exocrine insufficiencies. Address any drug or alcohol addiction.
  ∝ *Pain* – usually requires opiates; tailor medication and dosage to patient. NSAIDs may increase the risk of gastrointestinal hemorrhage. Celiac plexus blocks can be performed via EUS and can reduce opiate requirements, but is prone to recurrence of symptoms over time.
  ∝ *Exocrine insufficiency* – medications utilizing enteric coated microspheres prevent deactivation in the stomach and allow a normal fat intake, which is important for the maintenance of weight and correction of malnutrition. Fat-soluble vitamin supplements (A, D, E, K) are necessary.
  ∝ *Endocrine insufficiency* – diabetic control is usually obtained with oral hypoglycemics, but insulin may be necessary. Glucose control can be difficult in the presence of variable food intake due to the pain induced by eating. Therefore, careful monitoring is required.
✧ *Surgical*: Operations are considered mainly for the relief of pain; no surgical procedure can restore endocrine or exocrine function. Rehabilitation must be planned in advance, and there must be absolute avoidance of alcohol.

Indications for Surgery

✧ Intractable pain: Disruption to the patient's life, increasing requirement for narcotics needed to control the pain. Control of alcoholism, age and general condition of patient must be considered prior to surgery.

✧ Development of complications:

  ∝ Lower bile duct obstruction – ERCP to exclude other causes and cancer. Relief of obstruction may relieve the pain.

  ∝ Duodenal obstruction – rare in chronic pancreatitis. Exclude cancer by biopsy. Treat non-cancerous cases by gastrojejunostomy.

  ∝ Vascular involvement – pseudoaneurysms and portal hypertension.

  ∝ Pancreatic cysts, pseudocysts, abscesses, pancreatic ascites, and pleural effusions.

  ∝ Presence of a dominant mass leading to suspicion of cancer.

  ∝ Portal vein compression/mesenteric vein thrombosis.

  ∝ Pancreatic duct stricture with upstream dilatation with or without pancreatic duct stones.

  ∝ Colonic stricture.

✧ Therapy by location:

  ∝ Isolated pancreatic stricture – treated at ERCP, or if this fails and there is upstream duct dilatation, longitudinal pancreatico-jejunostomy.

  ∝ Pancreatic head mass – pylorus-preserving pancratico-duodenectomy, standard Whipple, or Beger's operation (duodenum-sparing pancreatic head resection – considered only if absolutely sure the lesion is not malignant).

  ∝ Inflammation restricted to the body and tail of the gland may be treated by distal pancreatectomy.

  ∝ Rare cases of whole-gland disease may be treated by total pancreatectomy with or without islet cell autotransplantation, depending on pre-operative endocrine testing.

✧ Open celiac plexus block can be combined with open procedures.

Follow-up

Arrange follow-up at short intervals (2–4 weeks) until pancreatic neoplasia is excluded. Afterward, proceed to long-term follow-up at regular intervals to monitor pain control, endocrine and exocrine insufficiency and abstinence from alcohol. Monitor weight and nutritional status, including vitamin deficiencies.

Post-operative Follow-up

Assess the patient for the success of the operation to relieve pain (approximately 70% of patients) and for the development of complications, both expected (endocrine and exocrine insufficiency) and unexpected (pancreatic fistula, small bowel obstruction). Follow-up is long term for detecting and managing endocrine and exocrine insufficiency. Gradually increase intervals as the patient stabilizes (1–6 months).

Neoplasms of the Exocrine Pancreas
Benign

Benign tumors of the pancreas are rare and are seldom of clinical significance unless they become very large and impinge on adjacent structures (CBD, duodenum, stomach, or main pancreatic duct). These include adenomas, cystadenomas, lipomas, fibromas, leiomyofibromas, myomas, hemangiomas, lymphangiomas, hemangioendotheliomas, and neuromas. These lesions usually need resection to confirm benign nature.

Pancreatic Cancer

Pancreatic ductal adenocarcinoma constitutes 80–90% of all primary malignant tumors arising from the gland and accounts for 10% of all cancers of the digestive tract. When cancer arises in the pancreatic head (70%), it must be differentiated from cancer arising in the ampulla, duodenum, or lower CBD, all of which have a much better prognosis than true pancreatic adenocarcinoma. The rare mucinous cystic neoplasms (mucinous cystadenoma/adenocarcinoma) have a good prognosis if completely resected.

Risk factors: Pancreatic cancer is more common in older people. It has an increased incidence in smokers, diabetics, alcoholics, and in patients affected by hereditary pancreatitis.

Cancer: Head of the Pancreas
History
The term "periampullary" does not differentiate between carcinomas of the duodenum, pancreas, common bile duct, or ampulla, but all of these tumors present with similar symptoms.

Jaundice presents in 90% of affected patients and is classically described as "painless," although abdominal pain can be present in up to 70% of cases. Severe pain radiating to the back is a sinister symptom suggestive of retroperitoneal tumor infiltration. Weight loss and anorexia is common even in the early stages. Nausea and vomiting, epigastric bloating, and change of bowel habits may be reported. Hematemesis and melena occur in late cases due to direct invasion of the mucosa or portal hypertension secondary to portal vein compression by the tumor. Chills and fever due to cholangitis can occur. Duodenal cancer can present with iron-deficiency anemia caused by occult GI bleeding or symptoms of gastric outlet obstruction. Fluctuating jaundice is a characteristic of ampullary tumors, as are silver stools representing steatorrhea combined with GI blood loss.

Physical Examination
✧ Perform a general examination.
✧ Examination may be normal; jaundice and a palpable gall bladder (Courvoisier's sign) are present in 25% of patients.
✧ The liver is enlarged on palpation in up to 80% of patients at presentation.

Cancer: Body and Tail of the Pancreas
History
There is pain and weight loss. Jaundice is uncommon and may indicate involvement of the porta hepatis. Pain is usually vague and dull, felt in the epigastrium or back; it can be episodic and related to meals, or constant and severe. Partial relief of pain may be obtained by flexing the trunk forward. Severe pain may indicate extension of the tumor into perineural tissues, lymphatics, and the posterior retroperitoneum. Weight loss may be severe and rapid. Early satiety and food aversion is common. Hematemesis and melena may occur.

Physical Examination
There may be evidence of weight loss, but otherwise examination is generally normal. Occasionally, there may be migratory thrombophlebitis (Trousseau's sign) indicating advanced cancer.

Early cases have few signs. Late signs are an abdominal mass or the stigmata of liver metastases. A rectal shelf may be evident on rectal examination in the rectovesical/vaginal pouch. Other late signs include ascites and enlarged lymph nodes in the supraclavicular fossa.

Diagnostics and Imaging

Ninety percent of patients are diagnosed in late stages. Always suspect pancreatic cancer in patients with seemingly recent symptoms, absent physical signs, and negative routine X-ray investigations.

CBC may reveal iron deficiency anemia. Blood glucose may detect diabetes mellitus or impaired glucose tolerance in 15% of patients. LFTs may indicate a cholestatic picture. Fecal elastase test may be abnormal.

Ultrasound is a good initial imaging technique and can usually identify a pancreatic mass, bile duct dilatation, liver metastases, ascites, extrapancreatic spread, and portal hypertension. Contrast-enhanced CT is the gold standard for diagnosis and accurate staging of the disease. ERCP enables biopsy for cytology and may be necessary to decompress the biliary tree. Alternatively, percutaneous needle biopsy under ultrasound/CT control for diagnosis in potentially incurable cases avoids a diagnostic laparotomy. In cases where this is not possible, a laparoscopic biopsy is less invasive than an open operation.

Markers for pancreatic cancer (e.g. Ca-19-9 and CEA) may be elevated and may fall to normal after resection, providing a means of monitoring recurrence if levels rise again.

Pancreatitis can coexist with all cancers and gallstones may be present – the occurrence of one does not exclude the other. Truly representative needle biopsies of the pancreas are often hard to obtain because of sampling error and confusion between tumor and associated pancreatitis.

Staging

✧ The main objective of staging is to detect unresectable disease, including tumors displaying vascular invasion (portal vein, SMA, celiac or hepatic artery) and metastases to the liver, peritoneal cavity, celiac nodes, or beyond. These can usually be detected by CT.

✧ Tumors larger than 3 cm, invasion of contiguous organs like the duodenum or colon, and enlarged lymph nodes within the resection field are not contraindications to surgery.

✧ EUS can provide detailed assessment of vascular involvement and, when combined with biopsy, can give histologic diagnosis.

✧ Staging laparoscopy can exclude liver and peritoneal metastases and, when combined with intra-operative ultrasound, can give further accurate staging.

Treatment

✧ *Pre-operative preparation*: Optimize the patient by ensuring a good state of nutrition and hydration supplemented with intravenous fluids, elemental diet, and multivitamins. Correct any clotting deficiency with vitamin K or FFP. If the serum bilirubin is high (>200 µmol/L), or in the presence of sepsis, hepatorenal failure, severe cardiopulmonary disease expected to respond to medical management, or severe malnutrition, a temporary percutaneous or transhepatic biliary decompression should be considered.

✧ *Exclusions for surgery*: Unresectable disease, very elderly or frail patients with multiple systemic disorders, or a life expectancy of less than 3 years.

✧ *Surgery*: For tumors of the head of the pancreas, duodenum, ampulla, and lower bile duct, Whipple pancreatico-duodenectomy, pylorus-preserving pancreatico-duodenectomy (PPPD), or total pancreatectomy. However, if the rest of the gland is severely affected by pancreatitis, total pancreatectomy may be the better option. If frozen section confirms cancer at the resection margin, a total pancreatectomy may occasionally be necessary. A suspected cancer of the body and tail is treated by a distal pancreatectomy with or without splenectomy.

✧ *Palliation*: If the cancer is unresectable or metastatic disease is found, a palliative biliary and gastric bypass can be performed if indicated.
- ∝ Relief of jaundice, pruritus, or impending cholangitis – ERCP/PTC and biliary stenting (metal stent if unresectable) or hepaticojejunostomy.
- ∝ Relief of duodenal obstruction – endoscopic or interventional stenting or open/laparoscopic gastrojejunostomy.
- ∝ Relief of pain – celiac plexus block. External beam radiotherapy.
- ∝ Unfit for surgery – ERCP sphincterotomy and biliary stent.

Post-operative Follow-up

Review the case to determine the success of the operation and to detect any complications. Review the pathology to determine whether the resection margins are clear of tumor.

Examine for the usual complications of a laparotomy and general anesthesia. Small bowel obstruction may be due to recurrent tumor or adhesions – laparotomy is indicated to establish the diagnosis and relieve obstruction. Biliary obstruction may be due to tumor recurrence or anastomotic stricture. Exclude endocrine and exocrine pancreatic insufficiency.

✧ *Monitoring for recurrence* – all patients should be referred for adjuvant chemotherapy following surgery. Single-agent gemcitabine has a survival benefit versus no chemotherapy. Patients with locally advanced disease may have a response to combination chemoradiotherapy, whereas patients with metastatic disease should be offered palliative chemotherapy. Tracking tumor marker levels (CA 19-9 or CEA) post-operatively may detect recurrence.
✧ *Management of pancreatic endocrine insufficiency* – insulin.
✧ *Management of pancreatic exocrine insufficiency* – pancreatic enzyme supplements, vitamins, and antibiotics.
✧ *Stent blockage* – indicated by recurrent jaundice and cholangitis. Perform ERCP and stent change.
✧ *Prognosis* – operative mortality is 1–5% in high-volume centers. Five-year survival is 10–25% for pancreatic ductal adenocarcinoma, 40–50% for ampullary carcinoma and distal cholangiocarcinoma, and higher for mucinous cystic neoplasms and neuroendocrine tumors. Most mortality occurs from 2 months to 2 years.

Lesions of the Endocrine Pancreas

Endocrine cancers are relatively slow-growing and many metastasize only to regional lymph nodes; this allows surgical cure in a sizeable proportion of patients.

Insulinoma

Hyperinsulinemia results in symptomatic hypoglycemia. It is caused by B-cell neoplasia (insulinoma) or, rarely, B-cell hyperplasia/microadenomatosis. In adults, 80% of insulinomas are benign solitary tumors, 10% are multiple and are part of the multiple endocrine neoplasia (MEN) 1 syndrome, and 10% are malignant. There is an even distribution of tumors in the head, body, and tail of the pancreas.

Differential Diagnosis

Brain tumor, epilepsy, alcoholism and drug abuse, fibrosarcoma and non-pancreatic tumors, glucocorticoid deficiency, diffuse liver disease, and factitious hyperinsulinemia due to insulin abuse.

Objectives
Diagnose cause, differentiate from other causes, localize tumor, treat hypoglycemia, treat tumor.

History and Physical Examination
Symptoms include weakness, sweating, hunger, palpitations, and trembling, and new neurologic findings. The median time from onset of symptoms to diagnosis is 2 years due to the rareness of the diagnosis and the non-specific nature of the symptoms.

Determine the relationship of symptoms to exercise and food; hypoglycemia may occur after fasting or soon after eating (reactive hypoglycemia). Fasting hypoglycemia is more typical of an insulinoma; reactive hypoglycemia occurring after meals is seen more commonly in alimentary disorders (e.g. post-gastrectomy). Examination may be normal.

Diagnostics and Imaging
To make a definitive diagnosis, measure simultaneous insulin and glucose levels at the time of hypoglycemia. A diagnostic inpatient 72-hour fast will detect all cases. Other causes of hypoglycemia, such as fibrosarcoma and non-pancreatic tumors, glucocorticoid deficiency, and diffuse liver disease, will not be associated with an elevated insulin level. Occasionally, provocative tests to induce hypoglycemia are needed, but these are second-line tests.

A positive diagnosis is based on three elements:
1. The recognition of the probable nature of a patient's symptoms.
2. The presence of Whipple's triad:
    - ∝ Hypoglycemic symptoms
    - ∝ Hypoglycemia documented during symptomatic episodes
    - ∝ Symptoms relieved by glucose intake.
3. Demonstration that plasma insulin concentration is inappropriately high for the existing levels of plasma glucose. An insulin (iu/mL) to glucose (mg/dL) ratio of greater than 0.3 indicates insulinoma.

Pre-operative Localization
Seventy-five percent of tumors are less than 1.5 cm and are not visible or palpable. EUS is particularly useful for endocrine tumors of the pancreas. Angiography is the most reliable localizing investigation, especially when combined with a calcium stimulation test. CT detects less than 60% of tumors; MRI may be more reliable.

If imaging is negative, selective venous sampling for insulin is necessary. However, at laparotomy, a complete examination of the whole gland is needed, including the use of intra-operative ultrasound to exclude multiple tumors.

Treatment
- ✧ *Benign disease*: Simple enucleation, Whipple's operation, or distal pancreatectomy, depending on the size and location of the lesion. Caution is advised in enucleating lesions close to the main pancreatic duct, as a pancreatic leak or fistula may develop.
- ✧ *Multifocal malignant disease*: Total pancreatectomy may be required; 95% of patients are cured, though 5–10% experience recurrent hypoglycemia requiring re-operation. Surgical mortality is less than 5%.
- ✧ *Medical therapy*:
    - ∝ Diazoxide – control of pre-operative hypoglycemia; needs careful monitoring.
    - ∝ Octreotide – infusion or long-acting depot preparation.
    - ∝ Streptozotocin – for metastatic insulinoma.

Follow-up
Follow-up is at short intervals (1–4 weeks) until diagnosis is achieved. Consider admission to the hospital for monitoring and treatment of hypoglycemia.

Post-operative Follow-up
Determine the success of the operation by the relief of symptoms. Check pathology to confirm complete excision. Long-term follow-up is required for management of pancreatic insufficiency.

Gastrinoma (Zollinger–Ellison Syndrome)
Gastrinomas frequently manifest with Zollinger–Ellison syndrome (ZE), consisting of intractable peptic ulceration caused by excess gastrin secretion. Twenty-five percent of patients with gastrinomas will have MEN 1; 60–90% of gastrinomas are malignant and 50–80% will have lymph node metastases at presentation; 66% of gastrinomas are located in the "gastrinoma triangle," which is defined by the junction of the cystic duct and CBD, the junction of the second and third portions of the duodenum, and the junction of the neck and body of the pancreas. These tumors are more often multiple than solitary.

Objectives
Diagnose gastrinoma, differentiate from other causes of recurrent ulceration, localize gastrinoma, treat gastrinoma, screen for MEN 1.

History and Physical Examination
While patients may present with symptoms of dyspepsia and/or severe diarrhea (5–7%), usually over the course of several years, physical examination is frequently normal.

ZE should be suspected in any patient with:
- ✧ Peptic ulcer disease refractory to treatment.
- ✧ Multiple ulcers or ulcers in unusual locations (distal duodenum or jejunum).
- ✧ Peptic ulcer disease with diarrhea.
- ✧ Ulcer recurrence after operation.
- ✧ Strong family history of MEN 1 or other features of MEN (e.g. hypercalcemia).

Diagnostics and Imaging
- ✧ *EGD* – perform to document the ulceration.
- ✧ *Gastric acid* – determine basal gastric acid output; evidence of acid hypersecretion, such as a basal level of more than 15 mmol/L, suggests gastrinoma. As a corollary, normal basal acid levels makes ZE unlikely.
- ✧ *Gastrin* – in patients with high basal acid levels, measure fasting serum gastrin levels. Gastrinoma is characterized by a basal gastrin level greater than 100 pg/L in the presence of acid hypersecretion. Note that this level must be measured without PPI medication, as they will increase gastrin levels. Levels greater than 500 pg/mL are almost diagnostic of gastrinoma, and levels from 100–500 pg/mL are highly suggestive. Basal gastrin levels are also raised in pernicious anemia, atrophic gastritis, and gastric cancer, but these conditions are not associated with acid hypersecretion. Conditions associated with both elevations in gastrin levels and acid hypersecretion include gastrinoma, retained gastric antrum after Billroth II, antral G-cell hyperplasia, and gastric outlet obstruction. Gastrinoma can be differentiated from these conditions by the secretin stimulation test. After injection of secretin, gastrin levels rise to over 200 pg/mL in gastrinoma patients only.

✧ Once gastrinoma is diagnosed, MEN syndrome needs to be excluded: serum calcium, phosphate and plasma prolactin levels need to be measured.

✧ *Tumor localization* – most gastrinomas can be localized by CT. However, tumors less than 7 mm are not detectable. MRI may improve visualization. Angiography is not useful, as gastrinomas are hypovascular. EUS is useful where available. Somatostatin receptor scintography (octreotide scan) can be positive in up to 80% of patients. Direct visualization can be conducted via exploratory laparotomy with intra-operative ultrasound and EGD to detect duodenal wall tumors by transillumination.

Treatment
Surgery
Patients with pre-operatively identified liver metastases or MEN 1 are treated medically with the control of ulceration by omeprazole. In the absence of liver metastases or MEN 1, medical therapy is used for 6–12 months; young and fit patients then undergo surgical exploration, after initial stabilization on medical therapy.

At operation, complete tumor resection is performed if feasible. However, if complete removal is impossible, the tumor should be grossly debulked, and medical therapy reintroduced post-operatively and continued for as long as symptoms are controlled; if medical therapy fails again, rarely, a total gastrectomy may be considered.

For patients in whom total tumor removal was performed, basal and stimulated gastrin levels are measured at intervals post-operatively. If gastrin levels are still elevated, medical therapy is reintroduced and gastrectomy is considered for poorly controlled patients.

Old or poor-risk patients are continued on medical therapy for as long as symptoms are controlled. If, at any stage, medical treatment ceases to be effective, the patients are explored surgically for the tumor. The tumor is resected if possible; otherwise a total gastrectomy is performed.

Palliation
In patients with liver metastases and advanced disease, the therapeutical modality is chemotherapy. Octreotide is used to control symptoms. Liver resection may be undertaken in carefully selected cases.

MEN 1
In cases of MEN 1, perform the parathyroid surgery first; this may relieve symptoms completely. However, this effect is often only temporary, and thus the patient should continue to be followed up in the clinic and should proceed to gastrinoma treatment if symptoms recur.

Post-operative Follow-up
Long term surveillance is needed as recurrences may manifest late. Successful removal of all gastrin-secreting tumor needs to be confirmed by serially negative plasma gastrin responses to secretin stimulation.

Vasoactive Intestinal Peptide Tumor (VIPoma)
The primary lesion in this exceedingly rare tumor is in the pancreas in 80% of cases; ganglioneuromas and neuroblastomas in the remaining 20%.

History and Physical Examination
VIPomas are characterized clinically with watery diarrhea. Examination may otherwise be normal.

Diagnostics and Imaging
Diagnosis is made by appreciating increased VIP levels, hypokalemia, achlorhydria and acidosis. The neoplasm is usually solitary and large, and can be detected by ultrasound, CT, or angiography.

Treatment
Initial interventions are usually medical, namely resuscitation with intravenous fluids and octreotide. Therapeutic options include surgical excision, debulking, and medical treatment. Metastatic disease is treated by chemotherapy.

Follow-up
Follow-up is long-term to detect recurrence and deterioration in condition.

Glucagonoma
A rare endocrine neoplasm arising in the A cells of islets. Seventy to eighty percent are malignant, with up to 50% of cases having already metastasized at the time of presentation.

History and Physical Examination
Glucagonomas are associated with a characteristic skin rash: necrolytic migrating erythema. Patients may also report weight loss, symptoms of diabetes mellitus, deep-venous thromboses (DVTs), anemia, hypoaminoacidemia, glossitis, and cheilitis. Diagnosis of the disease is based on the recognition of necrolytic migrating erythema in combination with diabetes mellitus in the setting of a chronic wasting disorder.

Diagnostics and Imaging
Glucagon levels exceed 1000 pg/mL. Other conditions associated with increased glucagon levels include diabetes, chronic renal failure, shock states (e.g. myocardial infarction, septicemia, burns), acute pancreatitis, cirrhosis, familial hyperglucagonemia, and exercise.
　　The tumors are usually large, thus ultrasound and CT are generally reliable.

Treatment
Treatment is topical steroids for the skin rash and intravenous amino acids. Octreotide is good at controlling symptoms in the pre-operative period and as chemical palliation. Ultimately, surgical excision is the primary therapeutic modality; debulking may be effective in symptom relief. If surgery is not an option, then treatment should consist of selective arterial embolization and chemotherapy.

Follow-up
Follow-up is long-term to detect recurrence or deterioration in clinical condition.

Multiple Endocrine Neoplasia 1
MEN 1 is an autosomal dominant familial disorder of the *MEN 1* gene characterized by the development of synchronous and metachronous endocrine and non-endocrine tumors, but with considerable phenotypic variability. The parathyroid glands are involved in 90% of cases and the majority of lesions consist of hyperplasia. Pancreatic islets (30–75%) are inevitably involved, and the most common pancreatic tumor is gastrinoma. Pancreatic tumors are usually multiple. Pituitary tumors are usually prolactinomas, with growth hormone tumors the second most frequently encountered (10–60%). Other occasionally associated tumors are adrenocortical lesions (25%), thyroid nodules, bronchial and intestinal carcinoids, and lipomas.

Diagnostics and Imaging

All patients with endocrine pancreatic tumors should be tested for serum calcium and phosphate levels, and have plasma assays of parathyroid hormone, insulin, gastrin, glucagon, somatostatin, pancreatic polypeptide, prolactin, growth hormone, ACTH and cortisol, and chromogranin A.

MRI scans of the pancreas, pituitary, and abdomen should be undertaken. All family members should be screened.

Multiple Endocrine Neoplasia 2

Stemming from a defect in the RET proto-oncogene, MEN 2 is an autosomal dominant familial cancer syndrome characterized by the development of medullary thyroid cancer (90%), pheochromocytoma (50%), and hyperparathyroidism (20–30%) with variable expression.

✧ Type A consists of hyperparathyroidism, medullary carcinoma of the thyroid, and pheochromocytoma, and can be associated with cutaneous lichen planus and Hirschsprung's disease.

✧ Type B is comprised of medullary carcinoma of the thyroid, pheochromocytoma, but a low incidence of parathyroid disease. However, MEN 2B manifests with multiple mucosal neuromas, intestinal ganglioneuromas leading to megacolon and constipation, a Marfanoid habitus, and characteristic facies with thickened lips and alae nasi.

Diagnostics and Screening

Calcitonin, CEA, both urine and serum metanephrine and normetanephrine levels, ionized calcium, and parathyroid hormone.

Questions and Answers

Q1 In which of the following conditions is alpha-fetoprotein not a marker?
  A Cirrhosis.
  B Hepatocellular carcinoma.
  C Biliary obstruction.
  D Pregnancy.
  E Germ cell tumors.

A1 C: All of the above conditions, except for biliary obstruction, can have an elevated alpha-fetoprotein (AFP). The immature liver cells of the fetus make AFP, and when born, babies have very high levels. Chronic liver disease and primary cancers of the liver can have elevated AFP. In hepatocellular carcinoma, only about 60% of patients will have an elevated AFP.

Q2 Which of the following is not associated with portal hypertension?
  A Hypersplenism.
  B Gastrointestinal hemorrhage.
  C Liver rupture.
  D Varices.
  E Ascites.

A2 C: Liver rupture is not associated with portal hypertension. Liver rupture is associated with trauma and some hepatic tumors. The effects of portal hypertension are related to the increased pressures in the portal system and the relative resistance to flow or reversal of flow in the vessels that drain into the portal system.

Q3   What is the condition that describes hepatic vein thrombosis?
- A   Budd–Chiari.
- B   Ehlers–Danlos.
- C   Zollinger–Ellison.
- D   Peutz–Jeghers.
- E   Child–Pugh.

A3   A: Budd–Chiari is the condition where there is obstruction of the hepatic veins. Causes of thrombosis include the use of oral contraceptives in women, ingestion of Bush teas, congenital diaphragm of the vena cava, or congestive right heart failure.

Q4   Which of the following is the least optimal treatment option for hepatocellular carcinoma?
- A   Intravenous chemotherapy.
- B   Liver transplant.
- C   Transarterial chemoembolization (TACE).
- D   Liver resection.
- E   Radiofrequency ablation.

A4   A: Intravenous chemotherapy is the least optimal treatment choice for hepatocellular carcinoma. The response rate is very low, and often the side effects of treatment limit the dose of chemotherapy that can be given. The best choice is liver transplant.

Q5   Which of the following is an absolute contraindication to pancreatico-duodenectomy for cancer of the head of the pancreas?
- A   Involvement of the duodenum.
- B   Resectable metastatic lesion to the liver.
- C   Involvement of the superior mesenteric vein.
- D   Biliary stent in place.
- E   Diabetes.

A5   B: If a patient is diagnosed as having a cancer of the head of the pancreas, a metastatic work-up needs to be completed which includes CT or MRI of the chest, abdomen, and pelvis. If there is tumor found in other sites, such as the liver, this needs to be confirmed as malignancy by biopsy. If it were confirmed, then the patient would not benefit from surgical resection. They can be palliated by stenting or bypass, depending on symptoms.

Colon, Rectum, and Anus
Kenneth R. Ziegler and Steven B. Goldin

Conditions affecting the colon, rectum, and anus range from the trivial to the life-threatening. The knowledge of these conditions among the public is complicated by embarrassment and folklore. Many patients seen in the outpatient surgical setting are concerned about the intimate nature of the examinations which they are likely to undergo, and require careful reassurance. Certain groups of patients become very preoccupied with the maintenance of a "regular bowel habit" and attend if there is any variation in what they perceive as normal; while reluctance to attend can result in others, who seek medical attention only when symptoms are severe and tumors may be advanced.

In addition to these difficulties, colorectal cancer is one of the most common malignancies in the United States and can mimic the presentation of nearly all other colorectal and anal disorders. The priority of investigation for many patients is to exclude colorectal malignancy, but the necessary tests are often unpleasant, invasive, and their application to all patients with colorectal symptoms would be impractical. However, the diagnosis must always be kept in mind, especially if minor conditions do not respond to treatment.

It is this combination of factors that make the assessment of colorectal disorders particularly difficult. After introductions and putting the patient at ease, it is important to ascertain what they are hoping for from their visit as, for many, tests to exclude malignancy are sufficient to satisfy patients who are then content to manage their own symptoms with simple advice.

Assessment of Colorectal Disorders
Colorectal History
This should include a basic history of the whole gastrointestinal (GI) tract, including questions about non-specific features such as malaise, weight loss, and vomiting. When the responses indicate a possible colorectal problem, a more detailed colorectal history is required.

Abdominal symptoms include pain (site, periodicity, aggravating factors, and nature: constant or colicky), distension or borborygmi (noisy bowels). Ask about any medications, in particular the long-term use of laxatives or antidiarrheal drugs. Ask about urgency, tenesmus, flatulence, incomplete evacuation, and weight loss. A history of recent exotic travel may be relevant, and a careful family history with particular attention to colitis, polyposis syndromes, and colorectal cancer is essential.

✧ *Abdominal pain*: Typically, abdominal pain in colonic disorders is colicky. Visceral midgut pain is generally felt in the periumbilical region, while hindgut pain tends to lead to suprapubic discomfort. The left iliac fossa is a common site for pain and this may be associated with diverticular disease, although other diagnoses are not excluded. Colicky colonic pain may equally be a feature of benign irritable bowel syndrome (IBS) or a stenosing carcinoma of the colon. Constant pain may indicate a complication of diverticular disease (e.g. localized or free perforation, abscess) or advanced bowel cancer with nerve involvement.

✧ *Alteration in bowel habit*: There is a wide variety of bowel habits which may be considered normal, but a change may be an important symptom of colorectal disease. Changes can suggest bowel cancer, and time should be taken to identify the previous bowel habit, the new bowel habit, the timing of the change, and the presence of constipation or diarrhea. Inquire about the consistency and frequency of stool and whether this is associated with the passage of blood or slime (mucous).

◇ *Rectal bleeding*: If rectal bleeding is part of the history, ask about the timing, any previous episodes of rectal bleeding, whether the bleeding is bright red, dripping into the toilet as in hemorrhoids, or mixed in the motion as with inflammatory bowel disease (IBD) or malignancy. Is the bleeding painful, as with an anal fissure, or painless? Does bleeding only occur at defecation or at times in between? Ask about the amount of blood, although patients commonly overestimate this. Does it drip into the toilet? Are there dark clots (suggests bleeding higher in the colon), or is there just a smear on the toilet paper? Note that the history is not totally reliable in excluding a cancer of the bowel which can present with any type of rectal bleeding.

◇ *Anal and perineal symptoms*: These include pruritus (itching), pain and its relation to defecation, discharge, and bleeding.

◇ *Prolapse*: Something "comes down" at defecation or on straining or coughing. These lumps may reduce spontaneously or require manual reduction.

◇ *Incontinence*: Ask about timing and severity – incontinence to flatus, liquid stool, solid stool. Inquire regarding urgency, tenesmus, flatulence, incomplete evacuation. A history of previous anal surgery or trauma is important, and in female patients, a careful obstetric history is essential, noting the number and nature of previous deliveries, obstructed and prolonged labor, instrument delivery and obstetric tears, or the need for episiotomy.

Colorectal Examination

General examination may reveal anemia associated with neoplasia or IBD. Dermoid cysts are associated with Gardner's syndrome, acanthosis nigricans and dermatomyositis with neoplasia, and pyoderma gangrenosum, arthropathy, uveitis, and finger clubbing with inflammatory bowel disease. Examination of the GI tract begins with the mouth, which may reveal oral Crohn's disease or the perioral pigmentation associated with Peutz–Jegher's syndrome.

Abdominal Examination

◇ Inspect the supine abdomen for stomas, scars associated with previous colorectal surgery and evidence of distension, visible peristalsis, a mass or other organomegaly.

◇ Palpation may reveal tenderness or a palpable sigmoid colon which is a common and normal finding, especially in constipation.

◇ Neoplasm or diverticular disease may be associated with a bowel mass.

◇ The liver may be enlarged due to secondary spread from a bowel neoplasm.

Rectal Examination

Explain the procedure to the patient, the justification for it, and obtain verbal consent. Place the patient in the left lateral position with the knees flexed as far as possible into the abdomen. Cover the patient's legs with a blanket to minimize exposure.

On inspection, look for evidence of pruritus ani, perianal warts, perianal abscess, perianal hematoma, prolapsing hemorrhoids, thrombosed hemorrhoids, skin tags, anal fistulas, anal fissures (and the frequently associated "sentinal tag"), anal cancer, rectal prolapse, fecal soiling of the perineum. Ask the patient to bear down as if defecating – look for abnormal perineal descent, eversion of the anus, prolapsing hemorrhoids, and other protruding lesions such as rectal prolapse or neoplasm.

The pulp of a gloved lubricated index finger is used to palpate for the thickened cord of a fistula track or other abnormalities around the anus. The finger is then pressed onto the anus until the sphincter relaxes and the finger is then slid into the rectum. Significant pain at this point may indicate an anal fissure, and the examination may have to be deferred until less painful following treatment of the fissure; or, if diagnostic concern is present, then examination should be performed under anesthesia.

Note the state of the resting anal tone, which largely reflects the condition of the internal anal sphincter. Ask the patient to contract the anus (examining the "squeeze pressure" provided by the external sphincter and hooking the finger over the puborectalis muscle. This indicates the uppermost limit of the external sphincters and can be used as a landmark to determine the position of lesions, e.g. lesions above this indicate supra-levator disease.

The rectum should be assessed in relation to three parts: the lumen and contents, the rectal wall, and structures outside the rectum. Note the contents of the rectum and the consistency of the feces. Consider the rectum in quadrants (front, back, left, right) and palpate each one in turn. Note the position of any abnormality in relation to a clock-face where the anterior wall is considered 12 o'clock and posterior 6 o'clock (as if the patient is viewed in the lithotomy position).

Withdraw the finger and inspect it for blood, mucus, pus, and the nature of the feces.

Extraintestinal Signs of Inflammatory Bowel Disease
There are various eye and skin signs which should be identified on examination in relation to Crohn's disease and ulcerative colitis.

✧ *Ophthalmic signs*: Generally seen in active disease and more common in Crohn's than ulcerative colitis.
  ∝ *Episcleritis* – redness and soreness of the eye similar to conjunctivitis, the most common ophthalmic manifestation of IBD.
  ∝ *Iritis* and *uveitis* – less common, associated with reduced visual acuity and a painful red eye.
✧ *Cutaneous signs*:
  ∝ *Erythema nodosum* – painful, raised red lesions often on the shins, most frequently associated with Crohn's disease, affecting 15% of sufferers. Mirrors disease activity, and biopsy shows subcutaneous septal panniculitis with neutrophil infiltrate.
  ∝ *Pyoderma gangrenosum* – affects around 2% of those with IBD, especially Crohn's colitis. Lesions are deep ulcers with a necrotic base and an undermined purple edge. They characteristically occur on the lower limbs and can be single or multiple, but are also seen around stomas and surgical scars. Histology reveals a neutrophilic dermatitis.

Examination of Colorectal Disorders
Laboratory Examinations
Blood Tests
✧ *Hematology* – complete blood count (CBC) for iron-deficiency anemia, white blood-cell count (WBC), and differential. Plasma viscosity, erythrocyte sedimentation rate.
✧ *Serum biochemistry* – liver function tests (LFTs) to test for metastases. Thyroid function tests may be useful in the assessment of constipation and diarrhea. C-reactive protein (CRP) for inflammatory conditions including colitis.
✧ *Immunology* – alpha-fetoprotein (AFP) and carcinoembryonic antigen (CEA) may be raised in colonic neoplasms.

Fecal Tests
✧ *Fecal occult blood test (FOBT)* – this guaiac-based test for peroxidise activity can be performed at home by the patient. The patient smears a fecal sample onto a

pre-prepared card, which is then returned to the laboratory where the presence of blood can be detected. The presence of blood can occur in normal individuals, but may be an indicator of GI pathology and a consistent finding requires further investigation. A simple and quick screening test, sensitivity is 50–70% and about two thirds of tumors are thought to bleed in the course of a week. False-positives caused by exogenous hemoglobin sources (e.g. ingestion of animal hemoglobin, nosebleeds) and dietary restrictions are required for 2 days prior to testing. False-negatives occur due to intermittent bleeding by the tumor. The test is of no use in patients with obvious rectal bleeding.

✧ *Microbiology* – in patients with diarrhea, potential infectious causes should be excluded by stool culture. Fresh fecal samples are required and, if parasites are suspected, these samples should be transported immediately to the laboratory for examination. Toxins produced by *Clostridium difficile* may be identified in patients with pseudomembranous colitis.

Imaging
Proctoscopy
A rectal examination is performed prior to insertion of the proctoscope.

The technique consists of the insertion of either a metal or a disposable plastic rigid tube fitted with a fiber-optic light source for inspection of the distal rectum and anus. The proctoscope is lubricated with water-soluble gel and inserted with the central obturator in place until the rectum has been entered; the obturator is then removed. The rectal mucosa is inspected as the instrument is slowly withdrawn. The patient is asked to bear down to demonstrate prolapsing mucosa and hemorrhoids.

This short instrument gives a good view of the distal rectum and anal canal and is particularly useful for the diagnosis of hemorrhoids. However, only the distal rectum can be observed. Injection or banding of the hemorrhoids can be performed through the proctoscope. Notably, the procedure may be unpleasant for the patient.

Rigid Sigmoidoscopy
A rectal examination is performed prior to insertion.

The sigmoidoscope is a rigid tube made of metal or disposable plastic with a removable central obturator. The longer length of the sigmoidoscope compared with the proctoscope enables more of the rectum and lower sigmoid colon to be inspected, although in practice only the distal two thirds of the rectum can frequently be assessed. In addition to a fiber-optic light source, there is also a connection for air insufflation using a rubber bulb.

The sigmoidoscope is inserted for a few centimeters through the anus, with anterior angulation of the scope being required to negotiate the 90-degree anorectal junction. The obturator is removed and the scope window secured to provide an airtight seal. The rectal ampulla is inspected and the lumen of the bowel identified. Air is introduced via a rubber bulb to open up the lumen ahead; the patient should be warned that air is being introduced and they may feel the need to pass flatus, but to try to retain the air if they can. The instrument is only advanced when the lumen ahead is visible.

More of the rectum and lower sigmoid can be inspected. The procedure can usually be performed in the outpatient setting without bowel preparation, although a phosphate enema can be administered if necessary. Biopsies can be taken from abnormal lesions; however, care should be taken when sampling mucosal lesions above 10 cm because of the risk of perforation, especially if the bowel is inflamed. There is a risk of bowel perforation if rigid sigmoidoscopy is not performed gently. The technique can be quite uncomfortable for the patient, especially if too much air is introduced.

Flexible Sigmoidoscopy

A 60 cm flexible fiber-optic sigmoidoscope is introduced via the anus and is frequently capable of evaluating the colonic mucosa as far as the splenic flexure. It is usually performed as an outpatient procedure involving bowel preparation with phosphate enema just prior to the examination. The steerable nature of the scopes enables the turns of the sigmoid colon to be negotiated. Air insufflation is used to open up the lumen ahead; the scope is advanced when the lumen is visible.

Approximately 70% of colorectal carcinomas are within reach of the flexible scope. Biopsies can be performed and polyps excised. Bowel preparation (with an enema) is necessary. Equipment is expensive and needs careful cleaning and maintenance. Not all of the colon is able to be inspected.

Colonoscopy

Similar to flexible sigmoidoscopy, colonoscopy involves a longer flexible fiber-optic scope that allows the whole of the colon to be inspected successfully by experienced operators in 90% of cases. Formal bowel preparation is required in the days prior to the procedure, using laxatives; intravenous sedation (usually with benzodiazepines and opiates) is used for the procedure itself, as it may be uncomfortable for the patient. Patients who are sedated should be warned not to drive or operate machinery for 24 hours after the procedure.

The scope is steerable and air insufflation is used. The whole colon can be visualized and biopsies taken for tissue diagnosis. However, the technique is very much operator dependent and one must trust the opinion of the operator who makes the report. Therapeutic procedures such as polypectomy can be performed. The major risks that colonoscopy patients should be warned about include colonic perforation in 0.1% (rising to 0.3–4% following biopsy/polypectomy) and hemorrhage rates quoted at 0.03% following diagnostic colonoscopy and 1.9% after polypectomy.

Double-contrast Barium Enema

Barium contrast is infused through a catheter into the rectum. The balloon on the catheter is inflated to prevent leakage. The patient is placed on a tilt table which is maneuvered through different positions to coat the whole bowel in barium. Air is insufflated after evacuation of most of the barium, to finely coat the bowel wall with barium and provide mucosal detail.

This procedure provides fine mucosal detail as well as visualizing gross anatomy and fistulas not easily visible on colonoscopy. However, it involves a significant dose of X-rays, bowel preparation is required, and rates of colonic perforation between 0.01 and 0.04% are reported.

Abdominal Ultrasound

Ultrasound is a useful non-invasive technique for the investigation of abdominal pain to detect pathology in visceral organs, although its ability to detect colonic pathology is somewhat limited. Pre-operatively it can be used to detect liver metastases in patients with colorectal cancer, although its accuracy in this respect is considered inferior to that afforded by computed tomography (CT). Ultrasound can also be used intra-operatively for the same purpose. It is highly operator dependent, and thus may be poor at defining bowel pathology.

Endoanal/Transrectal Ultrasound

A specially designed lubricated rotating probe, confined within a fluid-filled sheath to maintain tissue contact, is inserted into the rectum. Alternating bright and dark rings represent the anal sphincters and layers of the bowel wall; sphincter defects and the relationship of tumors or fistula tracks to the muscles can be assessed.

Transrectal ultrasound is a specialized technique, but in the centers where it is used it has proved useful in determining the local spread of rectal cancers and in the assessment of perianal fistulas and anal sphincters. As an ultrasound modality, its utility is operator dependent; it can be uncomfortable for the patient and may occasionally need to be performed under anesthesia.

Computed Tomography
CT can provide an accurate definition of anatomy. It is particularly useful for defining the extent of local spread of tumors and for investigating potential metastatic deposits. CT is commonly used to diagnose and assess for complications of diverticular disease. While it has become convenient, especially at large centers, it remains expensive and is associated with high doses of radiation. Equivalent information can often be obtained by other means with lower radiation exposure.

Magnetic Resonance Imaging (MRI)
MRI detects minute quantities of energy released by hydrogen ions when forced to change direction by a strong magnetic field. The resulting data provides detailed information useful in assessing the nature and extent of complicated perianal and other fistulas, and aids in the investigation of complicated anorectal sepsis. Reconstructions in multiple planes are possible, allowing excellent anatomical detail. MRI can be particularly useful in the assessment of rectal tumor encroachment on the mesorectal fascia, which can help to select those who would benefit from pre-operative radiotherapy.

Although expensive and time-consuming, MRI does not require exposure to ionizing radiation. Some patients find the experience intolerable, describing the scanner as noisy and claustrophobic.

Examination Under Anesthesia (EUA)
EUA may be useful for patients with very painful anal conditions preventing adequate examination and diagnosis in the outpatient setting, or in cancer to assess rectal resectability.

Diagnostic Laparoscopy
Although the technique is not as widespread as the practice of "staging laparoscopy" in the assessment of upper GI malignancies, it can potentially be used for the evaluation of a number of pathologies, including the appraisal of liver metastases when combined with intra-operative ultrasound.

Physiological Examinations
✧ *Anal manometry* – an air/water-filled balloon pressure-measuring system is inserted into the rectum. The pressure inside the rectum is recorded during different conditions. The maximum resting pressure reflects function of the internal sphincter, while the maximum squeeze pressure indicates function of the external sphincter. Pressures decrease with age and are commonly reduced in incontinence.
✧ *Rectal compliance* – a balloon is inflated in the rectum and the volume and pressure is recorded at first sensation and the maximum amounts tolerated. Compliance is decreased in IBD but increased in patients with chronic constipation used to harboring large volumes of stool in the rectum.
✧ *Electromyography* – fine electrodes are inserted into the anal sphincter muscles to

identify damage to the sphincters, although this is generally now regarded as a research tool rather than a clinical study.

✧ *Pudendal nerve latency* – this measurement is taken using a disposable electrode attached to a gloved finger. The nerve is stimulated as it crosses the ischial spine, and the time required for the impulse to travel to the sphincter is recorded. Prolonged latency is associated with fecal incontinence, rectal prolapse, solitary rectal ulcer syndrome, severe constipation, and sphincter defects.

✧ *The rectoanal reflex* – the normal reflex consists of an inhibition of sphincter contraction in response to inflation of a balloon in the rectum. The loss of this reflex is almost diagnostic of Hirshsprung's disease, but may also be absent in patients with rectal prolapse and incontinence if resting pressures are already low.

✧ *Anal sensation* – this is assessed in relation to a thermal or electrical stimulus applied to the anal mucosa. Reduced sensation may be an important factor in patients with incontinence, especially if they have had previous anal surgery.

✧ *Defecating proctogram* – barium suspension is infused into the rectum and the patients are recorded as they void this suspension. This simulates defecation and is useful for demonstrating abnormal anorectal angles in patients with pelvic floor weakness or prolapse, rectoceles, or for visualizing the function of ileoanal pouches. In patients with anismus or obstructed defecation, the acute anorectal angle may be maintained during attempted defecation due to paradoxical contraction of the external sphincter complex, and this can be demonstrated by the defecating proctogram.

✧ *Colonic transit time* – the patient ingests special radio-opaque markers, which can be followed by serial abdominal X-rays. Eighty percent of the markers should have cleared the bowel within 5 days for the study to be considered normal. This technique may be used to diagnose slow transit constipation.

Disorders of the Colon and Rectum
Rectal Bleeding
The majority of cases of rectal bleeding presenting to the outpatient surgical office are due to minor anorectal conditions, which are easily diagnosed and treated. However, these minor conditions may coexist with other, more serious, pathologies such as colorectal cancer. Thus, more serious causes of rectal bleeding should be excluded in middle-aged or older patients and in patients of any age where the symptoms fail to settle despite adequate treatment.

The causes of rectal bleeding, in decreasing order of incidence, include:
1. Benign anorectal disease:
    ∝ Hemorrhoids
    ∝ Anal fissure
    ∝ Fistula-in-ano
    ∝ Rectal prolapse
    ∝ Rectal varices
    ∝ Solitary rectal ulcer.
2. Diverticular disease.
3. Inflammatory bowel disease and colitis:
    ∝ Crohn's disease
    ∝ Ulcerative colitis
    ∝ Infective colitis
    ∝ Ischemic colitis.
4. Neoplasia:
    ∝ Benign polyps

      $\propto$ Adenocarcinoma.
5. Coagulopathy.
6. Arteriovenous malformation.
7. Radiation proctitis/enteritis.
8. Profuse upper gastrointestinal bleeding/small bowel bleeding, including gastroduodenal ulceration, jejunoileal diverticulae and Meckel's diverticulum.

History

Take a general colorectal history and anorectal history. Determine the type of bleeding, the timing, and the amount of blood. Determine whether the blood is separate from the stool or mixed into the feces. Is the blood bright red or dark? Is there pain associated with the passage of blood?

◇ *Hemorrhoids* are associated with bright red rectal bleeding. The blood is usually sepa-rate from the stool or coating it, located on toilet paper, or dripping into the toilet. Bleeding is usually painless and may be associated with prolapsing hemorrhoids.

◇ *Anal fissure* is associated with a smear of bright red blood on the paper and pain on defecation.

◇ *Rectal prolapse* is associated with serosanguinous discharge in addition to the prolapse.

◇ *Tumors* vary in their presentation depending on the site of the tumor and the rate of bleeding. Tumors near the anus tend to present with bright red bleeding similar to hemorrhoids. Proximal tumors may present with dark red bleeding, while cecal tumors may be insidious and only present with iron-deficiency anemia.

◇ *Inflammatory bowel disease* is associated with frequent, loose, bloody stools and the presence of mucus in more severe cases. Systemic disturbance, abdominal pain, malaise, and weight loss may also be features. In IBD, blood is usually mixed in with the stool, which may be loose or watery.

◇ *Diverticular disease or angiodysplasia* may present with a history of episodes of large amounts of brisk rectal bleeding or the passage of a large, dark red stool. This bleeding usually stops and stools return to normal before the next episode.

◇ *Ischemic colitis* is associated with left-sided abdominal pain and bloodstained diarrhea in elderly patients with evidence of atherosclerosis or previous aortic aneurysm repair.

◇ *Radiation proctitis* is associated with a history of radiotherapy, possibly following resection of a rectal carcinoma.

Physical Examination

Perform a general colorectal and anorectal examination. Examine for the presence of anemia and all causes outlined above.

Diagnostics and Imaging

CBC to detect anemia, inflammatory markers including erythrocyte sedimentation rate (ESR) and C-reactive protein, and stool cultures in the case of bloody diarrhea. Perform proctoscopy and rigid sigmoidoscopy in all patients. If indicated to exclude carcinoma or other underlying pathology, proceed to colonoscopy or flexible sigmoidoscopy and a barium enema to look for more proximal colonic lesions. Selective mesenteric angiogra-phy may be useful for identifying abnormal collections of blood vessels associated with angiodysplasia, but is more useful in identifying actively bleeding lesions in the acute situation where rates of bleeding of 0.5–1.0 mL/min can be detected. Bleeding as slow as 0.1mL/min can be detected by using radiolabeled red-cell scans.

Treatment

In young patients with hemorrhoids and no other suspicious features in the history, it may be justified to treat the minor anorectal condition and review at 4–6 weeks to assess whether the bleeding stops. If the symptoms are persistent, or there are any features in the history suggestive of malignancy, then direct visualization of the colon should be done early. Treat underlying causes as appropriate.

Follow-up

Following exclusion of serious underlying pathology, patients can be followed at 6-week intervals until the cause of the bleeding has been successfully treated.

Diarrhea

Diarrhea is defined as the passage of more than three loose stools a day or a stool mass greater than 200 g/day. Diarrhea can be classified as acute or chronic, and the causes fall into several groups:

Acute

1. Infectious or toxic diarrhea:
   - ∝ Viral – adenovirus, Norwalk, rotavirus
   - ∝ Bacterial – *Campylobacter, Escherichia coli, Shigella*
   - ∝ Toxins – *Clostridium difficile, Staphylococcus* spp
   - ∝ Parasites – *Entamoeba, Giardia.*
2. Drugs: angiotenin-converting enyzme (ACE) inhibitors, antibiotics, digoxin, fluoxetine, lithium, metformin, non-steroidal anti-inflammatory drugs (NSAIDs), proton-pump inhibitors (PPIs), ranitidine, statins, 5-aminosalicylate (5-ASA), alcohol, cocaine.
3. Ischemic colitis.
4. IBD.

Chronic

1. Infection: *Giardia, Campylobacter, Salmonella.*
2. Drugs (see above).
3. Malabsorption: lactose intolerance, chronic pancreatitis, bacterial overgrowth, short gut, celiac disease.
4. IBD: Crohn's disease, ulcerative colitis.
5. Metabolic disease: diabetes mellitus, hyperthyroidism.
6. Neoplasia: bowel cancer, pancreatic cancer, carcinoid, vasoactive intestinal peptide tumor (VIPoma), medullary thyroid cancer, Zollinger–Ellison syndrome (ZE).
7. Functional.
8. IBS.
9. Fecal impaction.
10. Anal sphincter damage.
11. Purgative abuse.

History

Obtain a general colorectal history. Ask about stool frequency and consistency. Ask about the duration of symptoms and associated blood or mucus. Differentiate from incontinence and the passage of frequent, small, hard stools with irritable bowel syndrome. How has the bowel habit changed, and over what period?

A short history may suggest an infectious cause, but may also be the first presentation of inflammatory bowel conditions such as Crohn's disease. Evidence should be sought regarding travel abroad, food poisoning, and diarrhea among other family members or close acquaintances.

✧ *Food poisoning* is usually obvious from the history, and onset within 12 hours suggests a toxic cause (e.g. *S. aureus* toxin, *Bacillus cereus*). *Vibrio parahemolyticus* is responsible for most seafood poisoning and may be associated with vomiting and severe abdominal pain. After 12 hours from ingestion and up to 3 days, *Salmonella enteritis* is the most common cause.

✧ *Viral gastroenteritis* is one of the most common infections of the small bowel and causes vomiting, abdominal pain, and diarrhea. Characteristically, the diarrhea is profuse and watery.

✧ *Bloody diarrhea* usually indicates large bowel infection (e.g. *Shigella* or *Entamoeba histolytica*).

✧ Crohn's disease or ulcerative colitis may be suggested by a positive family history, symptoms lasting longer than 1–2 weeks, or frequent bouts of diarrhea over time. Ask about other symptoms associated with these conditions (e.g. skin rashes, arthritis, iritis).

✧ *Previous surgery* on the stomach or small bowel, such as partial gastrectomy or small bowel resection, predisposes to conditions associated with diarrhea such as dumping syndrome or short gut syndrome.

✧ *Malabsorption* is suggested when chronic diarrhea is not associated with fever or blood in the stools, but is associated with weight loss and signs of nutritional deficiencies. Stools are often described as pale, have an offensive odor, and have oil droplets that float with the stool. Suspect exocrine pancreatic failure in these patients.

Ask about change of bowel habit and a pattern of alternating constipation and diarrhea that would suggest a possible colonic cancer. A long-standing history of alternating constipation and diarrhea associated with left iliac fossa pain in older patients is suggestive of diverticular disease.

Ask about symptoms of hyperthyroidism. Ask about diabetes mellitus – autonomic neuropathy can be associated with diarrhea. Tuberculosis (TB) is a rare cause of diarrhea and may be associated with travel to or from areas where TB is common. Lymphoma may be suggested by a chronic history of weight loss and night sweats.

A drug history is important; in particular, ask about antibiotic therapy and other drugs associated with diarrhea.

Rare causes such as carcinoid may be associated with other symptoms such as severe flushing and recent onset asthma. ZE with gastrinomas usually presents with severe peptic ulceration resistant to treatment.

Physical Examination

✧ Perform a general colorectal examination. Assess hydration and examine for pyrexia.

✧ Perform a rectal examination and proctoscopy/sigmoidoscopy to identify inflammatory mucosa or other lesions, and obtain a stool sample for microbiology. Perform a rectal biopsy for a diagnosis of inflammatory mucosa.

Diagnostics and Imaging

✧ Exclude infection and IBD. Food poisoning can be confirmed by sending stool and food samples for microbiology. If parasites are suspected, the stool sample should be transported to the laboratory immediately for inspection – ask for ova, cysts, and parasites.

✧ Consider rectal biopsy for histology to differentiate IBD from infectious causes of bloody diarrhea (*Shigella, Entamoeba histolytica*) and to differentiate between Crohn's disease and ulcerative colitis.

✧ An abdominal plain film can exclude a dilated colon (e.g. toxic megacolon) in severe ulcerative colitis.

✧ Colonoscopy/barium enema should be performed to exclude carcinoma if indicated. Care should be taken during colonoscopy for acute colitics due to the higher risk of perforation; in patients over the age of 45 with chronic diarrhea, imaging of the entire colon is mandatory to exclude malignancy.

✧ If malabsorption is suspected, perform a fecal fat estimation and if confirmed, investigate further to identify the underlying cause.

✧ Routine blood tests are *Salmonella* titers and amoebic serology if suspected, blood cultures if febrile, CBC, ESR/CRP, thyroid function tests, blood glucose, anti-endomysial or anti-tissue transglutaminase antibodies (for celiac disease), serum albumin, iron studies, folate and vitamin B12 levels.

Treatment

Food poisoning and infective diarrhea can be managed with isolation, fluid resuscitation, and other supportive measures until the episode subsides. Antibiotics are prescribed where indicated for severe infection with *Shigella* or *Campylobacter*. Traveller's diarrhea is most commonly caused by *E. coli* and can be treated with sulfamethoxazole/trimethoprim or ciprofloxacillin.

The management of Crohn's disease and ulcerative colitis, irritable bowel syndrome, colorectal carcinoma, diverticular disease, malabsorption, hyperthyroidism, carcinoid, and ZE will be described later under the relevant sections.

Follow-up

Appointments should be at short intervals until the cause is identified and serious causes excluded. There may be an indication for inpatient management in severe cases to avoid dehydration and facilitate prompt diagnosis.

Constipation

There is a wide range of what would be considered "normal" bowel frequency, from 2–3 times a day to once a week. The Rome III diagnostic criteria for constipation include symptoms that have lasted at least 3 months that began at least 6 months prior to diagnosis. Patients must have at least two of the following complaints with at least one quarter of their bowel movements: straining, lumpy or hard stool, the sensation of incomplete evacuation, the sensation of anorectal obstruction or blockage, or a requirement for manual maneuvers to facilitate defecation. Patients also have less than three bowel movements per week and rarely have loose stool without the use of laxatives. Irritable bowel syndrome should be excluded.

Severe constipation merits clinical consideration, as do a sensation of incomplete defecation and excessive time spent attempting to evacuate the bowels. Symptoms of constipation are said to have a prevalence of 2–28%. Most cases (50–60%) have simple/functional constipation with normal transit times and need no further work-up, as they respond to dietary manipulation and laxatives. Ten to fifteen percent have slow-transit constipation, which often requires long-term laxative use.

Causes of chronic constipation include:

1. Idiopathic slow transit constipation – the colon may be normal or have a variety of physiologic derangements.

2. Colorectal disease – underlying bowel disorder, the most important of which is cancer. Other conditions that can cause constipation are irritable bowel disease, diverticular disease, ischemic colitis, hernias, and volvulus.
3. Anal pathology – anal fissure, anal stenosis, anterior mucosal prolapse, hemorrhoids, descending perineum syndrome, perianal abscess, rectocele, anal cancer.
4. Neuromuscular disease or injury:
    ∝ Peripheral – Hirschsprung's disease, autonomic neuropathy, Chagas disease.
    ∝ Central – cerebrovascular accident, cerebral tumors, Parkinson's disease, meningocele, multiple sclerosis, paraplegia.
    ∝ Muscular – dermatomyositis, systemic sclerosis.
5. Metabolic disease (e.g. diabetes mellitus, hypothyroidism, hypercalcemia).
6. Psychiatric illness, depression, or disability.
7. Gynecologic pathology – large fibroids, ovarian cysts.
8. Drugs (e.g. codeine preparations, morphine, antidepressants, iron, anticholinergics).

History

Take a general colorectal history. Determine what the patient means by "constipation."

Determine the time course of the symptoms; sudden onset, especially in patients over 50 years old, is more suspicious of a serious underlying cause, as are other alarm symptoms including rectal bleeding and weight loss. Ask about the frequency of stool, the amount, and the consistency. The passage of small amounts of hard feces suggests constipation. Pain on passing feces suggests anal pathology.

Ask about a change in bowel habits: Is this a recent problem or has it been going on for years? Ask about abdominal pain and bloating or alternating bouts of diarrhea. Ask about medications. Ask about lifestyle; some work conditions or poor toilet facilities may lead to prolonged avoidance of defecation, which predisposes to constipation. Take an obstetric and gynecologic history to identify possible birth injury from instrumentation or gynecologic pathology associated with constipation (e.g. ovarian cysts). Ask about the other causes of constipation.

Physical Examination

✧ Perform a general examination. Examine for anemia, jaundice, hypothyroidism, and weight loss.
✧ Perform an abdominal examination; palpable masses may be fecal, diverticular, neoplastic, or gynecologic in origin.
✧ Perform a rectal examination and remember to examine for conditions such as fecal impaction, perianal scars, fissures, hemorrhoids, prolapse, and neoplasm. Assess perianal descent (the extent to which the anus descends on bearing down: normally 1–3.5 cm). Excessive descent (>3.5 cm or below the plane of the ischial tuberosities) suggests perineal laxity and can lead to the sensation of incomplete evacuation and/ or mucosal prolapse.

Diagnostics and Imaging

Proctoscopy, sigmoidoscopy, and abdominal plain film (dilated colon and fecal masses) should be performed on everybody. Patients with loss of haustral patterns or megacolon/ megarectum on X-ray are unlikely to respond to simple laxatives and further investigation is indicated. Gross structural abnormalities and colonic strictures can be excluded using a double-contrast barium enema. Colonoscopy should be reserved for those in whom colorectal cancer or inflammatory bowel disease need exclusion (alarm symptoms, sudden onset after 50 years of age, or a significant family history of colorectal neoplasia or IBD).

✧ Urea and electrolytes including calcium, blood glucose and, if indicated, thyroid function tests. Parathyroid hormone and serum porphyrins for metabolic and endocrine causes are performed where indicated.

✧ Colonic transit time studies are useful for those with normal-diameter colons and persistent symptoms.

✧ Anorectal physiology and electromyography of the puborectalis and the external anal sphincter are useful for suspected abnormalities of the defecation mechanism.

✧ Full-thickness rectal biopsy under general anesthesia is performed to exclude adult Hirshsprung's disease (absent anorectal reflex on anal manometry). Samples are sent fresh for immediate acetylcholine analysis.

Treatment

Older patients or patients who present with sudden-onset constipation need urgent investigation, including barium enema or colonoscopy, to exclude underlying cancer or other serious pathology. In younger patients with no other suspicious clinical features, or older patients where serious underlying pathology has been excluded, more time is available for assessment and trial of therapies.

Education regarding diet and exercise and what constitutes a normal bowel habit should be instituted. If the problem is simply straining at hard stools without abdominal or anal pain, simple advice regarding increasing fiber in the diet removes the need for further assessment unless the condition fails to respond. Increasing the amount of fiber in the diet may require a dietitian referral. Lactulose softens hard stools; senna increases bowel contractility to help expel the stool (take care in long-term use). Glycerin suppositories and oil enemas are useful to soften hard stool impacted in the rectum. Phosphate enemas can be useful to clear more stubborn stool extending into the sigmoid colon.

In those with established defecatory disorders, biofeedback may be useful; when established intractable constipation is present, an initial purge with potent osmotic laxatives may be required, followed by regular high doses of more gentle osmotic laxatives with or without stimulant laxatives. Care should be exercised, especially in the elderly who may require inpatient treatment and an intravenous drip.

Laxatives are unlikely to be effective if the haustral pattern of the colon has been lost or there is megacolon or megarectum. In these patients, anorectal manometry is useful to identify underlying disorders such as Hirschsprung's disease. Patients who have an absent rectosphincteric reflex and evidence of megacolon or megarectum should undergo a full thickness rectal biopsy to exclude Hirschsprung's disease.

Patients with severe idiopathic constipation should undergo colonic transit studies and anorectal physiology studies, as there are a number of abnormalities of defecation that can be diagnosed, including an increased anorectal angle caused by abnormal contraction of the puborectalis muscle at defecation, failure of the pelvic floor to relax on attempted defecation (outlet syndrome), abnormal perineal descent, and pudendal nerve neuropathy.

Surgery

✧ Hirschsprung's disease – short-segment disease can be addressed by anorectal myectomy, rectal myectomy, or anal sphincterotomy. Distal disease can be treated by a pull-through operation.

✧ Internal occlusive rectal prolapse can be treated with sigmoid colectomy and rectopexy.

✧ Anorectal myectomy may be effective in the "outlet syndrome"; it is contraindicated if marker studies indicate severe colonic inertia.

✧ Surgery is rarely used in severe idiopathic constipation except in the most serious and persistent cases, e.g. ileostomy, irrigating cecostomy, percutaneous endoscopic colostomy (PEC) with anterograde irrigation. In those with refractory slow-transit constipation and no defecatory disorder, colectomy and ileorectal anastomosis is occasionally indicated.

Follow-up
After the exclusion of serious underlying pathology, the majority of patients can be followed by the primary care physician (PCP) following simple advice on diet and laxatives. In those with refractory constipation, further follow-up should be guided according to the results of examinations.

Post-operative Follow-up
Review the pathology to confirm the diagnosis and determine the success of the operation. Detect any complications of general anesthesia and of the specific procedure. For "pull-through" operations, check the histology to confirm that normally innervated bowel had been reached. Residual Hirschsprung's disease can be a cause of residual constipation.

Chronic Megacolon
This is characterized on abdominal plain film as an abnormally dilated colon or rectum with loss of haustral pattern. Megacolon may affect the entire colon or partial segments. Causes are congenital (Hirschsprung's disease) or acquired.

Acquired causes include:
1. Obstruction – chronic anal stenosis, strictures (ischemic), annular neoplasms.
2. Chagas disease.
3. Hypothyroidism.
4. Neurologic disorders (spina bifida, cauda equina, paraplegia, Parkinson's disease).
5. Psychological disturbances.
6. Idiopathic, adynamic bowel syndrome – may affect colon only with normal rectum, or present as megarectum with variable colon in continuity. Rectal capacity and sensation are diminished but sphincteric responses and rectal biopsy are normal.

History
Take a general colorectal history. Patients may present with symptoms similar to chronic constipation, or with fecal incontinence due to overflow secondary to fecal impaction. Those with idiopathic megacolon may describe abdominal pain and distension in the context of chronic constipation.

Physical Examination
Perform a general colorectal examination, looking for the same abdominal and perianal conditions associated with chronic constipation.

Diagnostics and Imaging
✧ Proctoscopy, sigmoidoscopy, and abdominal plain film. X-ray reveals abnormally dilated large bowel and loss of haustral pattern.
✧ Colonoscopy/barium enema is performed to exclude underlying organic disease in older patients and other age groups where indicated.
✧ Anal physiology studies help identify Hirschsprung's disease and non-relaxation of the anal sphincter. Full-thickness rectal biopsies are required to exclude Hirschsprung's disease in selected patients.

Treatment

Treat underlying conditions. Otherwise, treat medically with colonic washouts, disimpaction of feces, and, in severely symptomatic patients, bowel resection. Generally, the longer the history, the worse the outcome; however, procedures including colectomy with ileorectal anastomosis and restorative proctocolectomy have good reported outcomes, with permanent stomas affording a generally good quality of life in those in whom initial surgery has failed.

Follow-up

Following the initial consultation, serious underlying causes suggested by the history and clinical examination should be excluded. Chronic and idiopathic causes can be reviewed at 3–4 month intervals to assess the efficacy of conservative treatments.

After organic causes have been excluded, continued follow-up should take place at the primary care level. Surgery can be considered in an appropriately counseled patient when all other avenues of treatment have failed.

Rectal Inertia

Occurs mainly in children, in whom the rectum is over-stretched repeatedly by inadequate evacuation.

History

Patients present complaining of chronic constipation despite being apparently healthy individuals. Mild abdominal distension and occasional perianal soiling may be reported. Older children and adults may have psychological problems. Differentiation from Hirschsprung's disease may be difficult, but Hirschsprung's normally presents with problems from birth while rectal inertia only presents after toilet training.

Physical Examination

The abdomen is usually flat but fecal masses may be palpable in the left colon. Rectal examination is needed to exclude underlying physical problem, e.g. anal fissure, anal stenosis. Evidence of soiling, poor anal tone and hard fecal masses may be found.

Diagnostics and Imaging

In cases that do not respond to medical treatment, EUA and full-thickness rectal biopsy may be warranted.

Treatment

Empty bowel by saline rectal washouts (as an inpatient if necessary). If indicated, perform manual evacuation then re-commence toilet training at regular intervals. For adults, continue the use of phosphate enemas or suppositories. Do not stimulate the proximal colon with laxatives – this may aggravate the condition.

Follow-up

Rectal inertia is usually chronic in nature, so there is no urgency for extensive work-up unless the history and examination suggest suspicious features. Diagnostics and trials of treatment can be performed at 1–3 month intervals until symptoms are controlled. Once stable on medication, defer patient to primary care.

Diverticular Disease

Despite the nomenclature, colonic diverticula are actually pulsion pseudodiverticula, consisting of mucosa and serosa. Colonic diverticula form at areas of structural weakness in the colonic wall where the vasa rectae penetrate the muscularis propria to supply the mucosa. The condition is thought to be a consequence of the Western diet, with a relative lack of vegetable fiber, although structural changes in the colonic wall associated with aging and disordered motility (hyperelastosis and altered collagen structure) are also thought to contribute.

Diverticulosis describes the presence of diverticula and is very common, affecting more than 60% of individuals over 70 years old, though around 90% of people are asymptomatic; thus, given the high prevalence, admissions for symptomatic diverticular disease are relatively infrequent. The term "diverticulitis" implies infection and inflammation in association with diverticula.

Right-sided diverticula are common in Asia, while in the West, left-sided diverticulosis is more typical. The condition typically starts after age 30 and peaks in the 60s to 70s, but younger patients do present acutely with complicated diverticular disease. Severity ranges from episodes of mild discomfort to the onset of complications that include perforation, abscess formation, intestinal obstruction, fistula formation into neighboring organs, and hemorrhage. Carcinoma of the colon can coexist with diverticular disease.

History

Take a general colorectal history. Symptoms may be episodic and recurrent, mild to severe left iliac fossa or lower abdominal pain, dull and constant, lasting hours to days, precipitated by diet or stress. Pellet-like ("rabbit dropping") feces with occasional mucus and diarrhea may be reported. Other symptoms may suggest the onset of complications:

✧ *Perforation* – severe constant pain in the lower abdomen and feeling systemically unwell.
✧ *Intestinal obstruction* – a history of increasing constipation and abdominal distension associated with colicky abdominal pain. Diverticular strictures are related to scarring following previous episodes of diverticulitis, and distinction from malignant strictures can often only be made after histologic examination of the resected specimen.
✧ *Fistula formation* can occur into the colon, small intestine, uterus, vagina, abdominal wall, and bladder. Fistulae form when an inflamed diverticulum adheres to an adjacent organ and a pericolic abscess ruptures into it. They may present with symptoms of chronic ill-health, low abdominal tenderness, intermittent diarrhea, pneumaturia and fecal vaginal discharge.
  ∝ Colovesical fistula – urgency and dysuria (recurrent urinary tract infection [UTI]), pneumaturia, and fecaluria.
  ∝ Colovaginal fistula – air and feces per vagina, much more common following a previous hysterectomy.
✧ *Hemorrhage* – there may be a history of episodes of brisk bright-red bleeding per rectum.
✧ *Cecal or right-sided diverticula* – occurs in one third of diverticulosis patients; presents with appendicitis-like symptoms.

Physical Examination

Perform a general examination. In acute attacks of diverticulitis, there may be a low-grade fever, tenderness and rigidity, and occasionally a mass in the lower abdomen. Localized perforation and abscess formation may be suspected if examination reveals a localized mass, while free perforation into the abdominal cavity generally presents as an emergency with generalized peritonitis. Vaginal examination may reveal a malodorous brown discharge. Abdominal distension and active bowel sounds may suggest intestinal obstruction. Rectal examination may reveal blood or pus.

Diagnostics and Imaging

Flexible sigmoidoscopy and barium enema are not advisable in the acute setting, due to the risk of perforation. Flexible sigmoidoscopy, however, if done shows multiple openings of the diverticula, and in acute attacks may reveal an inflamed mucosa and edema. Barium enema is useful for investigation of chronic symptoms. Barium shows the typical outpouchings and long constricted segments of bowel. Flexible sigmoidoscopy can exclude carcinoma within segments of diverticulosis. A midstream urine specimen is taken for microscopy and culture to detect subclinical fistula. CT is useful for assessment of adjoining organs for fistula, involvement of tissue planes, and the presence of an inflammatory phlegmon or abscess.

✧ *Perforation* – the presence of a localized mass or abscess can be confirmed on ultrasound, but CT is increasingly used in the acute setting as it provides more anatomic information. The Hinchey Classification is used to describe diverticular colonic perforations, with Hinchey I having a localized pericolonic abscess, Hinchey II a pelvic abscess, Hinchey III being characterized by purulent peritonitis with pus in the peritoneal cavity, and Hinchey IV being associated with feculent peritonitis.

✧ *Intestinal obstruction* – usually diagnosed by abdominal plain film. Gastrograffin enema can confirm the diagnosis and identify the level of obstruction.

✧ *Fistula* – barium enema can define the tract, but such connections are commonly not seen even when they exist. Cystography and cystoscopy can be used to confirm and define colovesical fistulas and exclude primary bladder neoplasms.

✧ *Hemorrhage* – differentiate from vascular ectatic lesions. Use sigmoidoscopy to exclude bleeding from hemorrhoids. Arteriography is performed to exclude vascular ectatic lesions and to potentially arrest bleeding in the case of massive diverticular bleeds.

Treatment

✧ *Diverticular pain* – colonic spasm rather than inflammation is relieved by fecal bulk-forming agents (e.g. Isogel, antispasmodics). Colonic resection is only for severe cases requiring repeated admissions, or those with complicated disease (local or free perforation, stricture, fistulae). Elective resections are increasingly being performed laparoscopically.

✧ *Uncomplicated disease* – acute attack settles over 4–5 days; only 30% of patients have recurrent symptoms. Five to ten percent become severe and need sigmoid colectomy.

✧ *Diverticular abscess* – CT-guided percutaneous drainage and intravenous antibiotics should be the first-line treatment in those with localized signs and a confirmed abscess, with emergency surgery reserved for those with generalized peritonitis.

✧ *Complicated disease and peritonitis* – Hartmann's procedure (resection and end colostomy) or colonic lavage, primary anastomosis and loop ileostomy depending on the extent of peritoneal contamination. If soiling is minimal, then consideration can be given to omission of the stoma.

✧ *Fistulae* – elective sigmoid resection with primary anastomosis and repair of the fistulous opening in the affected organ.

Follow-up

Initial work-up should be tailored to exclude serious underlying pathology. Colonoscopy should be delayed until recovery, but performed in patients over the age of 50 or in those with a strong family history of colorectal cancer or IBD. In most patients, the diagnosis can be confirmed by barium enema. Patients with uncomplicated diverticulitis can be given simple dietary advice. For those with complications, or multiple episodes of significant diverticulitis, surgical resection should be considered on an elective basis to prevent future emergency admissions and to reduce the likelihood of requiring a Hartmann's procedure.

Post-operative Follow-up
Review pathology to exclude coexisting carcinoma. Examine the patient for complications of laparotomy and general anesthesia. If a Hartmann's procedure was performed, determine the timetable for reversal or whether reversal is to be performed. Symptoms continue in 25% of patients after surgery and are thought to be due to underlying disordered bowel motility.

Polyps in the Colon and Rectum
A polyp is an abnormal overgrowth of the colonic mucosa and can be sessile (flat) or pedunculated (on a stalk):
1. *Inflammatory* – occur in ulcerative colitis, Crohn's disease, diverticulitis, chronic dysentery and, rarely, benign lymphoid hyperplasia.
2. *Hamartomatous polyps* – juvenile and Peutz–Jeghers syndrome (Peutz–Jeghers syndrome patients have significant malignant potential).
3. *Metaplastic polyps* – 1–2 mm in size, rarely greater than 5 mm; biopsy confirms the diagnosis and they need no ongoing observation.
4. *Adenomatous polyps* – benign tumors comprised of abnormal colonic glands. Classified according to the growth pattern of the glands. Seventy-five percent are tubular adenomas, 10% villous, and 15% tubulovillous adenomas. All have malignant potential.

There is a strong clinical relationship between polyps and cancer. Approximately 40% of patients treated for a polyp develop further polyps; only 3% of adenomatous polyps are malignant, but one third of villous papillomas are malignant. The risk of malignancy increases with size from 1% for polyps less than 5 mm, through 40% for polyps larger than 2 cm, to 60% for those greater than 3 cm.

Familial Polyposis Syndromes
✧ *Familial adenomatous polyposis (FAP)*: FAP is characterized by hundreds of adenomatous colorectal polyps present by the second or third decade of life. FAP has been linked to an autosomal dominant mutation of the *APC* gene at position 21 on chromosome 5q. In patients from affected families, screening should begin in the early teens. To prevent the almost inevitable development of colorectal cancer, prophylactic resection (restorative proctocolectomy or colectomy and ileorectal anastomosis, which necessitates ongoing rectal surveillance) should be performed as soon as practically possible following diagnosis, generally before the age of 25.
✧ *Hereditary nonpolyposis colorectal cancer (HNPCC, Lynch syndrome)*: Characterized by the early diagnosis of colorectal cancer (approximate age 45 years, compared with 65 for the general population), HNPCC is responsible for 2% of all colorectal cancers. Lynch syndrome is diagnosed according to Amsterdam Criteria II (Modified Amsterdam Criteria):
 ∝ At least three relatives with an HNPCC-associated cancer (colorectal, endometrial, small bowel, ureter, renal pelvis) of whom one should be a first-degree relative of the other two.
 ∝ At least two successive generations should be affected.
 ∝ At least one colorectal cancer should be diagnosed before the age of 50.
 ∝ FAP should be excluded.

Tumors should be verified pathologically.

History

✧ Take a general colorectal history and a careful family history.
✧ Polyps are usually asymptomatic and may present as anemia due to occult bleeding.
✧ Retrograde propulsion of large pedunculated polyps may produce abdominal pain, spasm, and colon, and cause colocolic intussusception.
✧ Rectal lesions can cause tenesmus or a change in bowel habit with diarrhea.
✧ Mucous discharge may occur, especially in cases of villous papilloma, which may lead to dehydration and electrolyte imbalance.
✧ Large papillomas may produce hypokalemia and metabolic acidosis, leading to symptoms of lethargy, muscle weakness, mental confusion, and renal failure.

Physical Examination

Perform a general examination. Examination may range from normal to signs of dehydration, anemia, mental confusion, and muscle weakness.

Diagnostics and Imaging

CBC may reveal anemia. Metabolic panel may indicate dehydration or hypokalemia. Rigid sigmoidoscopy may reveal the presence of rectal adenomas, which should prompt colonoscopic examination and polypectomy.

Treatment

✧ *Colorectal polyps and villous papillomas* – regular colonoscopy with intervals as specified by the American Cancer Society. CT colonography and barium enema are alternatives for patients in whom colonoscopy is technically challenging.
✧ *Malignant polyps* – following colonoscopic excision of a malignant polyp, a decision must be made as to whether radical resection of the excision site is required. Considerations include the likelihood of the cancer being completely excised and the chance of lymph node metastases being present.
  ∝ Favorable characteristics include: complete endoscopic resection with a margin of normal tissue, cancers confined to the head of a polyp, well or moderately differentiated tumors, and the absence of lymphovascular invasion.
  ∝ If doubt exists in patients fit for major surgery, then radical resection of the site is indicated. This is technically easier if the site of the polyp is "tattooed" with ink at the time of polypectomy to ensure that it is removed and examined histologically.

Follow-up

All patients are followed-up by regular colonoscopy according to American Cancer Society guidelines.
✧ Polyps and cancer:
  ∝ Flexible sigmoidoscopy every 5 years
  ∝ Colonoscopy every 10 years
  ∝ Double-contrast barium enema every 5 years
  ∝ CT colonography (virtual colonoscopy) every 5 years.
✧ Cancer screening only:
  ∝ Yearly fecal occult blood test (FOBT)
  ∝ Yearly fecal immunochemical test (FIT)
  ∝ Stool DNA test (sDNA), interval uncertain.

If flexible sigmoidoscopy, double-contrast barium enema, or CT colonography are positive, colonoscopy should be done. Fecal tests should be done as a multiple stool take-home study; single in-office exam is not adequate. If fecal tests are positive, colonoscopy should be completed.

Carcinoma of Colon and Rectum

The lifetime risk of colorectal cancer in the United States is around 5.1%, with 101,700 new cases of colon cancer and 39,510 new cases of rectal cancer expected in 2011. Colon cancer is responsible for 49,380 deaths annually. Eighty percent of cases occur within reach of the 60 cm flexible sigmoidoscope (i.e. distal to the splenic flexure). Rectal cancers, by definition, occur within 15 cm of the anal verge. Survival rate after colorectal cancer treatment is directly related to stage.

Conditions predisposing to the development of colorectal cancer include: genetics (including FAP, HNPCC), dietary factors (increased animal fat and proteins), colorectal polyps, radiation proctocolitis, previous ureterosigmoidostomy, and ulcerative colitis (especially total colon involvement >10 years – consider for prophylactic bowel excision).

The American Joint Commission on Cancer (AJCC) TNM staging classification is shown in Table 9.1.

✧ *Modes of spread* –intramural, transverse, lateral, and radial. Most consider a longitudinal clearance of 2 cm to be adequate. In rectal cancer, where "total mesorectal excision" is the recommended method of excision, a circumferential resection margin (distance from the tumor to the nearest radial cut edge) of >1 mm is considered to be adequate.

✧ *Extension to adjacent structures* – this applies more to the rectum than the colon:
   ∝ Anterior – seminal vesicles and prostate in the male, posterior vaginal wall in the female.
   ∝ Lymphatic spread – rectal cancer occurs in 50% of pararectal nodes and spreads to lower colic and inferior mesenteric nodes. Lateral lymph node spread is more common to the hypogastric lymph nodes (internal iliac nodes).
   ∝ Hematogenous spread – to liver in 18–20% of cases at presentation; to lung in 5%.
   ∝ Perineal spread, transperitoneal spread.

TABLE 9.1   AJCC TNM staging of colorectal carcinoma

Stage 0	Carcinoma in situ
Stage I	No nodal involvement, no distant metastasis
	Tumor invades submucosa (T1, N0, M0)
	Tumor invades muscularis propria (T2, N0, M0)
Stage II	No nodal involvement, no distant metastasis
IIA	Tumor invades into subserosa (T3, N0, M0)
IIB	Tumor invades into other organs (T4, N0, M0)
Stage III	Nodal involvement, no distant metastasis
IIIA–B	1-3 regional lymph nodes involved (any T, N1, M0)
IIIC	4 or more regional lymph nodes involved (any T, N2, M0)
Stage IV	Distant metastasis (any T, any N, M1)

History

Take a general colorectal history. The onset is often insidious; later, the development of symptoms depends on the site of the tumor. Inquire regarding predisposing conditions such as ulcerative colitis, Crohn's disease, and previous gastric surgery (associated with a twofold increased risk of colorectal cancer). In addition to the polyposis syndromes, a positive family history is an important risk factor for the development of colorectal cancer.

✧ *Cecal, ascending colon, and hepatic flexure* – insidious over a long period, may have occasional vague upper abdominal pain and flatulent distension, pallor, lassitude, and general ill-health. Alteration in bowel habit is less frequent. Occasionally presents with diarrhea.

✧ *Transverse and descending colon* – increasing constipation alternating with diarrhea. Occasionally associated with the passage of blood and mucous. May also present with fistula (e.g. gastrocolic – vomiting of feces.)

✧ *Sigmoid and rectal* – rectal bleeding is the most frequent presentation, usually slight, with alteration in bowel habit, tenesmus, spurious morning diarrhea – patient wakes and passes mucus in the presence of constipation. Severe pain may indicate extension into surrounding tissues and a poor prognosis. May also present with fistula (e.g. colovesical).

Identified risk factors for colorectal cancer include the following.

✧ *Static risk factors*:
  ∝ Age – 9 out of 10 patients diagnosed with colorectal cancer are older than 50 years.
  ∝ Personal history of colorectal polyps or cancer.
  ∝ Personal history of inflammatory bowel disease – dysplasia occurs in patients with long-standing IBD.
  ∝ Family history of colorectal cancer.
  ∝ Inherited polyposis syndromes – FAP, HNPCC, Turcot, Peutz–Jeghers, MUTYH-associated.
  ∝ Race and ethnicity – African Americans have the highest colorectal cancer incidence and mortality rates of all groups in the United States. Ashkenazi Jews have one of the highest risks for colorectal cancer of any ethnic group in the world.

✧ *Modifiable risk factors*:
  ∝ Diet – diets high in red meats and processed meats can increase colorectal cancer risk.
  ∝ Physical inactivity.
  ∝ Obesity.
  ∝ Smoking.
  ∝ Heavy alcohol use.
  ∝ Type 2 diabetes.

Physical Examination

✧ Perform a general colorectal examination. Examine for the presence of jaundice, anemia, and weight loss.

✧ On abdominal examination, look for palpable masses such as in the right iliac fossa due to a cecal lesion, or an enlarged liver indicating metastases.

✧ Perform a rectal examination: 75% of all rectal tumors and approximately a third of bowel tumors can be palpated. Determine the location, mobility, and extent of spread around the bowel and into surrounding tissues.

Diagnostics and Imaging

Carry out CBC, metabolic panel, LFTs, chest X-ray, and ECG and obtain a pre-operative CEA level. On proctoscopy, determine lesion size, site, extent, and distance from anal verge. Flexible sigmoidoscopy requires a bowel preparation with a phosphate enema. All patients suspected of possible carcinoma of the colon should undergo rigid sigmoidoscopy and barium enema or colonoscopy. Suspicious lesions detected on a barium study require a colonoscopy with a biopsy. CT scans of the chest and abdomen are used to stage the disease (looking for liver and lung metastases) and to look for local complications such as duodenal or ureteric involvement.

✧ *Barium enema* – the double-contrast method is more reliable, but still has a false-negative rate of greater than 2%. Features of malignancy are mucosal destruction, abrupt cut-off of barium and the visualization of a localized lesion with sharp demarcation from the involved areas ("apple-core lesions").

✧ *Colonoscopy* – generally considered the first-line investigation if there is a high suspicion of cancer, or if the barium enema is equivocal. Full examination of the colon is required to demonstrate additional pathology such as a synchronous carcinoma (present in 2–5% of cases) or diverticular disease. If colonoscopy cannot be performed pre-operatively due to a stenosing primary lesion, arrange for full examination of the colon within 3 months after resection of the primary lesion.

✧ *Endoluminal ultrasound* – EUS is useful in rectal tumors for defining the involvement of the rectal wall, extent of extra-rectal involvement, and spread to adjacent lymph nodes.

✧ *MRI* – increasingly used to locally stage rectal cancers, to determine their relationship to the mesorectal fascia, and to select patients likely to benefit from pre-operative radiotherapy.

Treatment

When available, all patients should be discussed at a multidisciplinary conference (involving surgeons, oncologists, radiologist, and pathologists) where potential alternative management strategies can be discussed. Pre-operative radiotherapy may be recommended in patients with large rectal tumors where the potential circumferential resection margin is threatened. Radiotherapy should also be considered in poor-risk patients where a local excision of a small rectal cancer is contemplated. Ongoing trials may suggest a survival benefit for all rectal cancer patients undergoing curative surgery.

Bowel Preparation

The necessity for and type of bowel preparation varies widely according to local policy, but there is a current trend away from the use of mechanical bowel preparation, its attendant side effects, and its negative impact on post-operative recovery. Exceptions are generally made when on-table colonoscopy is likely to be performed, or there is a high likelihood of forming a loop ileostomy, in which case many consider a column of feces between the stoma and anastomosis to be undesirable. Right-sided colonic lesions do not require preparation.

All bowel preparation agents can cause electrolyte disturbances and dehydration, and patients should be given concurrent intravenous fluids to prevent profound drops in blood pressure on the induction of anesthesia. Do not use in obstructing lesions; use on-table lavage instead.

Surgery

✧ *Abdominoperineal resection* (APR) – for situations where the tumor is very close to the anal verge or invading the anal sphincters. End colostomy in the left iliac fossa.

✧ *Low anterior resection* – preferred when the tumor situated more proximally in the rectum, such that adequate distal clearance can be attained with acceptable post-operative functional results. Sometimes a diverting colostomy/ileostomy is fashioned to mitigate the consequences of anastomotic leakage; it must be stated that stomas do not prevent leaks. Patients undergoing radical rectal surgery should be warned of the possibility of sexual and urinary dysfunction following surgery due to inadvertent damage to the pelvic nerves.

✧ *En bloc resection* – for locally advanced tumors. The radical approach can result in a survival rate of 50% at five years, depending on the stage.

✧ *Palliative transanal resection* – often performed with a urologic resectoscope (transanal resection of tumor [TART]). It can be used to palliate those with rectal cancers who are unfit for radical surgery.

Small Cancers of the Rectum

These neoplasms are often found mobile in the rectal mucosa, especially in the elderly. They can be treated with local excision with a 0.5–1.0 cm margin of healthy tissue. Transanal endoscopic microsurgery (TEM) allows accurate local full-thickness excision, but even T1 lesions may have lymph node metastases in up to 17% of patients if the tumors invade the lower third of the submucosa. Local radiotherapy is not widely accepted as a treatment.

Multiple Colonic Tumors (Synchronous Tumors)

The incidence of multiple synchronous tumors is 2–5%; therapy often requires total colectomy.

Hepatic Metastases

Even in the presence of liver metastases, the patient's best interests may be served by removal of the primary tumor. The aim of liver resection (resectability) is to remove all macroscopic disease with clear margins, leaving sufficient functioning liver. Considerations include:

✧ Patients with solitary, multiple, and bilobar disease who have had radical treatment of the primary colorectal cancer are candidates for liver resection.

✧ The ability to achieve clear margins (R0 resection) should be determined by the radiologist and surgeon in the regional hepatobiliary unit.

✧ The surgeon should define the acceptable residual functioning volume, approximately one third of the standard liver volume, or the equivalent of a minimum of two segments.

✧ The liver surgeon and anesthetist should make the clinical decision regarding fitness for surgery.

✧ If deemed medically unfit for surgery, patients should be considered for ablative therapy.

✧ Patients with extrahepatic disease that should be considered for liver resection include:

  ∝ Resectable/ablatable pulmonary metastases.
  ∝ Resectable/ablatable isolated extrahepatic sites – for example spleen, adrenal, or resectable local recurrence.
  ∝ Local direct extension of liver metastases to, for example, diaphragm/adrenal that can be resected.

Follow-up

In cases of suspected colorectal cancer, urgent endoscopic investigation should be performed and patients should be seen at regular appropriate intervals to give the results of biopsies and staging examinations and to formulate a treatment plan. If surgery is indicated, explain all possible procedures to the patient, including the possibility of a colostomy or loop ileostomy. Pre-operative referral to stoma care nursing may be helpful.

Regular colonoscopy screening should be undertaken in all patients with familial colonic polyposis, family history of colonic malignancy, previous colorectal cancer and adenomas, and inflammatory bowel disease.

In cases of inoperable and recurrent tumor, review the patient regularly, discuss palliative chemotherapy with an oncologist, and consider involving the palliative care team early as they can offer advice on the amelioration of symptoms as well as terminal care.

Monitor CEA levels; if increasing, this may indicate recurrence (assuming that a high pre-treatment level fell to normal following initial surgery). However, a large number of recurrences are associated with no rise in CEA levels.

Post-operative Follow-up

Review the pathology report to determine adequate tumor resection, for grading and staging of the tumor, and to discuss subsequent oncological follow-up, although this is increasingly arranged during a multidisciplinary team meeting.

Examine the patient for complications of laparotomy and general anesthesia. Complications of anterior resection include anastomotic leaks; these are usually detected as an inpatient but may present later as a pelvic abscess or collection. Investigate possible anastomotic leaks with a water-soluble enema and CT scan to define a collection. If the anastomosis has been protected by a diverting colostomy, the leak is small, and the patient is well, then conservative management can be pursued and resolution expected. Diverted patients should have a water-soluble contrast enema arranged 6 weeks following surgery to exclude "radiological leaks" prior to arranging reversal of the stoma.

Patients in whom direct evaluation of the entire colon was not possible prior to surgery (stenosing lesions, emergency surgery) should have a completion colonoscopy within 3 months after surgery to exclude a synchronous tumor not detected at operation. Opinion is divided as to the most appropriate follow-up strategy following colorectal cancer resection, with the benefits of intensive follow-up depending on the fitness of the patient to undergo subsequent hepatic or pulmonary resections should metastases be diagnosed. In some studies, the major benefit of following patients for five years following surgery has been psychological support, with very few asymptomatic recurrences being detected. Most patients currently followed-up after hospital discharge currently undergo abdominal palpation to look for hepatomegaly, rigid sigmoidoscopy to assess for anastomotic recurrence in the case of low anastomoses, and regular ultrasound or CT scans according to local protocols.

As adjuvant therapy for colorectal carcinoma, chemotherapy is generally considered for those with node-positive disease (stage III). Adjuvant chemotherapy for stage II disease remains controversial. Currently, FOLFOX (5-FU, leucovorin, and oxaliplatin) is the chemotherapy of choice.

Irritable Bowel Syndrome

Generally, IBS describes a syndrome of recurrent symptoms of abdominal pain, bloating and/or altered bowel habit with no underlying organic disease. However, the lack of organic disease does not diminish the distress that the symptoms can cause. Psychologic factors and stress play an important role in the symptoms, although most patients have no obvious psychologic or personality disorder.

In middle-aged and older patients, a diagnosis of IBS should only be made after carcinoma or other organic disease has been excluded by the appropriate investigations. In younger patients, cancer is less likely but not unknown and a difficult balance has to be obtained between unnecessary testing and missing the occasional tumor. The less experienced surgeon should probably err on the side of caution.

History
Take a general colorectal history. Classically, the IBS patient presents before the age of 35 years and gives a history of recurrent abdominal pain, which can occur at various sites around the abdomen. They may complain of abdominal bloating and describe some relief on passing flatus or feces. Feces are more frequent, smaller, and may be loose, string-like, or described as resembling rabbit droppings. There may be associated passage of mucus and a feeling of incomplete evacuation.

Typically, the symptoms seem out of proportion to the patient's apparent well-being. Take a careful dietary history and note the intake of fiber. Take a history of smoking, alcohol consumption, ongoing stress and psychological disturbances past and present.

Ask about other psychological symptoms – anxiety, stress, depression, drugs, and previous hospital visits to investigate similar anxiety-related symptoms affecting other body systems (e.g. difficulty swallowing).

Celiac disease is an important possibility in the differential diagnosis and should especially be considered in the presence of mild anemia.

Physical Examination
✧ Perform a general colorectal examination. Look to exclude underlying pathology. Determine the site of pain.
✧ Palpate for masses or a palpable colon in the left iliac fossa, which may indicate thickening or spasm.
✧ Rectal examination is mandatory to exclude rectal or anal pathology.

Diagnostics and Imaging
Proctoscopy, sigmoidoscopy, and abdominal X-rays. If insufflation of air at the sigmoidoscopy reproduces the pain, this is highly suggestive of IBS. Further investigation is only indicated if underlying pathology is suspected (e.g. colonoscopy/barium enema, ultrasound scan, or in the presence of alarm features including onset after age 50, bleeding, and weight loss). In patients without such features, testing should be kept to a minimum as they may simply increase the patient's anxiety.

Treatment
Explanation of symptoms, empathy, and reassurance. A high-fiber diet may improve symptoms or may make them worse, but is often tried initially. Sorbitol and caffeine may exacerbate symptoms. A trial of peppermint oil may be used to reduce gut spasm, as may anticholinergic drugs such as dicycloverine and hyoscine butylbromide, but there is no convincing trial evidence to suggest that they are better than placebo. Tricyclic antidepressants in low doses have been shown to be beneficial, possibly working via gut serotonin receptors. Some patients have had good results from cognitive behavioral therapy.

Follow-up
Once organic disease is excluded, further investigation should be kept to a minimum. Time should be given for dietary manipulations or other treatments to work; but if these fail, then patients may benefit from referral to gastroenterologists with a special interest in IBS.

Pneumatosis Coli

Pneumatosis coli is characterized by gas-filled cysts found in the subserosal and submucosal planes of the large intestine. It is thought to result from lymphatic stasis; the dilated channels secondarily fill with gas.

History

Patients may be asymptomatic or present with colicky abdominal pain. A fulminant form exists, where patients may present with abdominal pain and bloody diarrhea associated with pneumoperitoneum.

Physical Examination

Examination may be normal or there may be evidence of abdominal distension.

Diagnostics and Imaging

Pneumatosis coli is often detected as an incidental finding on abdominal plain film and barium enema.

Treatment

No active treatment is necessary. The cysts can be induced to disappear by oxygen therapy over 3–4 days. In fulminant disease, the patient should be treated symptomatically, but if they deteriorate to a point requiring laparotomy, the outlook is bleak and surgery generally involves excision of the affected segments and exteriorization of both bowel ends (stoma and mucus fistula).

Volvulus of the Large Bowel
Sigmoid Volvulus

Anatomic features that predispose to sigmoid volvulus include a long, redundant loop of sigmoid colon with a narrow base of attachment of the sigmoid mesocolon. This is classically seen in those with a long history of constipation and laxative abuse, and often found in patients in long-term care facilities who have neuropsychiatric disorders. Patients may present with an anticlockwise torsion of 180 degrees which reverts spontaneously, leading to intermittent symptoms of abdominal pain, distension, and constipation; if rotation of 360 degrees or more occurs, then reduction is required to prevent perforation secondary to closed-loop obstruction. The chronic form may cause symptoms over many years.

History

Take a general colorectal history. In the chronic form, patients may present with a history of recurrent episodes, colicky central abdominal pain associated with distension, and complete constipation. Motility disorders such as Hirschsprung's and Chagas diseases may predispose to sigmoid volvulus.

Physical Examination

Perform a general examination. Examination may be normal between episodes; during episodes, there may be abdominal distension, tinkling bowel sounds, and an empty rectum with blood found on rectal examination.

Diagnostics and Imaging

Abdominal plain films will reveal a markedly distended loop of colon originating from the left iliac fossa and extending into the right upper quadrant ("coffee bean"). A metabolic panel may reveal dehydration and other electrolyte abnormalities. A CBC may reveal anemia. Between episodes, a barium enema may reveal a large redundant sigmoid loop, which suggests the diagnosis.

Treatment
Begin with resuscitation if the presentation is acute. Colonoscopic reduction is successful in 80% of cases, but recurrence occurs in 90% and therefore should be considered a temporary measure prior to definitive surgery.

Follow-up
Review for need for surgery. Because of the high rate of recurrence and the risks of emergency surgery, all but the most unfit should be considered for elective repair. Options include resection with or without stoma, or a novel minimally invasive treatment such as percutaneous endoscopic colostomy (PEC), which involves fixation of the colonic loop to the anterior abdominal wall using percutaneous endoscopic gastrostomy (PEG) tubes.

Cecal Volvulus
Cecal volvulus usually occurs in the setting of a congenitally mobile cecum, which twists up into the left upper quadrant of the abdomen. This often occurs in younger patients than those affected by sigmoid volvulus, and can be precipitated by pregnancy, recent surgery, left colonic obstructions, and congenital malrotation and bands. The majority are really ileocolic; only 10% are purely cecal. Eleven percent of people have a failure of fusion.

History
Patients may present acutely or with indolent obstructive symptoms with recurring vague indigestion and cramp-like abdominal pain.

Physical Examination
Examination may be normal between episodes or present with abdominal distension arising from the right iliac fossa.

Diagnostics and Imaging
During acute episodes, an abdominal plain film will reveal a large bowel loop arising from the right iliac fossa to the left upper quadrant. Between episodes, a barium enema may reveal a chronically enlarged cecum, which suggests the diagnosis.

Treatment
Unlike sigmoid volvulus, colonoscopic decompression is not effective and surgery is required. Options include right hemicolectomy, cecopexy, and cecostomy.

Follow-up
Review test results, which may or may not suggest the diagnosis but should exclude other causes (e.g. cancer). Decide on the need for surgery.

Post-operative Follow-up
Review histology to exclude the presence of coexisting carcinoma or other pathology. Detect any complications of laparotomy and large bowel resection.

Vascular Lesions of the Colon
The major vascular conditions affecting the colon can be classified into:

1. Ischemic lesions of the large bowel.
2. Angiodysplastic lesions of the colon (vascular ectasia).

Ischemic Conditions of the Colon

The primary causes of large-bowel ischemia include:

1. *Thrombosis* – arterial or venous, caused by arteriosclerosis, polycythemia rubra vera, portal hypertension, malignant disease of the colon, hyperviscosity syndromes due to platelet abnormalities, or high-molecular-weight dextran infusion.
2. *Emboli* – left atrium (atrial fibrillation), left ventricle (myocardial infarction), atheromatous plaque in the aorta.
3. *Vasculitides* – polyarteritis nodosa, systemic lupus erythematosus (SLE), giant cell arteritis (Takayasu's arteritis), Buerger's disease, Henoch–Schönlein purpura.
4. *Surgical trauma to vessels* – aortic reconstruction (with an inadequate marginal artery), resection of adjacent intestine.
5. *Non-occlusive ischemia* – shock (hypovolemia or septic), congestive cardiac failure. An uncommon but frequently fatal complication of cardiopulmonary bypass.
6. Spontaneous ischemic colitis.

Ischemic colitis tends to present in one of three forms: gangrenous, transient, and stricturing.

1. *Gangrenous colitis* presents with several days of abdominal pain and rectal bleeding. There is mild to moderate abdominal tenderness. Proctoscopy shows bleeding above the level of the proctoscope ("red-currant jelly"). Disease occurs most commonly at the splenic flexure ("Griffiths' point": the watershed area between the superior and inferior mesenteric artery territories). On abdominal X-ray, patients with ischemic colitis will show thumb printing, picket-fence thickening of folds, and sacculation. Thumb printing is due to submucosal edema and hemorrhage. Arteriography may show complete occlusion of the vessel. Colonoscopy may reveal hemorrhagic nodules and ulceration, but should be performed with care due to the risk of perforation. Treatment is initially supportive with total parenteral nutrition (TPN) and, if the patient deteriorates, surgery with resection.
2. *Transient ischemic colitis* generally occurs in patients who are middle-aged with known peripheral vascular disease; in these patients, it is often noted that collateralization has occurred.
3. *Stricturing colitis* may present with symptoms of chronic obstruction in patients with a history of vascular disease (cardiac or peripheral). Strictures form due to scarring following an episode of acute ischemia.

Vascular Ectasia of the Colon

Colonic vascular ectasias are acquired disorders also known as angiodysplasia or arteriovenous malformations that tend to affect patients over 60 years of age. They tend to produce anemia from chronic blood loss, generally of venous origin, but may also hemorrhage suddenly. Ectasias are usually small and may possibly be detected by colonoscopy or angiography. They occur most frequently in the cecum and right colon. The cause is unknown, but there is a 20% correlation between aortic stenosis and angiodysplasia. There is also an association with microaneurysms and collagen diseases.

History

Patients will present with obscure colonic bleeding. There may be a history of intermittent episodes of fresh rectal bleeding.

Physical Examination
Chronic cases may present with anemia and otherwise normal examination findings. Acute cases may present with shock and fresh rectal bleeding.

Diagnostics and Imaging
EGD and colonoscopy should be done to rule out other causes of bleeding. Radiolabeled red-cell scans or selective mesenteric angiography can help to identify the site of bleeding, and therapeutic angiography can be used to embolize the affected vessel.

Treatment
Angiographic embolization or segmental colectomy as guided by imaging studies.

Follow-up
Follow-up is at short intervals (1–4 weeks) until the cause is identified.

Inflammatory Bowel Disease: Ulcerative Colitis and Crohn's Disease
IBD describes conditions associated with inflammation of the large bowel. The main differential diagnosis is between ulcerative colitis (UC) and Crohn's disease. However, other conditions which enter the differential diagnosis include TB infections, amoebic dysentery, bilharzial infestations of the colon, *Salmonella* enteritis and colitis, *Campylobacter* infections, antibiotic-associated pseudomembranous colitis, necrotizing enterocolitis, radiation-induced colitis and enteritis, ischemic colitis (rare under age 60), complicated diverticular disease (especially with internal fistula), pneumatosis cystoides intestinalis (early stages), and primary cytomegalovirus colitis (can simulate or complicate UC). Diseases that mimic Crohn's disease and exhibit similar radiologic signs include small bowel adenocarcinoma, lymphomas, and small bowel phytobezoar.

Differentiation between Ulcerative Colitis and Crohn's Disease
Crohn's disease can affect the entire GI tract, from mouth to anus, and is characterized by discontinuous "skip" lesions. UC only affects the colon, except in cases of backwash ileitis in patients with diffuse and severe disease who have an incompetent ileocecal valve, and tends to do so in a confluent manner from the rectum extending variable distances proximally (note that in some patients with UC there is relative "rectal sparing"). UC and Crohn's disease describe a spectrum of disease, and those patients with colitis that cannot be differentiated into either category are labeled "indeterminate colitis."

Serology using a Prometheus test that includes c-ANCA (antineutrophilic cytoplasmic antibody), p-ANCA, and anti-*Saccharomyces cervisiae* antibody (ASCA), among others, can also be helpful in both diagnosing IBD and discriminating between UC and Crohn's disease. IBD is covered in full in the section describing disorders of the small bowel (*see* page 115).

Pseudomembranous Colitis
A specific form of infective colitis generally seen in hospitalized patients receiving antibiotics. It is caused by *Clostridium difficile*. It occurs more commonly in elderly patients, after surgical intervention, in patients with intestinal neoplasm, and in patients with atherosclerotic ischemia.

History and Physical Examination
Mild cases present with watery mucoid diarrhea, which is malodorous. Severe cases result in toxic dilatation of the colon and a risk of perforation.

Diagnostics and Imaging
Diagnosis is by colonoscopy and biopsies, where an off-white slough of necrotic mucosa and exudates (the "pseudomembrane") is characteristic. Stool culture is carried out to identify *C. difficile* or its exotoxin.

Treatment
Oral vancomycin for 1–2 weeks or intravenous metronidazole.

Neutropenic Colitis
Neutropenic colitis may develop in patients undergoing chemotherapy and other immunosuppressed individuals due to superinfection (e.g. *Clostridium septicum*).

Rectal and Anorectal Disorders
Proctitis
Proctitis is an inflammation of the bowel similar to ulcerative colitis, but the inflammation is initially confined to the rectum and anal canal. The causes of proctitis include:
- *Sexually transmitted infections* – include gonorrhoea, herpes, *Chlamydia*, and lymphogranuloma venereum, which are common in those engaging in unprotected receptive anal intercourse.
- *Non-sexually transmitted infections* – including group "A" streptococcus.
- *Inflammatory bowel disease* – a non-specific variation of UC accounts for many cases of non-infective proctitis. While most cases run a benign course, the condition may result in late rectal strictures. Crohn's disease and UC may also present initially with isolated proctitis.
- *Trauma* – often related to the insertion of foreign bodies into the rectum for sexual gratification, or radiation injury following radical radiotherapy for prostate cancer (*see* p. 250).

History
Take a general colorectal history. Affected patients are mainly young adults who present with rectal bleeding, diarrhea, tenesmus, and passage of mucus or mucino-sanguinous discharge. Take a sexual history to identify possible infective or factitious causes.

Physical Examination
Perform a general examination. Examination may be normal, but be sure to look for general features of ulcerative colitis. During rectal examination, look for other perianal conditions.

Diagnostics and Imaging
On sigmoidoscopy, mucosa will appear edematous and hyperemic. Take biopsies for histology. Colonic involvement is excluded by colonoscopy.

Treatment
Bowel sedatives and stool softeners, prednisolone suppositories and enemas, sulfasalazine tablets or enemas. Any coexisting perianal disease (fissure, abscess, fistula, hemorrhoids) is treated by the appropriate surgical procedure.

Neutropenic Anorectal Infections
There is a high incidence of anorectal bacterial infections in neutropenic patients caused by *E. coli*, *S. aureus*, and *Klebsiella* spp. Diagnosis can be late in patients who are unable to mount a white-cell response, and the development of large abscesses or necrotizing fasciitis is possible.

Infections are treated with intravenous antibiotics, drainage of pus, limited debridement of necrotic areas, and formation of colostomy in cases where the condition progresses and medical management fails.

Radiation Proctitis

Rectal bleeding following pelvic irradiation has been reported in up to 95% of patients in retrospective studies, with symptoms peaking at 1 year from treatment and tending to resolve after 18 months. Some authors have suggested that up to 5–10% of patients require surgery for complications of radiation proctitis. There is an increased incidence of radiation proctitis in diabetics and those with significant cardiovascular disease. Symptoms may appear within 2 weeks of treatment.

History

Affected patients may report frequency, diarrhea, rectal blood and mucus, and tenesmus. Occasionally symptoms are delayed and the patient is found to have a large rectal ulcer, which requires biopsy to exclude cancer. Other symptoms may result from rectal fistulization into the vagina or urinary tract. There may also be damage to small bowel and transverse colon.

Physical Examination

Patients may have lower abdominal tenderness; rectal examination may be normal or an indurated area may be palpable. There may be blood on the digital rectal examination.

Diagnostics and Imaging

Sigmoidoscopy with biopsy for diagnosis and to determine the extent of the disease.

Treatment

Initial interventions are medical: 5-ASA and steroid enemas if symptoms are persistent or troublesome. Severe symptoms warrant consideration of topical formalin solution (requires anesthesia) or laser coagulation. Formalin is effective in 80% of patients after 1–2 applications, but 30% develop recurrent symptoms.

Surgery is reserved for those with severe complications (perforation, fistula, stricture) and often requires a diverting sigmoid loop colostomy for 6–12 months. However, hemorrhage and tenesmus may continue. Alternatively, a Hartmann's procedure can be performed, although acceptable leak rates are reported in those with isolated segments of radiation injury undergoing primary anastomosis.

Follow-up

Flexible sigmoidoscopy and biopsy are needed to make the diagnosis, define the extent of affected bowel, and exclude other causes such as cancer. Trial of medical treatment can be attempted in those with debilitating symptoms, but close review is required to monitor response. In severe cases, consider admission for inpatient care.

Post-operative Follow-up

Review pathology to confirm the diagnosis and detect complications of the procedure. Determine if the surgical procedure has been successful in relieving the symptoms and review accordingly.

Decide whether to reverse an ostomy at 6–12 months. Symptoms should have settled completely before this is performed.

Involvement of the Colon by Gynecological Pathology

Involvement of the sigmoid colon by ovarian carcinoma can present with symptoms suggestive of bowel cancer. Endometriosis can implant onto the serosa of the sigmoid colon and rectum and cause characteristic symptoms.

Endometriosis of the Bowel

Although endometriosis (defined as the presence of functioning endometrial tissue outside of the uterus) occurs in 4–17% of women of reproductive age, only 5–10% of these women will have colorectal involvement.

History

Obtain a general colorectal and gynecological history. Dysmenorrhea, dyspareunia, cyclical rectal bleeding (occurs in up to one third of patients but very few have involvement of the bowel mucosa), and painful defecation just before menstruation are characteristic of bowel endometriosis. Pain is relieved once menstruation starts. Occasionally, bowel obstruction is caused. Differential diagnosis includes malignancy (primary or metastatic), diverticulitis, IBD, pelvic inflammatory disease (PID), and radiation colitis.

Physical Examination

Perform a general examination including full abdominal and pelvic examination. Usually examination is normal and the diagnosis is suspected on the history.

Diagnostics and Imaging

Sigmoidoscopy. Laparoscopy and biopsy for histological diagnosis; joint care with gynecologists.

Treatment

Hormone manipulation initially (combined oral contraceptive pill, GnRH analogues). Hysterectomy, oophorectomy, and rectosigmoidectomy may be required for cases that do not respond to medical therapy. In younger patients, excise endometrial implants.

Follow-up

Follow-up is at short intervals until diagnosis is confirmed.

Post-operative Follow-up

Review pathology to confirm diagnosis. Recurrence requires further laparoscopy.

Rectovaginal Fistulas

Causes include:

1. Obstetric injury.
2. IBD (Crohn's disease).
3. Radiation injury.
4. Infection (cryptoglandular, Bartholin's gland, lymphogranuloma venereum).
5. Neoplasm (anal, rectal, vaginal).
6. Trauma (foreign body, iatrogenic: vaginal or anorectal surgery).
7. Congenital.

History

Take a general colorectal and gynecologic history. History will include the occurrence of a foul vaginal discharge resistant to normal therapy progressing to the passage of flatus or feces per vagina. Symptoms may be intermittent or constant. Recent prolonged labor preceding the onset of symptoms may be a feature. There may be recent perineal irradiation.

Physical Examination
Perform a general examination including abdominal, rectal, and vaginal examination.

Diagnostics and Imaging
Rigid sigmoidoscopy may reveal the fistula. Some recommend the rigid sigmoidoscope to examine the vagina as well in this circumstance, and it is better than the speculum at identifying the vaginal component of the fistula. A fistula may also be demonstrated by barium enema or vaginal contrast study. EUA may be required in difficult cases. Inserting a tampon into the vagina and instilling methylene blue into the rectum can help to prove the existence of a fistula, which is hard to demonstrate.

Treatment
Depends on the cause and location of the fistula. All abscesses should be adequately drained before definitive repair. Very superficial tracks can sometimes be treated by simple fistulotomy; medical treatments such as infliximab may be useful in Crohn's fistulae. Diverting stoma should be considered for recurrent fistulae and complex cases.

✧ *Transanal repair* – rectal advancement flap, sleeve (circumferential) advancement flap (used if defect is large).

✧ *Transperineal repair* – laying open of fistula, immediate overlapping sphincter repair, transverse transperineal repair (fistula track divided along with perineal body; vaginal and rectal defects closed separately).

✧ *Transvaginal repair* – inversion of fistula (into rectum), vaginal advancement flap.

✧ *Transabdominal repair* – dissection of rectovaginal septum, interposition of omental or gracilis muscle flap, with or without limited rectal excision.

Follow-up
Follow-up is at short intervals until cancer is excluded. Prompt treatment is required to avoid complications from sepsis.

Post-operative Follow-up
Review pathology to exclude cancer. Determine the success of the procedure and decide a date for possible closure of any covering colostomy.

Recto-urinary Fistulas
Most recto-urinary fistulas result from injury, mainly as a result of prostatic or urethral instrumentation. Other causes include diverticulitis, Crohn's disease, carcinoma, irradiation of the bladder, and TB of the prostate. Retroprostatic fistulas are rare and result from complications of transrectal needle biopsy of the prostate.

History
Take a general colorectal and urologic history. Patients usually report recurrent urinary tract infections or the passage of flatus (pneumaturia) or feces (fecaluria) in the urine. Other features of the history may be suggestive of one of the causes above.

Physical Examination
✧ Perform a general examination.
✧ Examine for evidence of sepsis, anemia, and renal impairment.

✧ Examine for features of the underlying causes.

Diagnostics and Imaging
CBC, electrolytes, BUN, creatinine, and urine and blood cultures. Sigmoidoscopy may identify the fistula and help identify any underlying disorder. Contrast studies of the bowel may identify the fistula. CT scan may give more detailed information for planning definitive surgery.

Treatment
Insertion of a urinary catheter and definitive diagnosis and treatment of the underlying pathology. Post-traumatic fistulas are amenable to direct repair either by perineal, transanal or transsphincteric approach.

Follow-up
See the patient at short intervals until the cause is identified. Treatment should be arranged promptly to avoid the development of sepsis and deterioration in renal function.

Post-operative Follow-up
Review the pathology to confirm the diagnosis. Determine the success of the operation and detect any complications of the procedure.

Disorders of the Anorectal Musculature
Rectal Prolapse
A partial prolapse involves the mucosa only, whereas a complete prolapse involves the entire thickness of the rectal wall. In children under 2 years, prolapse is not uncommon (often associated with a diarrheal illness or prolonged coughing), but usually resolves spontaneously; it is, however, associated with cystic fibrosis, so a sweat test should be performed. The differential diagnosis in adults includes hemorrhoids and large polypoidal tumors.

History
Take a general colorectal history. In children, the prolapse is usually incomplete and comes to clinical attention after being noticed by the parent. Adults tend to complain either of the prolapse itself and resulting soiling of underclothes from mucus, blood, and feces, or a varying degree of fecal incontinence. The prolapse will tend to be noticed at defecation or on coughing or straining.

Physical Examination
Perform a general examination. In children, the prolapse can be viewed when sitting the child on a potty. In adults, the anus may be patulous with decreased tone. Active contraction of the anal sphincter onto the examining finger is weak. The patient experiences no discomfort on rectal examination and anal and rectal sensation is decreased. Bearing down produces the prolapse. If complete, two thickness layers of bowel wall are palpable between the fingers. Generally, a prolapse of greater than 5 cm in length is complete; less than 5 cm needs careful examination to differentiate complete from incomplete.

Procidentia of the uterus may often coexist and a combined approach to treatment between a gynecologist and surgeon is required.

Diagnostics and Imaging

Proctoscopy and sigmoidoscopy are performed to exclude underlying rectal disorders. Anorectal physiology is useful for detecting any underlying pathology, investigating the incontinence aspect of the disorder, and planning appropriate treatment.

Treatment

Treatment will vary by age.

✧ *Infants*: Watchful waiting; prolapse in this population will generally resolve spontaneously.
✧ *Children*: Usually experience incomplete prolapse with a self-limiting clinical course. Therapy consists of laxatives and regular defecation with or without enemas.
✧ *Older children*: Injection of sclerosants into the lower rectal mucosa.
✧ *Adults*: If anal sphincter function is satisfactory and the prolapse partial (i.e. anterior mucosal prolapse), then a careful mucosal excision similar to a hemorrhoidectomy can be done. In cases of poor sphincter tone, sphincteric exercises are recommended. Otherwise, surgery may be required.

A multitude of surgical interventions exist in the treatment of rectal prolapse:

✧ *Perineal procedures*: Delorme's (mucosal stripping and muscle placation), Altemeier's (perineal rectosigmoidectomy).
✧ *Abdominal procedures*: Include laparoscopic/open suture rectopexy, Ivalon sponge/mesh rectopexy, resection rectopexy.

Transabdominal rectopexy has a 90% success rate, but is a major abdominal procedure. There is a risk of sexual dysfunction, which needs to be included in the consent process. For frail or elderly patients, a Delorme's procedure may relieve symptoms and does not preclude a second procedure, but has a high recurrence rate.

Follow-up

Intervals are short until serious underlying pathology has been excluded. Thereafter, a decision on surgical treatment or expectant management should be made.

Post-operative Follow-up

Patients are reviewed to determine the success of the procedure and to detect any complications. After transabdominal rectopexy, the most common complication is constipation, which occurs in a third of patients. If prosthetic mesh has been used, there is the risk of deep-seated infection, which may require removal of the mesh. Some patients may complain of sexual and urinary disturbances due to disruption of the pelvic nerves.

Descending Perineum Syndrome

Excessive straining leads to a prolonged reflex inhibition of musculature with an abnormal descent of the perineum and bulging of the anterior rectal wall toward the anal canal.

History

Take a general colorectal history. Generally there are non-specific symptoms of difficulty passing feces, tenesmus, and incontinence. Associations include a long history of constipation, vaginal deliveries, previous rectal/perineal surgery, rectoceles, and enteroceles.

Physical Examination

Perform a general examination. On straining, the anus descends to 1cm below the inter-ischial line.

Diagnostics and Imaging

Sigmoidoscopy to exclude rectal disease and detect complications (e.g. solitary rectal ulcer). Anal physiology studies may be helpful in difficult cases, as may defecating proctography.

Treatment

Avoid straining, bisacodyl suppositories, and bulk-forming laxatives. Inject sclerosants or surgically excise any mucosal prolapse. Biofeedback may be beneficial.

Follow-up

Non-urgent review is carried out to determine the success of the treatment in helping defecation. When condition is stabilized, defer to primary care for follow-up.

Post-operative Follow-up

Review to determine the operative success and detect any complications. Otherwise, follow-up is the same as in non-operative disease.

Solitary Rectal Ulcer

Symptoms result from an internal rectal prolapse or intussusception, which causes trauma to the rectal wall. Persistent rectal symptoms are due to rectal ulceration, which is commonly situated 7–10 cm from the anal verge on the anterior or anterolateral wall. Rectal ulcers are identified as having well-defined indurated edges with a gray base; surrounding mucosa may be normal or edematous and nodular. The mechanism of ulceration may be rectal prolapse, failure of relaxation of puborectalis muscle, or insertion of foreign bodies.

History

Obtain a general colorectal history. This condition is characterized by a long history of multiple, prolonged visits to the toilet associated with drawn-out, unproductive straining, although rectal bleeding and passage of mucus during and between defecation may occur. There may be a deep-seated perineal pain, and the sensation of a need to defecate may be so strong that the patient becomes desperate and inserts fingers or other objects into the rectum in an attempt to empty the already empty rectum.

Physical Examination

General examination may be normal with some lower abdominal discomfort. Rectal examination reveals rectal soreness and an indurated area internally.

Diagnostics and Imaging

Sigmoidoscopy and biopsy. Sigmoidoscopy reveals hemorrhage, edema, or, in 50%, an ulcer adjacent to a valve of Huston on the anterior surface approximately 5–8 cm from the anal verge. This may look like a rectal carcinoma, but repeated biopsy reveals only non-specific inflammatory changes or fibromuscular hyperplasia of the lamina propria. A defecating proctogram may reveal an internal intussusception.

Treatment

Explain the condition to the patient. There is no definitive medical therapy, although rectal steroids have been used. Biofeedback has been proposed to modify the harmful toilet habit. In patients who experience severe symptoms, abdominal rectopexy to treat prolapse or rectal excision and end-colostomy can be used, although less than two thirds of patients derived a benefit from rectopexy in some series.

Follow-up

Follow-up is at short intervals (1–2 weeks) until cancer is excluded. Thereafter, see every 1–3 months to try different therapies and assess severity of symptoms and decide on the need for surgery.

Post-operative Follow-up

Review to determine the success of the procedure in relieving symptoms and to detect complications. Complications of rectopexy are described on p. 254.

Fecal Incontinence

Fecal incontinence is defined as the involuntary passing of flatus or stool. The incidence is underestimated, but may be upwards of 1–2%. Causes include old age, childbirth, chronic constipation, anal dilatation or fistula surgery, dementia and fecal impaction, low rectal tumors, and autonomic neuropathy associated with diabetes mellitus. Generally, classification can be considered etiologically as:

✧ *Traumatic* – obstetric, surgical, accidental/war.
✧ *Colorectal disease* – hemorrhoids, rectal prolapse, IBD, tumors.
✧ *Congenital* – spina bifida, surgery for imperforate anus, Hirschsprung's disease.
✧ *Neurologic* – cerebral, spinal, peripheral.
✧ *Miscellaneous* – behavioral, fecal impaction.

Anal continence depends on a variety of mechanisms including stool consistency, rectal capacity and compliance, sphincter function, anal sensation and an intact rectoanal inhibitory reflex. The underlying mechanisms in incontinence may include either damage to the anal sphincter or perineal descent, often due to excessive straining over many years leading to a traction neuropathy of the pudendal nerve.

Severity of Fecal Incontinence

Of the many scales used to objectively measure fecal incontinence severity, the most commonly used in the United States is the Cleveland Clinic Florida (Wexner) fecal incontinence score. This metric is easy to use and assigns each of five parameters a score of 0 (absent) to 4 (daily), which are based on the frequency of incontinence to gas, liquid, or solid contents, the need to wear a pad, and lifestyle changes. The overall sum is the objective measure. A score of 20 indicates complete incontinence, while a score of 0 means that the patient has complete control over continence.

History

Take a general colorectal history. Ask about the above causes and the severity of incontinence; rate the severity of incontinence using a standard metric.

Physical Examination

✧ Perform a general physical examination.
✧ Examine for perineal scars from obstetric injury or fistula surgery.
✧ Note the degree of perineal descent at rest and on straining and any associated prolapse.
✧ Exclude an abnormality of lumbosacral plexus.
✧ On rectal examination, feel for fecal impaction or rectal tumors, and test sphincter integrity at rest and on contraction.

Diagnostics and Imaging

Proctoscopy and sigmoidoscopy. If recognized causes of fecal incontinence are not found, the patient is said to have idiopathic fecal incontinence. Less severe cases require no further investigation, but can be treated symptomatically with loperamide.

In more severe cases, additional work-up is aided by:

✧ Anal manometry – measures the presence of and relaxation after rectal distension by balloon. Anal canal pressures at rest reflect activity of the internal sphincter (50–80 cm H_2O), and voluntary contraction of the external sphincter (squeeze pressure) will increase the pressure of the anal canal to 150 cm H_2O. This is used to diagnose a short and weak sphincter.

✧ Sphincter electromyography (EMG) – can detect silent areas of a sphincter defect and localize the ends of the muscle pre-operatively. In traction neuropathy of the pudendal nerve, some muscle fibers lose their innervation.

✧ Rectal compliance balloon or thermal stimulation to test anorectal sensation.

✧ Transanal ultrasound to image defects in the sphincter.

✧ Defecating proctogram to detect prolapse.

Treatment
In cases of mild incontinence, treatment should start with counseling, with the addition of constipating agents if loose stool is present. Physiotherapy can be instituted with anal sphincter and pelvic floor exercises or biofeedback methods. Leakage after stooling may indicate incomplete evacuation, which can be treated by a glycerine suppository after each bowel movement or a daily phosphate enema.

Severe fecal incontinence may require operative treatment, for example sphincter repair when defects are identified. Reconstructive options include graciloplasty or the insertion of artificial neosphincters.

Sacral nerve stimulation has emerged as a potential treatment, though research is still ongoing.

Follow-up
Follow-up is at short intervals initially to assess the severity of incontinence and review tests. Mild cases can be deferred to primary care once serious underlying pathology has been excluded. Severe cases need a decision made regarding surgery when appropriate testing has been completed.

Post-operative Follow-up:
Review to assess the success of the procedure and to detect any complications of the procedure. Recurrence not amenable to further surgery may require a stoma.

Other Anorectal Disorders
Anorectal Suppuration and Abscesses
Suppuration and abscesses can be caused by both aerobic (*Staphylococcus* sp., *Streptococcus* sp., *E. coli*, and *Pseudomonas aeruginosa*) and anaerobic (*Clostridium perfringens* and *Bacteroides* sp.) bacteria. Particularly susceptible are leukopenic patients, diabetics, and patients with ulcerative colitis (15%) or Crohn's disease (25%). Perianal skin infections are generally caused by *S. aureus* and nearly all heal with simple incision and drainage.

Perianal abscesses of bowel origin start internally in glands in the inter-sphincteric space (cryptoglandular). When these infections spread to the skin immediately adjacent to the anus, they are termed "perianal abscesses." If they spread laterally into the buttock, they are termed "ischiorectal abscesses"; these may originate from high intersphincteric infections or from pelvirectal disease. These abscesses can be considered as perianal fistulae in which the internal openings are small, cannot be found at operation, and will heal spontaneously in the majority. In a minority, the fistulous track will persist and require formal fistula surgery.

History

Patients report a severe throbbing perianal pain that is worse on sitting and coughing. Ask about a history of predisposing factors (e.g. malignancy, chemotherapy, UC, Crohn's disease, or diabetes). Patients will often present as emergencies rather than to the outpatient clinic.

Physical Examination

These will present as erythematous (variable), tender rounded swellings in the perianal area; there may be some degree of induration and, later, some fluctuation. Ischiorectal abscesses occupy a larger area to one side of the anus and sometimes may be bilateral.

✧ *Submucousal abscess* – dull aching pain in the rectum with usually no external evidence of infection. Rectal examination may reveal a rounded smooth area of induration on one side of the upper anal canal and lower rectum. Pus may be seen draining from an internal opening.

✧ *Pelvirectal abscess* – normally a complication of pelvic sepsis. There are signs of infection with pyrexia, rigors, diarrhea, weakness, and lower abdominal tenderness, or even a mass. On rectal examination, patients will be tender high in the rectum and may have a boggy swelling in this area.

Diagnostics and Imaging

CBC to detect underlying leukopenic condition. Blood glucose to detect diabetes mellitus. Perform EUA. Pus should be sent for microbiology, and a sample of the abscess cavity wall should be sent for microbiology and histology.

Treatment

EUA, incision and drainage. Perform rigid sigmoidoscopy and proctoscopy; biopsies of inflamed mucosal lesions are taken if appropriate. Examine for the internal opening of a perianal fistula. If the internal opening of a fistula is seen, it should be noted and left. Attempts to probe cavities for fistula tracks in the acute setting are likely to be rewarded only by the creation of new tracks through the friable indurated tissue, rather than the identification of an existing track. Otherwise, incise and drain the abscess cavity. Treat underlying disorders appropriately.

Post-operative Follow-up

Review the results of the microbiological studies of the pus. Infections by *S. aureus* will heal provided the wound is clean; these patients can be discharged to primary care after the initial post-operative check.

Those with organisms of bowel origin should be followed up until complete healing is confirmed. The majority will heal normally, but some may experience a long recovery course or have recurrence within a short time. These patients should be investigated for possible perianal fistula by EUA.

Anorectal Fistulas

Anorectal fistulas usually have only one internal opening, but there may be more than one external opening. These usually start as a perianal abscess, but the internal opening persists or perianal gland infection persists as a source of sepsis. This is particularly likely to occur in the presence of some underlying disorder such as UC or Crohn's disease, or in the setting of chronic infections such as TB, actinomycoses, and lymphogranuloma venereum. Occasionally, carcinoma of the rectum can present as a fistula.

The differential diagnosis for anorectal fistulas includes colloid rectal carcinoma, proctocolitis, small intestinal fistula secondary to Crohn's disease, TB, actinomycosis, lymphogranuloma venereum, and local conditions such as pilonidal sinuses, suppurative hidradenitis, a chronically infected Bartholin's gland, and vaginal and urethral fistula.

Classification

Goodsall's rule: Fistulas with external openings anterior to the interischial line have their internal opening in a straight line to the rectum. External openings posterior to the interischial line form a horseshoe to open in the posterior midline. Exceptions include anterior openings more than 3 cm from the anus (which may be anterior extensions of posterior horseshoe fistulas), and anterior fistulas associated with other diseases such as Crohn's disease and malignancy.

Relation to the anal sphincters: Fistulas are also classified according to height and relation to the anal sphincters:
1. Subcutaneous.
2. Low intersphincteric – goes underneath the subcutaneous part of the external sphincter.
3. Transsphincteric – track extends through the external sphincter.
4. Anorectal – opening between the rectum and exterior.

History

Take a general colorectal history. There may be a history suggesting an underlying disorder or a previous acute perianal abscess followed by intermittent or persistent discharge or recurrent abscess.

Physical Examination

Perform a general examination. Rectal examination may reveal the presence of single or multiple external openings. Granulation tissue may mark the opening or there may be the presence of pus. The external opening may have temporarily healed and be indicated by an area of reddish-brown induration. Induration may also be palpated inside the rectum, indicating the site of the internal opening. Try to determine the course of the track between the internal and external openings.

Ask the patient to squeeze the inserted finger to determine the relation of the primary track to the puborectalis sling, which correlates to the upper extent of the external sphincters, and then advance the finger to identify any induration above the levator muscles.

Diagnostics and Imaging

The main test for anorectal fistula is EUA. However, in complicated disease or in cases complicated by other diseases, fistulography may provide useful information as to the course of the track, especially if an internal opening has not been identified. MRI has an increasing role in identifying the course of fistulas and excluding other disease. In experienced hands, endoanal ultrasound (often with hydrogen peroxide contrast) can give valuable anatomic information.

Treatment

Therapy for anorectal fistulae is surgical – EUA and treatment of the fistula.
1. Opening of the fistulous tract – fistulotomy for tracts that do not involve the sphincter.
2. Anal fistula plug for fistula that traverse the sphincter.

3. Mucosal advancement flap for high fistulas.
4. Seton insertion.
5. Chronic cases – long-term metronidazole treatment.
6. In cases of TB, treat the TB before addressing the anatomic defect.
7. Similarly, in UC and Crohn's disease, get control of the primary disease first. However, even resection of the ileocecal region in Crohn's with no other apparent disease of the bowel often fails to heal perianal fistulas. Long-term treatment with metronidazole, salazopyrine, or azathioprine is needed. Patients with UC may experience amyloid deposition and death from amyloid renal and cardiac failure; therefore rectal excision and colostomy are acceptable alternatives. Infliximab may be used for Crohn's treatment in an attempt to heal a fistula once any associated abscess has been drained.

Follow-up
If a fistula is suspected, EUA is warranted for formal assessment. If symptoms are atypical, it may be prudent to perform a flexible sigmoidoscopy first, or at the time of the EUA, to exclude coexisting colorectal conditions.

Post-operative Follow-up
Examine the seton if inserted (some patients are left long-term with a loosely tied drainage seton to control their symptoms of sepsis). Examine for evidence of ongoing sepsis or recurrent discharge, which may suggest unrecognized extensions of the original disease and require either repeat surgery or an MRI to diagnose.

Hidradenitis of the Perianal Skin
While hidradenitis is not a condition of bowel origin, it tends to be referred to colorectal surgery attention because of the location. The condition consists of the chronic inflammation of sweat glands, leading to recurrent infection and abscess formation. Affected areas begin as induration and may progress to sinus formation. The majority of cases occur in the axillae, but 30% are perianal.

Differential diagnosis in these cases includes pruritus ani and perianal fistula.

History
Obtain a general colorectal history, which will usually be normal. There is a history of recurrent infections of the area, sometimes progressing to boils/abscess formation.

Physical Examination
Perform a general examination. Examine the axillae to detect any disease. The groins and perianal area may be indurated and have evidence of scarring and chronic inflammation. There may be multiple small boils with white heads and small amounts of pus in the sweat area of the groins and perianal area. Rectal examination is normal.

Diagnostics and Imaging
Few laboratory tests are needed for a diagnosis. Bowel imaging is indicated only if the history/examination suggests a coexisting bowel condition. Microbiology of any pus should confirm skin bacteria only. Test urine to exclude glycosuria; test blood sugar.

Treatment
In mild cases, long-term antibiotics (e.g. erythromycin) may be effective in reducing the rate of infection when combined with conservative measures such as wearing loose airy clothing, daily washing, etc. More severe cases require excision of affected skin and

subcutaneous tissue to deep fascia with or without a split skin graft (plastic surgery referral).

Follow-up

Mild cases can be reviewed after 1–6 months to determine the effect of conservative measures. Failure of medical treatment or severe disease is an indication to consider surgery.

Post-operative Follow-up

Review histology to confirm diagnosis. Detect recurrence or any complications of surgery (e.g. skin necrosis). Unless severe, skin necrosis can be treated conservatively with antibiotics and dressings. Extensive skin necrosis may require a plastic surgical consultation.

Pruritis Ani

Pruritis ani is described as an "itchy" and irritated anus. Secondary causes include anorectal and dermatologic disorders, but in many, the underlying problem cannot be found. It is thought that in many patients, minor degrees of fecal soiling lead to irritation and scratching or overzealous cleaning and the application of inappropriate topical preparations. This in turn results in damage to the delicate perianal skin and further irritation, and a vicious circle results. Dysfunction of the internal anal sphincter allows anal leakage, and skin tags and perianal warts prevent adequate cleaning of the anus. There may be a mucous discharge from hemorrhoids, benign or malignant rectal tumors, anal fissures and fistulas. All may be made worse by the ingestion of spicy foods and caffeine.

Secondary causes can be classified as:
1. *Fungal infection* – secondary infection due to candida, trichomonas, or tinea crura.
2. *Parasitic infestation* – threadworms, scabies.
3. *Other infections* – gonococcal proctitis, condyloma acuminatum, herpes simplex.
4. *Dermatological disorders* – contact dermatitis, psoriasis, lichen planus, eczema.
5. *Neoplasia* – rectal adenoma, rectal adenocarcinoma, squamous cell anal carcinoma, malignant melanoma, Bowen's disease, Paget's disease.
6. *Benign anorectal* – hemorrhoids, fistula, fissure, prolapse, sphincter dysfunction, incontinence, radiation proctitis, ulcerative colitis.

History

Take a general and colorectal history to detect any of the causes outlined above. Perianal and anal itching may be severe and worse when warm. Ask about the length of symptoms, change of bowel habit, diet, and recent travel. In children, suspect *Enterobius* infestation. Inquire about an itchy or irritating rash elsewhere on the body.

Physical Examination

Perform a general examination to detect any general skin conditions. Long-standing irritation causes excoriation and icthyosis; the perianal skin is corrugated, making removal of fecal particles difficult. In advanced cases, the skin becomes atrophic and excoriated with edema and thickening of the underlying dermis.

Examine the anus resting and straining. On rectal examination, assess the anal tone and squeeze pressure. Palpate for polyps, fissures, fistulas, and neoplasms.

Diagnostics and Imaging

Urinalysis, blood glucose, and CBC. Examine the affected area under a Wood's light. *Corynebacterium minutissimum* is diagnosed by the presence of bright pink-orange fluorescence. (Note: Anusol fluoresces purple.)

Perform proctoscopy and sigmoidoscopy to detect any underlying colorectal condition (e.g. neoplasm, hemorrhoids, prolapse). Perform biopsies and arrange colonoscopy as indicated. Biopsy affected skin if suspicious. Skin scrapings are taken for fungal elements.

In children, test for the presence of pinworms: Scotch tape is applied to the anus and then stuck onto a clean glass slide; this is repeated twice in the morning. Microscopy reveals the ova deposited on the perianal skin overnight.

Treatment
The aims are to decrease leakage, improve hygiene, and prevent injury to the perianal skin.
- *Treat underlying conditions* such as hemorrhoids, fissures and warts.
- *Treat fungal infections* with nystatin or chlortrimazole. Treat threadworms with piperazine.
- *Advice on hygiene* – gentle washing with water only; no soap. Wet wiping after defecation is more efficient at cleaning the anus than dry wiping. Advise to avoid vigorous rubbing, wear cotton underwear, do not wear tights.
- *Decrease leakage* – modify diet to avoid spicy foods and fiber, reduce or abstain from alcohol and caffeine. Prescribe loperamide or codeine.
- *Pruritus* – avoid scratching. Hydrocortisone cream can be applied for 10 days to break the cycle, but excessive use can cause skin atrophy and itching on withdrawal of the cream.

Follow-up
Review at regular intervals (1–3 months) once diagnosis is achieved to gauge the effect of therapies.

Hemorrhoids
Hemorrhoids are enlargements of the venous tissue in the rectum, which can cause symptoms by prolapsing or bleeding. Hemorrhoids are very common and are a common cause of perianal bleeding. However, the presence of hemorrhoids does not imply that they are the only cause of the perianal bleeding; hemorrhoids can coexist with cancers or other serious pathology and should not be assumed to be the cause of rectal bleeding, especially in those over 50. Internal hemorrhoids may be classified as follows:
- *First degree* – bleeding but no prolapse.
- *Second degree* – prolapse but reduce spontaneously.
- *Third degree* – prolapse requires manual reduction.
- *Fourth degree* – irreducibly prolapsed.

History
Take a general colorectal history. Usually, patients will complain of prolapse and bleeding. The bleeding is bright red on the toilet paper or dripping into the toilet. Pain is uncommon, but can be present in up to 20% of cases. Prolapse may be associated with a mucoid discharge and perianal wetness.

Physical Examination
Perform a general examination. External inspection of the anus may be normal or the hemorrhoids may already be visible. Alternatively, there may be skin tags visible, which are an indicator of previous episodes of prolapsed hemorrhoids. Occasionally, a pea-sized blue swelling is present on the anal margin, which represents a thrombosed perianal hematoma; these are often confused with hemorrhoids. Ask the patient to strain down and the hemorrhoids may appear. Digital examination may be normal.

Diagnostics and Imaging

Sigmoidoscopy to exclude higher carcinoma. Proctoscopy is the best way to demonstrate the hemorrhoids, which will prolapse into the lumen of the scope. Despite a history of bleeding, hemorrhage is often not visualized on proctoscopy.

Treatment

Conservative measures include laxatives, bulk-forming agents, and advice to avoid straining while stooling.

✦ *Injection sclerotherapy* – useful for all first-degree and smaller second-degree hemorrhoids. Contraindicated in third-degree hemorrhoids, thrombosed hemorrhoids, or associated anal fissure. There is a small risk of pelvic sepsis or prostatitis if the injection is misplaced. Repeat in 3–4 weeks after first treatment.

✦ *Rubber band ligation* – bands are placed at the base of the hemorrhoids, which strangulate a disc of tissue that will slough and leave an ulcer that scars and fixes the mucosa in place, preventing the mucosa from becoming engorged and prolapsing.

✦ *Hemorrhoidectomy* – used if the hemorrhoids fail to respond to injection sclerotherapy or rubber banding. Late complications include pain, fissure, and fistula formation along the tracks of cutaneous wounds. Stenosis may develop by 3 weeks; treat with an anal dilator. Advances in treatment include the introduction of "stapled hemorrhoidectomy," in which a circular stapler is introduced via the anus and fired, removing a circle of mucosa.

✦ *Thrombosed hemorrhoids* – conservative treatment (ice, analgesia, bed rest) or immediate operation (can be technically difficult and bloody).

✦ *Perianal hematoma* – presents as a blue pea-sized swelling at the anal margin. Can be managed conservatively with analgesia and ice, or incised and drained with instant relief of discomfort.

✦ *Hemorrhoidal Artery Ligation Operation (HALO)* – a new procedure claimed to have minimal pain. A miniature ultrasound probe is used to localize the arteries to the hemorrhoid, which are then ligated with a stitch; the hemorrhoid eventually atrophies.

Summary of treatment options for hemorrhoids

✦ *First degree* – dietary modification.
✦ *Second degree* – rubber band ligation, sclerotherapy (hemorrhoidectomy).
✦ *Third degree* – rubber band ligation (hemorrhoidectomy).
✦ *Fourth degree* – hemorrhoidectomy.

Follow-up

Once the diagnosis is made (and concurrent pathology is excluded), review at 6-week intervals to gauge the effect of injection or banding. Defer to primary care once the patient is symptom-free, with advice to avoid constipation and straining with bowel movements, or book for hemorrhoidectomy if not responding to repeated outpatient management.

Post-operative Follow-up

Review to determine the success of the operation and to confirm healing. Complications include prolonged healing and anal stenosis. Anal stenosis can be treated with anal dilators. In cases of prolonged healing, exclude any coexisting pathology or infection and allow 1–2 months before further EUA.

Incontinence may occur due to anal stretching, loss of the anal cushions, or overuse of laxatives. Most cases settle with conservative measures, but anal physiology studies may be required for persistent cases.

Anal Fissure

Anal fissures are common and represent up to 10% of referrals to colorectal clinics. They are longitudinal tears in the anoderm, which typically are seen at the posterior midline but may be seen anteriorly, especially in women. They are often seen in association with a "sentinel pile," a skin tag at the distal extreme of the fissure. Patients enter a vicious cycle in which pain causes fear of defecation, leading to constipation and the passage of hard stool, which exacerbates the problem. Spasm of the internal sphincter (the white fibers of which are often visible in the base of a chronic fissure) reduces the blood supply to the anoderm (vessels penetrate the muscle and are occluded by sphincter spasm), further reducing the ability of the sphincter to heal.

Differential diagnosis: Atypical ulceration of the perianal margin may be caused by miliary tuberculosis or syphilis (if suspected, requires biopsy and culture of tissue). With gross fissures, suspect UC or Crohn's disease. If indurated, suspect malignancy – send tissue for histology.

History

Patients may report severe pain for 20–30 minutes after defecation. Bleeding is noticed on paper; there may be a slight mucoid discharge. There may be history of proctocolitis or Crohn's disease.

Physical Examination

Check to see if there is a sentinel pile (a perianal skin tag in the posterior midline). The distal extent of the fissure may just be visible as the perianal skin is gently distracted, and the white, transverse fibers of the exposed internal sphincter in the base of a chronic fissure may be visible. Rectal examination is frequently not possible due to the pain.

Diagnostics and Imaging

Usually no testing is necessary, but the following can be performed if atypical features are present: CBC and CRP for IBD, serological tests for syphilis, rectal biopsy, biopsy of the ulcer edge with tissue for bacterial and viral cultures if infective cause suspected, and histology if there is any suspicion that the fissure is atypical and may in fact be a malignancy. Perform anal manometry if disordered defecation is suspected.

Treatment

Most acute fissures heal spontaneously in 2–3 weeks with laxatives and fiber supplements. Five percent lidocaine cream applied well within the anal canal may offer symptomatic relief in the interim. Nitroglycerin ointment applied to the anal region decreases sphincter tone and enables healing; topical diltiazem is an alternative, notably in those who cannot tolerate the headache frequently associated with nitroglycerin.

For those that fail to heal, botulinum A toxin (Botox) can be injected in the outpatient setting, with either local, sedation, or general anesthesia as needed. Initial healing rates of 70–96% have been reported, but the effect of the blockade wears off after about 3 months and recurrences do occur even after this time.

Surgery is required both to exclude more serious conditions (fissure biopsy) and to speed recovery. Operation consists of EUA (rectal examination, sigmoidoscopy, and biopsy if indicated) and lateral internal anal sphincterotomy (healing rates of up to 85–95%, but incontinence to flatus occurs in up to 35% of patients). Uncontrolled manual anal dilatation ("the four finger stretch") is no longer recommended due to the unacceptable high risk of sphincter injury.

Follow-up
Review at short intervals (1–4 weeks) to determine the success of conservative measures in relieving symptoms. Failure is an indication to consider surgery.

Post-operative Follow-up
Review pathology if biopsy taken. Determine the success of the operation in relieving symptoms and confirm healing (this may take 4–6 weeks). Continued pain or non-healing may require further EUA to reconsider the diagnosis or expand further treatment such as advancement skin flaps (V-Y advancement flaps). Mild degrees of incontinence usually recover or respond to constipating agents.

Carcinoma of the Anal Canal and Anus
Squamous cell carcinoma of the anus is rare: In 2009, about 5,300 new cases were diagnosed in the United States, with an estimated 710 deaths from the disease. Differential diagnosis includes anal fissure, simple papilla, anal condyloma, prolapsed hemorrhoids, and Crohn's disease.

Adenocarcinoma of the rectum may spread down and invade the anal canal; these lesions tend to be softer and more mucoid, but are differentiated on the basis of biopsy and histology. Predisposing factors include human papillomavirus (HPV) infection, HIV, and immunosuppression.

History
Take a general colorectal history. Patients may complain of painful defecation, rectal bleeding, or bloody discharge and/or a lump. Occasionally, they may complain of symptoms relating to a rectovaginal fistula. Patients presenting with inguinal lymphadenopathy should always have anal cancer excluded.

Physical Examination
Perform a general examination. Anal carcinoma may present as a warty protuberance, flattened plaque, or penetrating ulcer. Rectal examination may be difficult due to pain. Examine for the presence of enlarged inguinal nodes.

Diagnostics and Imaging
All suspicious lesions need an examination under anesthesia and biopsy. Perform a fine needle aspiration (FNA) of enlarged inguinal lymph nodes. Local staging is clinical, by MRI and/or endoanal ultrasound. The presence of distant metastases (affecting 40% of patients in the chest or abdomen) is diagnosed by CT.

Treatment
The primary treatment of anal cancer is not surgical, but uses the Nigro protocol or modification of this protocol with 5-fluorouracil, mitomycin C, and radiation therapy. Small lesions at the anal margin can, however, still be treated by local excision alone with equally good results.

Inguinal lymph node involvement is seen in 10–25% of those with anal cancer and may be treated by radiotherapy, although some advocate radical groin dissection (histological proof of nodal involvement should be obtained before embarking on this).

Surgery may be required in four main scenarios:
1. Residual disease.
2. Complications of primary treatment.
3. Incontinence or fistula after tumor resolution.

4. Subsequent tumor recurrence (salvage abdominoperineal excision).

Follow-up
Follow-up is at short intervals (1–2 weeks) until the diagnosis is achieved and treatment initiated. Lymph nodes not thought to be involved should be examined every month for the first 6 months after treatment of the primary lesion, then every 2 months for the next 18 months. Suspicious lesions require FNA or lymph node biopsy.

Post-operative Follow-up
Review wide local excision results. Overall, anal cancer has a 55% survival at five years. If lymph nodes are involved at presentation, the prognosis is 0% survival at five years. Delayed involvement of inguinal lymph nodes is associated with a 60% survival at five years.

Lymph nodes not thought to be involved should be examined every month for the first 6 months after treatment of the primary lesion, then every 2 months for the next 18 months. Suspicious lesions require FNA or lymph node dissection.

Rare Lesions of the Anal Region
✧ *Basal cell carcinoma* – a small raised and indurated lesion, occasionally ulcerated. Usually only 1–2 cm in diameter. Good results are obtained from wide local excision.
✧ *Bowen's disease* – a rare intraepidermal cancer of the anal region. Usually diagnosed after biopsy of an unusual anal lesion. Treated by wide local excision with or without skin grafting.
✧ Other rare tumors of the anal canal include *basiloid (cloacogenic) carcinoma* and *malignant melanoma*. Malignant melanoma may mimic a perianal hematoma due to its color, although amelanotic lesions can occur. Its prognosis is even worse than that at other sites, so radical surgery is generally avoided.

Perianal Papillomas (Condyloma Accuminata)
Papillomas represent one of the most common sexually transmitted diseases, especially among homosexual men, of whom as many as 50–75% will harbor asymptomatic condylomas. It is caused by HPV, and is important because of the association with malignant change and the development of anal carcinoma. Differential diagnosis includes condyloma latum, molluscum contagiosum, squamous cell carcinoma of the anus, and hypertrophied anal papillae.

History
Obtain a general colorectal and sexual history. Symptoms include bleeding, discharge causing permanent wetness, pain, and pruritus ani.

Physical Examination
Perform a general examination. Appearance may vary from a few pink spots to a confluent mass or a sheet of warts.

Diagnostics and Imaging
Proctoscopy and sigmoidoscopy may reveal papillae within the anal canal, which also require eradication if treatment is to be successful.

Treatment
Principles of treatment include the complete eradication of all lesions and biopsy of lesions to detect malignant change.

✧ EUA and electrocautery excision or fulgeration of perianal and intra-anal lesions.
✧ Podophyllin – requires multiple treatments. Can cause histological changes similar to carcinoma in situ, which reverses 4 weeks after treatment.
✧ Bichloroacetic acid – multiple, weekly treatments are required.

Follow-up
Review histology to exclude carcinoma in situ and confirm healing. Recurrence requires further treatment. Carcinoma in situ requires further follow-up and repeated biopsies.

Pilonidal Sinus Disease
Pilonidal sinuses are often characterized as "nests of hairs." The disorder is commonly referred to colorectal clinics, although it is not strictly a disease involving the bowel but a disorder of the skin near the anus: the natal cleft occurs in men and hirsute women. It is a disease of chronic inflammation involving the presence of hairs within sinuses in the skin. It can be confused with perianal fistula disease. In rare cases, a congenital sinus can be found originating from the spinal cord.

History
Take a general colorectal history, which is usually normal. The onset of the disease is after puberty and presence of sinuses in childhood should raise concern for a congenital spinal sinus. The disease can present either as an acute abscess or as a chronic sinus periodically discharging pus. There may be a history of previous surgery in the area.

Physical Examination
Perform a general examination, which is usually normal. Examination of the perianal area reveals usually one or more midline pits within the skin of the natal cleft. Some of these pits may have lateral extensions. Some sinuses may be inflamed and indurated. Pressing may produce some pus from the pits or hairs may exude from them. There may be scars or unhealed wounds from previous surgery.

Diagnostics and Imaging
Testing is usually not required, apart from urinalysis to exclude glycosuria. Imaging such as CT or MRI may be required if a congenital spinal abnormality is suspected.

Treatment
✧ Asymptomatic pits do not require treatment.
✧ *Acute abscess* – if possible, repeated aspiration and antibiotics allows the disease to settle, enabling definitive surgery at a later date. If incision and drainage is required, the preferred approach is to make the incisions away from the midline and to achieve definitive treatment of the sinus once the acute infection has resolved.
✧ *Chronic abscess* – usually requires a surgical procedure, but mild chronic disease may settle if the area can be maintained hairless by regular shaving or the use of depilatory creams. Brushing of the pits and injection with sclerosant has also been attempted with variable success.

Surgery
A variety of surgical options exist, and the choices include:
1. Excision and packing (healing by secondary intent: often, prolonged time to healing).
2. Excision and midline closure (frequent wound breakdown).
3. Pit excision and lateral drainage (Bascom procedure).

4. Excision with asymmetric closure – aims to keep the wound out of the midline to allow better healing and is often combined with an approach which flattens the natal cleft to reduce recurrence.
5. Complex plastic surgical reconstructions (including z-plasties and myocutaneous flaps).

Follow-up
Review within weeks after the acute episode and arrange definitive treatment as soon as possible. If the disease is chronic, decide whether or not surgery is indicated.

Post-operative Follow-up
Review pathology to confirm diagnosis and monitor healing. Healing can take a long time after incision and drainage or definitive surgery using midline wounds. Aim to keep the area free of hair by regular shaving until and after healing occurs.

The most common complication is the chronic non-healing midline wound. This may be due to recurrent disease, but generally is due to the problems of healing at this site. Further lateral surgery may be indicated. For large wounds, plastic surgical procedures may be required.

Intestinal Stomas
A stoma is a surgically constructed opening of the bowel (or urinary system) onto the skin of the abdomen. Stomas can be permanent or temporary. The aim with temporary stomas is to restore bowel continuity at a later date. End stomas have one end of the bowel sutured to the skin. Loop stomas are usually temporary, where a loop of bowel is brought through the abdominal wall and the anterior wall opened so that two orifices, proximal and distal, are visible but only the proximal end discharges. Over time the distal orifice may shrink so that it is barely visible. The double-barrelled stoma is similar except that two ends of bowel are brought out together, usually after the segment of bowel between has been resected. Double-barrelled stomas are usually temporary.

Ileostomies are constructed from the terminal ileum.

Complications of Stomas
Many problems may arise with stomas, which can present to the outpatient office. Many issues can frequently be improved by a stoma care nurse using different appliances. One of the first considerations is to determine whether the stoma is temporary or permanent. If significant problems arise in a temporary stoma, the correct management may be to bring forward the operation to restore bowel continuity. Most centers have experienced stoma care nurses who should be involved in most management decisions.

✧ *Constipation and diarrhea* – management may depend to a certain extent on the underlying disorder, but this can usually be treated with appropriate drugs.
✧ *Prolapse of stoma* – a common problem that often occurs when an originally dilated obstructed bowel returns to normal caliber. It is unsightly and uncomfortable but rarely dangerous, although ulceration and ischemic changes at the apex can occur. If surgery is indicated, this usually involves revising the ostomy and excising redundant bowel.
✧ *Stenosis of stoma* – a stoma should usually admit a gloved index finger easily. If not, dilators can be used, but are seldom a long-term solution. Surgical revision is usually necessary.
✧ *Skin rashes* – rashes are usually due to irritation of the skin resulting from a failure of the bag to fit snugly around the stoma. Occasionally, it is caused by the adhesive (contact dermatitis) and a different appliance is required. Involve the stoma nurse for advice regarding appliances.

✧ *Parastomal hernia* – weakness in the abdominal wall predisposes to hernia formation and a bulge underneath the stoma. If asymptomatic, this can be treated conservatively. If troublesome, hernia repair via either surgical re-siting or local repair is required. Recurrence rates are high. Laparoscopic repair using a prosthetic mesh is a potential solution to prevent the need for relocation of an otherwise acceptable stoma. Some surgeons are now using biologic mesh at the time of stoma formation to try to prevent the formation of parastomal hernias post-operatively.

✧ *Bleeding stoma* – this may be due to lesions on the edge of the mucocutaneous junction or lesions further up the GI tract. Superficial granulations respond to silver nitrate cauterization, but unusual lesions may need to be biopsied, especially if the primary surgery was for malignancy. More troublesome bleeding requires further investigation, including proctoscopy/sigmoidoscopy or flexible endoscopy down the stoma. Pyoderma gangrenosum may bleed and complicate skin surrounding ostomies of patients with IBD.

Questions and Answers

Q1   A 30-year-old female presents to your office complaining of bright red blood on her toilet paper when she wipes. She has no family history of colon or rectal cancer. She has obvious hemorrhoids on digital rectal examination. The appropriate treatment for this patient includes:

    A   Careful history about bowel habits, reassurance of the patient that everything is OK, high-fiber diet.

    B   Careful history about bowel habits, digital rectal examination, flexible sigmoidoscopy.

    C   Careful history about bowel habits, digital rectal examination, barium enema.

    D   Careful history about bowel habits, digital rectal examination, barium enema and colonoscopy.

    E   Careful history about bowel habits, digital rectal examination, fecal occult blood testing and colonoscopy.

A1   B. All patients with rectal bleeding require a careful history. In addition to this, a rectal examination is required. Fecal occult blood testing is unnecessary since she has gross blood present. Due to her age and lack of a family history of colon cancer, flexible sigmoidoscopy is appropriate.

Q2   A 51-year-old female complains of constipation. She moves her bowels once every 10 days with laxatives. Stool softeners do not help. Her symptoms all began after her hysterectomy. A colonoscopy was normal. What additional studies are required to evaluate this patient?

    A   Colonic transit.

    B   Defacography.

    C   Anal manometry.

    D   Rectal and pelvic examination.

    E   All of the above.

A2   E. Anatomic and functional causes for severe constipation include non-relaxation of the anal sphincter, colonic inertia, and internal occlusive rectal prolapse. The evaluation of these disorders includes all of those tests listed above.

Q3 A 63-year-old male is admitted to the hospital with his first episode of left lower quadrant pain. A CT scan demonstrated inflammation in the sigmoid colon consistent with diverticulitis. There was no drainable collection identified. How would you manage this patient?

    A Perform a sigmoid colectomy 6 weeks after treatment with antibiotics when the inflammation has resolved.

    B Obtain a colonoscopy the following day.

    C Obtain a barium enema the following day.

    D Place him on antibiotics and obtain a colonoscopy in 6 weeks once the inflammation resolves.

    E Perform a sigmoid colectomy during this hospitalization.

A3 D. Diverticulitis can be classified as complicated or uncomplicated. This is a case of uncomplicated diverticulitis. All cases of diverticulitis involve at least a microperforation of the colon. Therefore, procedures that increase intraluminal pressure like colonoscopy or a barium enema are contraindicated in the acute setting. Surgery is not indicated for a single episode of uncomplicated diverticulitis.

Q4 A 22-year-old male presents with a draining sinus in the right gluteal area. Three weeks ago, he developed severe pain in this area that spontaneously drained purulent material. He feels better now, but the drainage has continued. On examination you see a reddish opening in the lateral gluteal region on the right side. This patient has a:

    A Hemorrhoid.

    B Fistula-in-ano.

    C Perirectal abscess.

    D Anal fissure.

    E Anal condylomata.

A4 B. Hemorrhoids, anal fissures and condyloma are located in the anal canal or perianal region. This patient had a perirectal abscess that has subsequently resulted in a fistula-in-ano since there is now a draining sinus tract.

Q5 A 37-year-old female complains of rectal bleeding for two years following bowel movements. She feels a mass extend from her anus that requires her to push it back into the anal canal. Her colonoscopy demonstrated only hemorrhoids. By definition she has:

    A First-degree internal hemorrhoids.

    B Second-degree internal hemorrhoids.

    C Third-degree internal hemorrhoids.

    D Fourth-degree internal hemorrhoids.

    E External hemorrhoids.

A5 C. Internal hemorrhoids are classified from first- to fourth-degree. First-degree hemorrhoids do not prolapse. Second-degree hemorrhoids prolapse but reduce spontaneously, third- degree require manual reduction, and fourth-degree cannot be reduced.

Vascular
Michael J. Collins and John A. Curci

TEN

Vascular Surgery
Vascular surgery covers both interventional and medical management of a large number of disorders affecting the arterial, venous, and lymphatic systems. The majority of arterial disorders leading to vascular insufficiency are caused by the effect of atherosclerosis; however, some, such as Raynaud's, are vasospastic in nature while others, e.g. thoracic outlet syndrome, result from extrinsic compression. Arteries are also vulnerable to aneurysmal change, vasculitis, connective tissue disorders, and chronic degeneration. Venous insufficiency can occur due to primary varicose veins or venous thrombosis and can cause problems ranging from edema to ulceration and even phlegmasia. A cross-section of the common disorders referred to a vascular clinic will be described.

Disorders of the Arterial System
Many of the disorders seen by vascular surgeons are arterial and the result of atherosclerosis causing ischemic symptoms of an end-organ. However, because atherosclerosis is very common the vascular surgeon must be very familiar with the physiology of a large number of organ systems in order to be able to develop appropriate differential diagnoses of the patient's symptoms. For example, symptoms affecting the lower limb may be due to musculoskeletal or neurologic pathologies and not vascular disease, even though some element of vascular dysfunction is present. Identifying the dominant pathology can be a difficult clinical challenge.

Patients afflicted by severe atherosclerotic disease which impairs perfusion to any vascular bed must be recognized to be at increased risk of vascular disease in any other vascular bed. For example, the natural history of patients presenting with intermittent claudication is dominated by events such as myocardial infarction (MI) and stroke, rather than progression of the lower extremity arterial insufficiency itself. In every patient presenting with peripheral arterial disease, management must include modification of risk factors such as smoking, dyslipidemia, control of hypertension, and diabetes.

General Evaluation of the Patient with Arterial Insufficiency
The history of a patient with vascular insufficiency must be comprehensive and include a complete and thorough review of systems. Particular attention should be paid to specific questions related to the presenting complaint and general questions related to general cardiovascular status, risk factor analysis, family and drug history, etc.

Concomitant coronary atherosclerosis is an important cause of morbidity in patients undergoing peripheral vascular interventions; therefore, a careful assessment of the cardiac status is important. Enquire regarding angina or previous MI, cardiac valve disease, arrhythmias, and heart failure.

✧ After *MI*, the mortality/morbidity of any peripheral vascular procedure is increased within 3 months of a myocardial infarct, especially if this is associated with any degree of heart failure.

✧ *Cardiac valve disease* should be noted, as the consequences of cardiac valve disease are heart failure, embolization, and arrhythmias.

✧ *Heart failure* may impair oxygenation of the blood and impair the delivery of this blood to the tissues. The presence of heart failure exacerbates ischemic symptoms and increases the morbidity/mortality of peripheral vascular interventions.

Risk Factors

Much can be done to improve the prognosis and symptoms of patients presenting with peripheral vascular disease through the modification of cardiovascular risk factors. Some risk factors, such as age and family history, are important to the epidemiology of the disease but are not modifiable. Several of the most important modifiable/controllable risk factors for the development and progression of vascular disease are listed below:

✧ *Hypertension* is a significant risk factor in stroke, heart failure and ischemic heart disease. Appropriate identification of secondary causes of hypertension should be made, including that related to renal artery stenosis (discussed on p. 285). Primary hypertension should be appropriately controlled with a medical regimen.

✧ *Smoking* is associated with a substantial increase in the risk of peripheral vascular disease (PVD), as well as up to a 10-fold increased risk for aortic aneurysm disease. The natural history of all arterial vascular pathology can be beneficially altered by smoking cessation.

✧ *Diabetes mellitus* is associated with a threefold increased risk of PVD in men and a fivefold higher risk in women. Good diabetic monitoring in the form of glucose control, foot care, and neuropathy are important factors in the prevention of serious complications of PVD.

✧ *Hypercholesterolemia* can significantly increase the risk of developing PVD. High low-density lipoprotien (LDL) levels and low high-density lipoprotein (HDL) levels are associated with an increased risk of PVD. High serum triglyceride levels are also associated with the development of PVD.

Vascular Examination

In addition to a comprehensive physical examination, all peripheral pulses are palpated and the volume and character of each pulse is recorded – radial, brachial, axillary, subclavian, carotid, aortic, femoral, popliteal, dorsalis pedis, and posterior tibial. The dorsalis pedis or posterior tibial pulse may be absent in 10% of normal individuals. The blood pressure is measured with the patient semi-reclined. Examine for radio-radial delay and radio-femoral delay. Listen for carotid, subclavian, aortic, iliac, femoral, and popliteal artery bruits.

Examine the respiratory and cardiovascular systems. Examine for signs of heart failure and cardiac valve disease. Examine the abdomen and palpate for any aortic aneurysm. It should be recalled that the abdominal aorta bifurcates at about the level of the umbilicus, therefore abdominal aneurysms are typically palpated above this, and iliac aneurysm below this. Auscultate for an aortic bruit – this may indicate aortic, renal, or iliac stenotic disease. A machinery-type murmur associated with an aneurysm may indicate an aorto-caval fistula, especially if associated with swelling of the legs.

In the legs, examine for limb swelling, ulceration, or the presence of varicose veins. Port-wine stains or differing limb size may indicate underlying arteriovenous malformations. Examine for signs of ischemia – relative skin temperatures, venous guttering, delayed (>2 s) capillary refill, hair loss, red shiny skin on the toes, patches of infarction/gangrene on the toes.

Perform Buerger's test. Raise the legs and note the angle at which the soles of the feet turn pale. After 1 minute, hang the legs down and note the time for the feet to develop a brick red color and the veins to refill. A brick red color is indicative of ischemia.

Laboratory Investigations

The differential diagnosis will guide the appropriate laboratory studies. These may include urinalysis and general biochemical tests to screen for underlying renal disease/

renovascular disease, diabetes mellitus, etc., which may influence vascular treatment. Evaluation may also include quantification of fasting serum lipids as well as screening for anemia or coagulopathies.

Imaging Techniques
The past 20 years have seen a great increase in the variety and quality of imaging technologies available for the diagnosis of vascular abnormalities. These are summarized below. The proper technique to be used for any individual will depend on the specific vessel to be evaluated as well as the patient-specific risks of any test.

Ultrasound Techniques
Ultrasound uses high-frequency sound waves which enter the tissues and are reflected in different amounts from structures of different composition. The reflected waves are detected and used to construct representative images of the underlying tissues. This is known as the B-mode image. When ultrasound waves reach moving objects such as the blood cells within a vessel, analysis of the reflected waves allows the direction and speed of travel to be determined using the Doppler equation. In its simplest continuous wave form the output can be either an audible output – the typical whoosh, whoosh of the ultrasound machine – or a visual output displayed as a waveform on the screen.

The B-mode image and the Doppler waveform can be combined; the widely used trade name for this combination is "duplex." The use of pulsed Doppler allows the ultrasound to be sampled from a particular depth within the tissues so that the artery can be visualized and Doppler signals measured at different points within it. The velocity and direction of the Doppler information can be color-coded and superimposed on the B-mode image, giving the impression of blood moving within the artery in real time. This is known as color duplex.

Continuous Wave Doppler (CWD)
✧ *Technique* – CWD is the simplest form of ultrasound and is ideal for use by the doctor in the outpatient clinic to detect flow within blood vessels – most frequently in the extremities. The device is typically handheld and portable. In the head of the probe is a transmitter and a receiver which are continuously active. The probe is moved over the area of interest, and when flow is detected the typical whoosh-whoosh sound becomes audible.
✧ *Advantages* – simple, quick, and easy to use. It is more sensitive than the physical exam for flow in vessels. Good for longitudinal evaluations of patients with arterial insufficiency.
✧ *Disadvantages* – limited information is provided other than the presence or absence of flow.

Ankle–Brachial Pressure Index (ABI).
✧ *Technique* – in a healthy patient the systolic blood pressure at the ankle should be the same as or slightly higher than in the arm. Since atherosclerosis usually affects the leg vessels severely and spares the arm vessels, this test provides a means to quantify lower-extremity perfusion. To measure the ABI (also known as the ankle–arm index [AAI]), a blood pressure cuff is placed on the upper arm and the radial pulse is detected at the wrist using CWD. The cuff is then inflated until the CWD signal disappears. The cuff is deflated slowly until the signal returns. The procedure is then repeated for the lower limb with the cuff applied just above the ankle and the probe placed on the dorsalis pedis, posterior tibial, and/or peroneal arteries. The

pressure at which the signal returns is compared for the arm and the leg and expressed as a ratio – the ABI. An ABI of 0.9–1.0 is normal; less than 0.9 indicates vascular disease.

✧ *Advantages* – ABI is a quick and easy technique that provides a reasonably reproducible measurement which corrects for variations in systemic blood pressure between patients and in the same patient on different occasions.

✧ *Disadvantages* – ABI can be unobtainable in the presence of incompressible arteries. As a CWD signal can always be detected, even at very high cuff pressures, the patient will have a falsely elevated ABI (>1). This phenomenon commonly occurs in diabetic patients. Other testing modalities are necessary to quantify perfusion; the toe pressure is often relatively reliable in this patient population.

Resting ABI may miss well collateralized arterial disease. In these situations, the disease can be detected by repeating the ABI after a period of exercise (see below).

Toe-pressure Measurement

✧ *Technique* – an alternative method in patients with incompressible arteries. A small cuff is inflated around the big toe until the arterial signal in the digital arteries disappears. Smaller arteries in the digits are usually not affected by calcification and provide a more reliable toe–brachial pressure index (TBI). TBI <0.8 indicates ischemia; an absolute pressure measurement of less than 30–35 mmHg indicates critical ischemia.

✧ *Advantages* – provides an objective alternative to ABI in patients with incompressible arteries.

✧ *Disadvantages* – does not provide level of disease.

Treadmill Exercise Testing

✧ *Technique* – lower-extremity exercise partnered with the ABI is particularly useful in detecting well-collateralized arterial disease of the legs. The commonest method utilizes a treadmill. The resting ABI is measured initially. The patient walks on the treadmill at a pace of 3.5 km/h and at a grade of 10 degrees for 1 minute or until the symptoms are experienced. The ABI is then measured immediately on stopping the exercise. In the presence of vascular disease, the ABI falls after exercise. A normal ABI after exercise which has precipitated the symptoms strongly mitigates against a vascular cause.

✧ *Advantages* – exercise testing is more sensitive than resting ABI in detecting or excluding significant vascular disease.

✧ *Disadvantages* – not all patients are capable of walking on a moving treadmill.

Ankle Flexion/Extension Exercise Testing

✧ *Technique* – this is another technique to stress the legs and evaluate the ABI. The patient sits reclined and repeatedly flexes and extends the ankle of the affected limb against a fixed resistance device, thereby exercising the calf muscle. The ABI is measured before and after exercise and is interpreted in the same way as the treadmill exercise.

✧ *Advantages* – this alternative exercise may be useful for patients who are unable to walk on the treadmill.

✧ *Disadvantages* – simulates rather than replicates the action of walking. This technique is less reproducible than the standardized treadmill testing.

Color Duplex Ultrasonography

✧ *Technique* – color duplex ultrasonography is the combination of B-mode images and color-coded pulsed Doppler information which has become the dominant non-invasive investigation in vascular practice. Acoustic water-based gel is applied to the skin overlying the area of interest, and the probe applied. The depth and power of the signal is adjusted until the artery is visualized. Doppler waveforms are then sampled from different parts of the artery. Color coding allows high-velocity signals and turbulence within the artery to be identified, indicating the site of possible stenoses. This technique is particularly powerful in determining the presence of carotid stenosis, but is used less frequently in distal vessels owing to the difficulty in visualizing vessels completely.

✧ *Advantages* – provides non-invasive structural and hemodynamic data.

✧ *Disadvantages* – it is very much operator dependent, taking years to develop expertise. It is difficult to confirm vessel occlusions, and difficult in very calcified arteries.

Radiologic Techniques

Nearly all vascular imaging techniques rely on a contrast agent to enhance the imaging of blood flow in vessels to allow for adequate definition of areas of stenosis or occlusion. It is critical to recognize the risks and benefits of each agent and technique, and to determine which imaging technique provides the best anatomic detail at the lowest risk.

Diagnostic Arterial Angiography

✧ *Technique* – direct intra-arterial injection of contrast agent into the vascular tree of concern is generally considered the gold-standard imaging technique. Typically, iodinated contrast agents are used, with attendant risks of anaphylaxis and renal dysfunction. The risk of contrast-induced nephropathy (CIN) is related to the pre-procedural degree of renal dysfunction, therefore creatinine clearance should be evaluated prior to the procedure. The risk of CIN is also associated with dehydration and providing sufficient hydration will reduce this risk, particularly in those with borderline renal dysfunction. The oral hypoglycemic metformin has also been shown to be associated with lactic acidosis and renal dysfunction in individuals receiving iodinated contrast and should be stopped at least 48 hours prior to the procedure.

✧ Digital subtraction angiography (DSA) is a computerized technique for improving the image quality obtained at angiography. X-ray images are digitalized and the images of soft tissue and bone suppressed while the image of contrast within the blood vessels is enhanced. The technique is frequently a part of modern angiography.

✧ *Procedure* – entry to the vascular system is typically through the femoral artery, although the axillary and brachial arteries can also be used. Under local anesthesia and utilizing the Seldinger technique, the artery is punctured using a hollow needle through which a floppy-ended wire is passed. The needle is then removed and a plastic sheath is passed over the wire into the artery. A variety of catheters are used to enter the vessel of interest in order to inject contrast. Radiologic images are taken as the contrast is displaced through the distal vasculature, utilizing arterial digital subtraction imaging. At the end of the procedure the wire, catheter, and sheath are removed and direct pressure is applied at the puncture site for 15–20 minutes. The patient then remains supine on absolute bed-rest for 2–4 hours after the procedure.

✧ *Advantages* – provides an accurate map of the arterial tree, identifying stenoses and occlusions. Diagnostic angiography can be combined with therapeutic interventions for the treatment of a variety of vascular problems.

✧ *Disadvantages* – angiograms require the direct puncture of an arterial vessel. Complications include bleeding, trauma to the artery, hematoma, pseudoaneurysm, embolization, arterial dissection, allergic reactions to the contrast, and renal failure. Angiography also does not image the vessel wall, and aneurysms can be easily missed with this modality.

Computed Tomography Angiography (CTA)
✧ *Technique* – a CT scan with "thin cuts" is performed together with injection of intravenous contrast. The data obtained can be processed in a number of ways to obtain images similar to those obtained with DSA, without the requirement for direct arterial injection of the contrast.
✧ *Advantages* – excellent imaging of vascular structures and post-processing can allow for a number of creative imaging projections, including three-dimensional. Unlike DSA, the walls of the vessels, as well as the luminal contrast, are imaged.
✧ *Disadvantages* – CTA is somewhat technically demanding, and there are a number of pitfalls in the technical performance of the procedure and the reconstructions which can lead to misleading or uninformative results. There is potential for allergic reactions and CIN secondary to the large volume of contrast required.

Magnetic Resonance Imaging Angiography
✧ *Technique* – MRI scans are performed; moving blood acts as its own contrast and no additional contrast needs to be given. For imaging of small vessels, additional small coils are placed over the area concerned. Improved images can be obtained with the intravenous injection of gadolinium and T1 acquisition.
✧ *Advantages* – contrast can be avoided; it is a non-invasive investigation.
✧ *Disadvantages* – not applicable to patients with significant metal implants. Images are still not accurate enough for small vessels.

Lower Extremity Arterial Insufficiency
Atherosclerosis is the major cause of lower limb ischemia – the most common reason for patients to require vascular surgery evaluation. Therefore, the overwhelming majority of patients presenting with intermittent claudication or rest pain suffer from atherosclerosis. Other causes of lower limb ischemia are more common in younger patients and may also need to be considered. These include cystic adventitial disease, popliteal entrapment, fibromuscular dysplasia, and Buerger's disease.

Intermittent Claudication
Intermittent claudication occurs when stenosed arteries cannot supply sufficient blood to the muscles during exercise. In the lower limbs the patient describes cramp-like symptoms in the legs, most commonly the calf muscles, occurring at a predictable distance and which is quickly relieved by rest. Once the pain is relieved the patient may then describe the ability to walk further the second time before the pain returns. These symptoms need to be differentiated from other causes of pain in the legs when walking, such as arthritis or sciatica.

The decision to treat is based on the severity of the symptoms and the effect on the patient's lifestyle. Severity is not decided purely on the distance walked. A claudication distance of 400 yards may be an occasional inconvenience to a retired patient but may be job-threatening to a manual worker.

✧ *Calf claudication* – commonly associated with femoral artery disease. A typical history of vascular calf claudication is pain in one or both calves which occurs after walking a certain distance and is relieved by rest. The distance tends to be constant but may lessen over weeks and months as the disease progresses. The pain is quickly relieved by rest (1–2 minutes).

✧ *Buttock claudication* – commonly associated with aorto-iliac disease. It has a slightly different character to calf claudication. Patients describe more aching and weakness or complain of their hip giving way. However, the pain is exacerbated by exercise and relieved by rest. Male patients with bilateral aortoiliac disease may admit to impotence on questioning.

✧ *Foot claudication* is very rare and occurs only in patients with Buerger's disease and occlusive disease, which affects the distal arteries first and spreads proximally. Patients describe pain and numbness which affects the forefoot with exercise. This is often diagnosed as an orthopedic pain and may have progressed to persistent rest pain by the time a vascular opinion is sought.

Other common causes of pain in the calf or leg include:

✧ *Arthritis* – arthritis of the knee or ankle may cause referred pain to the calf. Similarly, arthritis of the spine or hip may produce symptoms similar to buttock claudication. However, arthritic symptoms tend to vary in severity from day to day or with weather conditions. The pain may occur at rest or start with exercise. The amount of exercise necessary to produce symptoms varies and the pain may persist for hours after the exercise stops.

✧ *Nocturnal cramp* – pain in the calf which typically occurs in bed and wakes the patient, and is relieved by massage of the calf or getting out of bed and walking around.

✧ *Spinal stenosis* – there is usually a history of arthritis; the condition is caused by osteophytes narrowing the spinal canal. The pain occurs on walking and is relieved by rest but especially by bending forward. However, this pain can also be precipitated by prolonged standing. There may be associated numbness and paresthesia, especially around the perineum.

✧ *Chronic compartment syndrome* – often affects athletes with large calf muscles. The symptoms are similar to claudication but require a large amount of exercise to produce the symptoms.

History
If the symptoms are typical of vascular claudication, determine the distance walked before symptoms start. Determine how this affects the patient's lifestyle. If the walking distance is very small (<50 yards) ask about rest pain (pain in the toes at rest), especially at night in bed. The patient should also be asked about other signs of chronic ischemia such as non-healing wounds, hair loss, and chronic cold/cool feet or toes.

Examination
Palpate all the pulses and auscultate for bruits. Look for general stigmata of vascular insufficiency, e.g. loss of hair in the lower leg, atrophic skin, etc. Claudication is usually but not always associated with absent pulses – pulses may be present at rest but disappear with exercise.

Try to determine the site of the arterial disease, e.g. absent femoral pulse suggests iliac artery disease.

Investigations
Routine atherosclerotic screen – urinalysis, complete blood count (CBC), chemistries, serum lipids, and electrocardiography (ECG). An ABI <0.9 indicates underlying vascular

disease. The treadmill test may reveal ankle pressure drop after exercise. CTA or conventional angiography can identify the precise site and guide the choice of treatment (i.e. angioplasty versus surgical intervention).

Treatment

◆ *Mild claudication not interfering with patient's lifestyle* – correct any underlying disorder such as hyperlipidemia. Advise daily walks, losing weight, stopping smoking, to improve cardiac and respiratory function. Patients should be encouraged to develop a regular exercise program to improve the distance the patient may walk prior to onset of claudication.

◆ *Moderate claudication affecting the patient's lifestyle but not severely so* – as for mild disease, but review earlier and proceed to active treatment if conservative measures fail. Some centers advocate a supervised exercise program under the control of a physiotherapist. Results may be comparable to angioplasty without the risk of complications and represent a non-interventional alternative.

◆ *Severe claudication severely affecting daily living* – more active treatment is indicated. Angioplasty with or without stenting is frequently the first choice, providing the lesion is amenable. Long, diffuse disease lesions, or patients who have failed prior angioplasty, are typically considered for arterial bypass surgery (operations are described under critical ischemia).

Follow-up

◆ *Mild claudication* – depending on the duration and progression of symptoms, patients with mild claudication should be followed at 6-month to 1-year intervals to evaluate symptom progression. Yearly ABI may also assist the clinician to document disease progression.

◆ *Moderate claudication* – follow at 3 to 6-month intervals to assess patient compliance and success with risk-factor modification. A patient who continues to experience worsening claudication despite risk-factor modification will often undergo a CTA to determine whether angioplasty or bypass are warranted or possible.

◆ *Severe claudication* – review after angiogram/angioplasty to decide whether further angioplasty or surgical intervention is indicated.

Critical Ischemia, Rest Pain, Gangrene

Ischemic rest pain occurs when not enough blood is reaching the foot to maintain the viability of the foot at rest, and represents critical ischemia. Therefore, the pain tends to start at areas of the lower limb furthest away from the heart and may spread proximally. If critical ischemia is not reversed, then dry gangrene ensues.

Gangrene also occurs when a small injury occurs in a severely ischemic foot. Healing tissue requires up to 10 times the blood supply of normal tissue in order to heal. Failure to meet these oxygen requirements results in tissue back-progressing proximally to the point of adequate blood supply. In this way a relatively small wound sustained to the tip of the big toe of a critically ischemic foot can result in gangrene affecting a much wider area.

Ischemic rest pain needs to be differentiated from other causes of pain in the foot at rest, e.g. arthritis of the toes or metatarso-phalangeal joints.

History

Take a general and vascular history. Rest pain may first start at night when the foot is lifted on to the bed thereby losing the help of gravity to supply blood to the foot. Patients may describe gaining relief from the pain by dangling the foot over the side of the bed. With progression of ischemia, pain is present at all times. Pain starts at the point furthest away from the heart and spreads proximally.

Other causes of constant lower limb pain include:

✧ *Embolization* – distal embolization (from cardiac, aortic, or iliac lesions) may result in rest pain affecting the toes but the foot appears well perfused and foot pulses may be palpable.

✧ *Arthritis* – causes pain in the foot or ankle at rest but tends to be localized to the joints or areas proximal to the toes. Pain in the metatarsals can occur at night and is relieved by standing; this can be confused for vascular night pain. However, metatarsal pain tends to run a fluctuating course, causing symptoms for several days or weeks with similar asymptomatic periods.

✧ *Painful peripheral neuritis* – tends to occur in diabetics and is characterized by a constant burning pain affecting both lower legs. The pain is worse at night when the legs become warm.

✧ *Reflex sympathetic dystrophy* – produces a burning pain. The condition is ill-defined but there may be a history of preceding trauma which may be relatively minor. The limb becomes swollen and is initially warm and dry, but later becomes cool, mottled, and cyanotic. However, the arterial tree is normal.

✧ *Neuralgia* – results from incomplete nerve injury and produces a similar constant burning pain.

Examination
Palpate all the pulses and listen for bruits. Look for signs of peripheral ischemia – loss of hair, thin shiny skin, atrophic musculature. The foot may be edematous from chronic dependency. Note that a critically ischemic foot may actually appear erythematous with good capillary return when dependent – this is known as *dependent rubor* and may be confused with infection. Elevation of the foot will reveal a very pale foot. Examine for evidence of distal embolization, e.g. focal spots of skin infarction in an otherwise well-perfused foot.

Investigations
Routine atherosclerotic screen of urinalysis and blood tests. Perform ABI test – a ratio of less than 0.9 indicates peripheral vascular disease, and less than 0.5 indicates severe ischemia. The majority of these patients are sent for angiography, CTA, or MRI angiography to plan for revascularization.

Treatment
In order to salvage the leg and foot, active intervention is indicated. Patients usually require admission for adequate pain relief, elevation of the limb to reduce tissue edema, and intravenous antibiotics if indicated. Optimize cardiac and respiratory function.

Vascular reconstruction procedures will vary depending on the site of the disease and the presence of suitable proximal and distal anastomosis targets. As a general rule, the most proximal lesion is corrected first and ischemic skin lesions have the best chance of healing if there is a continuous channel of blood from the aorta to the pedal arch. Many different operations are available; only the commonly performed procedures will be described. It should be noted that for critical limb ischemia, it is generally necessary to correct disease at at least two of three levels (aorto-iliac, femoro-popliteal, tibial).

✧ *Angioplasty/stenting* – angioplasty and stenting for critical limb ischemia should generally be limited to short-segment occlusions in large vessels. This can often be used as an adjunct to femoro-popliteal reconstructions in patients with ipsilateral iliac disease.

✧ *Aorto-bifemoral bypass* – occlusive disease of the iliac arteries can be bypassed using a prosthetic bifurcated graft from the aorta to both femoral arteries. The patient must be fit enough to withstand clamping of the aorta; in unfit individuals, an axillo-bifemoral graft is a less invasive alternative. However, it is unusual for gangrene or rest pain to be associated with aorto-iliac occlusions alone; critical limb ischemia is usually associated with multi-level vascular disease.

✧ *Femoro-popliteal bypass* – occlusive disease of the superficial femoral artery can be by-passed by using either a prosthetic graft or the patient's own vein, usually the saphenous vein. The choice of conduit (vein versus prosthetic material) depends on many factors, including the length of the required bypass, availability of vein, and other considerations. Vein has superior patency, especially when the graft must cross a joint, but results with prosthetic graft to the above-knee popliteal artery are accept-able. Patency of prosthetic grafts to the below-knee popliteal artery may be improved when a segment of vein is interposed between the graft and the artery.

✧ *Femoro-distal bypass* – bypass operations performed to the distal run-off vessels (pos-terior tibial, anterior tibial, and peroneal) typically require autologous vein to be used to obtain reasonable long-term patency due to the small calibre of the vessels.

✧ *Amputation* – amputation may be necessary for an unretrievably gangrenous extrem-ity/digit or for one where there are no viable revascularization options. Options for amputation can include digital amputations to transtibial, transfemoral or hip dis-articulation. The best amputation is the least amputation which allows for adequate healing of the extremity.

Post-operative Follow-up

When angioplasty and/or arterial bypass operations have been performed for critical ischemia, long-term regular follow-up is indicated to detect recurrence, progression of disease or vessel/graft thrombosis.

✧ *Vein-graft surveillance* – when autologous vein has been used to bypass occlusions in the leg arteries, many hospitals follow patients with regular duplex ultrasound scans of the vein to detect subclinical stenoses. Significant vein-graft stenoses are treated by urgent angioplasty or operative vein-patch angioplasty. Between scans patients are advised to seek urgent medical attention if the leg turns white, cold, numb, or painful, as the graft may have occluded and may be salvaged if operated on early. Surveillance using duplex is generally performed on all patients for the first year and extended for a second year for grafts which are considered at risk. Thereafter patients are followed with duplex scans at 6–12 months and discharged when symptom-free.

✧ *Complications* include wound infections, hematomas, and graft failure. Superficial infections should be treated aggressively with antibiotics and close follow-up. Deeper infections may require inpatient treatment and intravenous antibiotics, especially if prosthetic grafts have been used. If the wound near an anastomosis becomes infected or opens up, inpatient therapy is mandatory as there is a real risk of secondary hem-orrhage. Wound hematomas and lymph collections can be managed conservatively provided they do not become infected. Limb swelling is normal after arterial bypass surgery and can be treated conservatively if deep-venous thrombosis (DVT) and cel-lulitis have been excluded.

Non-atherosclerotic Causes of Lower Extremity Arterial Insufficiency

Cystic Adventitial Disease (CAD)

This is an uncommon cause of lower limb ischemia in younger patients. The adventitia of the popliteal artery undergoes a degenerative process and develops a cyst. When the pressure of the contents of the cyst exceed arterial pressure, the cyst may compress the artery causing sudden-onset ischemia.

The differential diagnosis includes popliteal aneurysm, popliteal entrapment, and simple knee joint cysts. Excludes cardiac source for emboli, vasculitis, and/or connective tissue disease (CTD).

History
Patients are usually young and complain of claudication of recent onset. Symptoms may be severe due to the lack of collateral development. Patients may describe ischemic neuropathy symptoms of burning, paresthesia, and cold.

Examination
There is usually a lack of atherosclerotic signs in other body sites. All pulses in the affected limb may be present at rest, but foot pulses disappear on flexion of the knee. Palpation of the affected artery may simulate a popliteal aneurysm. A popliteal bruit may be audible. Later, if occlusion of the popliteal artery occurs, pulses are lost.

Investigation
ECG may be indicated to exclude a cardiac source of emboli. Color duplex may demonstrate the compression of the artery and also identify the cyst and exclude a popliteal aneurysm. CT and MRI may better define the lesion in relation to other anatomical structures. Arteriography demonstrates a smooth localized stenosis behind the knee.

Treatment
Angioplasty tends *not* to be successful because the walls are compliant and cyst content may embolize distally. Aspiration of cysts under CT guidance can be attempted, but lesions tend to recur. Surgical evacuation of the cyst is effective treatment; however, if the artery has progressed to occlusion, then resection and interposition graft repair is required.

Post-operative Follow-up
If aspiration has been performed, medium-term follow-up may be required to detect recurrence. Follow-up of bypass procedures is described under critical ischemia.

Popliteal Entrapment Syndrome
Popliteal entrapment is an uncommon disorder but should be excluded in all young patients complaining of lower limb symptoms consistent with arterial insufficiency. Popliteal entrapment results from compression of the popliteal artery (or other popliteal neurovascular structures) by a congenital abnormality of the medial head of the gastrocnemius muscle. There are five types of popliteal entrapment, based on the specific anatomic abnormality found in the popliteal fossa.
- ✧ *Type I*: Popliteal artery has aberrant medial course around the medial head of the gastrocnemius muscle.
- ✧ *Type II*: Medial head of the gastrocnemius inserts laterally, artery not displaced.
- ✧ *Type III*: Accessory slip of muscle around the artery.
- ✧ *Type IV*: Artery trapped deeply by popliteus muscle or a fibrous band.
- ✧ *Type V*: Both popliteal artery and vein are involved.

History
Most patients are young and active and describe typical symptoms of claudication associated with physical exercise. Patients may describe atypical features such as numbness of

the foot, blanching, paresthesia, or pain on walking but not running, etc. Enquire regarding cardiac abnormalities and arrhythmias or possible vasculitic pathologies, CTD, etc.

Examination
Exclude cardiac or other sources of embolization. There is usually a lack of atherosclerosis affecting other arteries. Pulses may be palpable at rest but disappear on dorsiflexion or forced plantar flexion of the foot. Later cases may have absent pulses due to popliteal occlusion. Alternatively, some patients may have post-stenotic aneurysmal degeneration of the popliteal artery.

Investigation
Consider ECG to exclude cardiac source of emboli. Duplex ultrasound may demonstrate compression of the artery and identify aneurysmal dilatation. MRI is being increasingly used to identify the soft-tissue abnormalities associated with this condition. Angiography is used to confirm the diagnosis and exclude any arterial abnormality. In cases of occlusion, angiography defines the distal run-off vessels in preparation for surgery.

Treatment
All confirmed cases are treated surgically with release of the constricting band or muscle and/or reconstruction of the artery. The specific conduct of the procedure is based on damage to the vessel and the specific altered anatomy of the popliteal musculature.

Post-operative Follow-up
Review to determine the success of the procedure and detect any complications. If a vein interposition graft has been used, then regular vein-graft surveillance is appropriate to detect stenoses and prevent occlusion.

Popliteal entrapment tends to be bilateral and the contralateral leg should be considered for evaluation and release of compression prior to the development of arterial damage and significant symptoms.

Cerebrovascular Arterial Disease
Carotid Artery Disease
A common location for the development of significant atherosclerotic plaque is at the bifurcation of the carotid artery. The risk of this carotid atherosclerotic disease is cerebral ischemia, nearly always due to embolic events of the plaque or thrombus which has developed in ulcerated plaque. The risk of a cerebrobascular event due to carotid atherosclerotic disease is proportional to the degree of stenosis and the prior history of ipsilateral cerebrovascular events. Most of the high-quality data on the safety and efficacy of surgical treatment of carotid artery disease is well over a decade old. However, current recommendations are based on that data and subsequent, less well controlled studies.

Objectives
Detect severe carotid stenosis, identify neurologic symptoms ipsilateral to the stenosed artery, exclude non-specific neurologic symptoms.

History
The focus of the history is on any symptoms which may indicate an embolic neurologic event ipsilateral to the diseased vasculature. Non-specific or non-hemispheric symptoms such as blackouts, drop attacks, fainting, dizziness, double vision, vertigo, etc., are more suggestive of cardiac neurologic or ear, nose, and throat (ENT) disease, and further

investigation or referral to the relevant specialty should be considered. However, some of these symptoms may indicate vertebrobasilar ischemia (VBI) which may have a primary vascular cause, and this should be excluded (*see* p. 284).

Examination

✧ Perform a general and vascular examination. Listen for bruits over the carotid and subclavian arteries. Note that the absence of a carotid bruit does not exclude the presence of a severely stenosed carotid artery, nor does the presence of a bruit assure that there is significant disease of the internal carotid artery.
✧ Perform a general neurologic examination and record any existing neurologic deficits.

Perform a cardiac examination – in particular, examine for arrhythmias, valve abnormalities, and heart failure.

Investigations

The non-invasive technique of color duplex ultrasonography is used most frequently to evaluate the carotid arteries to determine the degree of stenosis, and this is reliable when performed by an experienced operator. It should be noted that the primary diagnostic criteria is the Doppler-measured velocities of the internal carotid artery. B-mode imaging can be very misleading. Carotid angiography is useful in situations where the Doppler evaluation is unreliable or to identify aortic arch, brachiocephalic or subclavian artery disease. CT/MRI brain scan may be indicated to exclude neurologic disease or define the extent of a recent stroke.

Treatment

The decision to intervene on a patient with carotid stenosis is based on the risks of the procedure and the anticipated future risk of stroke in the absence of intervention. It follows that carotid intervention should only be undertaken by interventionalists who have demonstrated extremely low rates of peri-procedural events. For patients with ipsilateral symptoms, any stenosis >50% may benefit from carotid endarterectomy. For those patients confirmed to have a severe symptomatic carotid stenosis, carotid endarterectomy is most effective within 3 months of the onset of symptoms, and even earlier interventions may be best. For patients without ipsilateral cerebral symptoms and stenosis, surgical intervention should be considered for anyone with stenosis greater than 70–80%. Benefits will be limited in patients with severe comorbidities and limited life expectancy.

✧ *Carotid endarterectomy (CEA)* is the current standard of care for carotid atherosclerotic disease. In experienced hands, the risk of peri-procedural stroke is very low and the durability of the procedure is well documented. CEA may be associated with higher risk in patients with severe coronary disease, radiation to the ipsilateral neck, or in recurrent stenosis.
✧ *Carotid angioplasty/stenting* has been shown to demonstrate reasonably good results in patients with complicated carotid disease who may be at high risk for CEA. The value of this modality in patients who are asymptomatic or otherwise at good risk for CEA remains an area of considerable discussion.

Post-operative Follow-up

Patients are seen 4–6 weeks after operation to check on local complications related to the wound. In some centers a further duplex scan is performed on the operated artery to identify re-stenosis or asymptomatic occlusion. Re-stenosis is usually due to intimal hyperplasia.

Other complications following CEA include cranial nerve lesions, infection (superficial and deep), and false aneurysm. Transient cranial lesions occur in up to one third of patients and usually resolve within 6–12 months.

Vertebrobasilar Ischemia (VBI)

Symptomatic VBI is less common than symptomatic carotid disease and the criteria for surgical treatment are less well defined. Symptoms of VBI may be embolic or hemodynamic, and may arise from disease of the vertebral artery itself or from the subclavian artery proximal to the origin of the vertebral artery. The cause of symptoms may be intrinsic or extrinsic, e.g. the vertebral arteries may be compressed by osteophytes associated with cervical spondylosis. Other neurologic pathologies, orthostatic hypotension, cardiac arrhythmias, ENT, and other non-vascular causes may need to be excluded.

Objectives

Diagnose vertebrobasilar ischemia, differentiate from other pathologies, treat VBI.

History

Determine exactly the circumstances when symptoms occur. There is a very large differential diagnosis for posterior cerebral circulation or global cerebral insufficiency.

The simultaneous occurrence of at least three of the following vertebrobasilar symptoms is required for diagnosis of vertebrobasilar syndrome; isolated symptoms are less significant. The symptoms are: unilateral or bilateral simultaneous motor/sensory deficits, ataxia, diplopia, dysarthria, dysphagia, bilateral homonymous hemianopia, vertigo, tinnitus, transient global amnesia. Drop attacks or loss of consciousness may be the result of subclavian steal syndrome (SSS) if they coincide with vigorous use of the arm.

Enquire regarding other neurologic, ENT, or cardiac pathologies.

Examination

Perform a general, neurologic and vascular examination. Listen for supraclavicular and carotid bruits. Examine the neck for tenderness and range of movement. Always check bilateral upper extremity blood pressures and make note of significant discrepancies. Examine for cardiac abnormalities.

Investigations

If indicated, perform a general atherosclerotic screen of urinalysis and blood tests. Color duplex of the carotid subclavian and vertebral arteries is sensitive enough to detect significant disease. Definitive identification of lesions requires angiography. CT brain scan may be required to exclude brain tumors producing similar symptoms. A 24-hour Holter monitor may be required to investigate cardiac arrhythmias.

Treatment

Embolic symptoms are usually successfully treated with correction of vascular risk factors and low-dose aspirin. For hemodynamic lesions in the subclavian artery (typically the left), angioplasty or bypass of subclavian stenoses/occlusions may be undertaken.

Indications for surgery include severe (>70%) symptomatic stenoses of the vertebral artery, short occlusions of both vertebral artery origins, or stenosis of one remaining or dominant artery causing symptoms. Surgical reconstruction of the vertebral artery is a specialized technique performed mainly for recognized embolic or hemodynamic disease, and consists of carotid to vertebral artery bypass or transposition of the vertebral artery to the carotid.

Visceral Arterial Disease
Renal Artery Stenosis

Renal artery stenosis (RAS) is a potentially curable cause of hypertension and deteriorating renal function. There are two main disease processes, atherosclerosis and fibromuscular dysplasia (FMD). Other less common causes include Takayasu's arteritis, renal artery aneurysm, arteriovenous malformation, neurofibromatosis, Marfan's syndrome.

✧ Atherosclerosis tends to be associated with an atherosclerotic aorta and affects mainly the ostia of the renal arteries.

✧ FMD is more common in women and affects the more distal renal artery and its branches.

✧ FMD is a particularly common cause of renovascular hypertension in children.

Objectives

Diagnose RAS, differentiate between atherosclerosis and FMD, identify those patients suitable for intervention, treat suitable patients, detect recurrent disease.

History

Take a general and vascular history.

Patients may be referred to the vascular surgeon from other specialties with hypertension that is difficult to control – often requiring 3–4 antihypertensive agents. There may be episodes of flash pulmonary edema causing sudden heart failure and breathlessness occurring at night.

Alternatively, patients may be referred because of deteriorating renal function. Most of these patients will have had some investigation which suggests RAS. Some patients will have experienced a deterioration in renal function after starting an angiotensin-converting enzyme (ACE) inhibitor as treatment for their blood pressure. In RAS, contraction of the efferent glomerular arteriole is a protective mechanism maintaining glomerular filtration. ACE inhibitors prevent this and thus renal function deteriorates.

Examination

Perform a general and vascular examination. Measure the blood pressure. Evidence of general atherosclerosis suggests RAS as the cause of hypertension. There may be absent pulses and audible abdominal and flank bruits.

Investigation

Carry out a dipstick urine test and perform routine hematology, biochemistry, and serum lipids. Measurement of plasma renin may also suggest the diagnosis.

Abdominal ultrasound is used to measure the length of the kidneys. A renal length less than 8–9 cm suggests an irretrievable loss of renal parenchyma, and correction of the RAS may not provide significant salvage of renal function. Duplex scan of the renal arteries may identify stenosis, but is technically difficult.

Functional testing, such as captopril renography or selective renal vein renin measurements, may be helpful in selective cases but their utility is limited by bilateral renal artery disease and other technical details. The sensitivity and specificity of these studies is also limited.

Contrast arterial angiography is the gold standard, using lateral and oblique views to define the RAS. FMD gives the classical "string of beads" appearance of alternating stenoses and microaneurysm formation. Angiography also demonstrates ostial disease and atherosclerotic aorta. Ask for lateral views of superior mesenteric and celiac arteries as well, in case extra-anatomical bypass is to be considered. Angiography may also demonstrate renal artery aneurysms.

Treatment

✧ *Angioplasty* is the treatment of choice for FMD – recurrent and renal artery branch lesions also respond well. Angioplasty is less successful for atherosclerosis. There is considerable debate about the value of angioplasty/stenting of atherosclerotic RAS. This modality should only be employed in carefully selected patients.

✧ *Surgical treatment – nephrectomy* may be indicated for a small, scarred kidney producing significant amounts of renin (renal vein renin ratio >1.5) causing hypertension with a normal kidney on the contralateral side.

✧ *Revascularization* procedures are particularly appropriate where there is coexisting aortic disease or angioplasty has failed, and for bilateral RAS caused by atherosclerosis. Surgery is the first-choice option for the solitary failing kidney. Procedures are divided into aortic and extra-anatomic bypass. The choice depends on the patient's ability to withstand aortic clamping.

   ∝ Extra-anatomic bypass may be considered provided there is a suitable disease-free donor artery; splenic artery on the left, common hepatic artery on the right.

   ∝ Procedures requiring aortic clamping include aortic replacement and bypass grafting, aortic replacement and renal artery endarterectomy, and renal artery endarterectomy and patch angioplasty.

   ∝ Direct aorto-renal grafting is also performed.

✧ *Branch renal artery disease* – complex disease involving the branches of the renal artery, such as FMD, renal artery aneurysm, dissection, diffuse atheroma, and arteritis, may require removal of the kidney, bench surgery to correct the abnormality, and reimplantation (autotransplantation).

Post-operative Follow-up

Long term follow-up is required to detect recurrent disease causing deterioration in renal function or hypertension so that secondary procedures can be instituted. Renal artery duplex may be a good modality to follow renal artery reconstructions in patients with an appropriate body habitus.

Intestinal Vascular Disease

Intestinal ischemia may be encountered as an acute emergency caused by mesenteric artery embolism or thrombosis or mesenteric venous thrombosis. Acute mesenteric insufficiency should be considered a surgical emergency. In the outpatient clinic, patients may be referred for chronic episodic abdominal pain and weight loss.

The blood supply of the intestinal tract is particularly rich in collaterals. Therefore, mesenteric ischemia only occurs if two out of the three main intestinal arteries are occluded or severely stenosed. Isolated mesenteric artery disease is unlikely to result in mesenteric ischemia unless previous abdominal surgery has been performed and the collateral pathways have been disrupted. The most important artery for intestinal blood supply is the superior mesenteric artery (SMA). Therefore, isolated stenosis of the celiac or inferior mesenteric artery (IMA) rarely cases intestinal ischemia.

Objectives

Diagnose mesenteric ischemia, exclude other pathology, define lesion, treat lesion.

History

Take a general, gastrointestinal (GI), and vascular history. Typically, patients describe a constant history of severe epigastric or periumbilical pain developing 30–45 minutes after food every time they eat. The pain is increasing in severity but the patient may have learned to reduce the pain by eating smaller meals, inducing vomiting before the 30–45 minutes, or avoiding eating completely. There is usually a history of severe weight loss.

There may be other symptoms of atherosclerosis, e.g. claudication, angina. The patient is commonly female and a heavy smoker. There may be a history of extensive investigation for GI or psychiatric disease.

Examination

Perform a general, GI, and cardiovascular examination. There may be evidence of severe weight loss – calculate body mass index (BMI) and skin-fold thickness. There may be evidence of generalized atherosclerosis. Abdominal bruits may be audible.

Investigation

◇ Routine atherosclerotic screen, hematology, biochemistry including liver function tests (LFTs), and serum lipids.
◇ Exclude more common causes of abdominal pain and weight loss, e.g. carcinoma of the tail of the pancreas – CT or MRI is recommended if not previously performed.
◇ Duplex ultrasonography may identify mesenteric stenoses, but examination is difficult and a negative result does not exclude disease.
◇ Mesenteric angiography with lateral aortic views is the gold standard. This may reveal ostial occlusions, stenoses, and disease of the aorta, renal arteries, and other branches.
◇ MRI and spiral CTA may also demonstrate disease.

Treatment

Acute mesenteric ischemia is a surgical emergency requiring urgent revascularization and resection of all non-viable bowel. A "second-look" procedure is mandatory. Initial medical management of chronic mesenteric ischemia consists of correction of pain, fluid, and electrolyte disturbances and malnourishment. Consider parenteral nutrition until lesions can be treated.

Definitive treatment of mesenteric ischemia consists of angioplasty or surgical revascularization. Angioplasty in select situations may be the best first option, and carries a lower morbidity than surgical revascularization.

Surgery is indicated in otherwise fit patients or after failed angioplasty. Procedures consist of transaortic endarterectomy, mesenteric artery bypass, or reimplantation of the SMA. Revascularization procedures should always revascularize the SMA and more than one mesenteric artery if possible. Prolonged parenteral nutrition may be required in the post-operative period.

Follow-up

Once the diagnosis of mesenteric ischemia is made, revascularization should be promptly performed.

Post-operative Follow-up

Recovery of bowel function can be prolonged, and patients may spend a long time in hospital after any procedure. Successful revascularization will typically result in recovery of at least some of the lost weight. Long-term follow-up with regular duplex scans is indicated to detect recurrent disease.

Arterial Lesions of the Upper Limb

Atherosclerosis occurs less frequently in the arm compared with the leg, but is still the most common cause of ischemia, though not the most common cause of ischemia-like symptoms (*see* thoracic outlet syndrome, p. 308). Atherosclerosis affects the aortic arch, the brachiocephalic and subclavian artery proximal to the origin of the vertebral artery, and may give rise to ischemic and embolic symptoms in the arm. The source of emboli to the upper limb may be the arterial lesions, but they are more commonly from the heart originating from atrial fibrillation or mural thrombus associated with MI.

Emboli can present with an acutely ischemic arm, or chronic microembolization may present with a Raynaud's type picture affecting the one hand. If untreated this may eventually lead to occlusion of the radial and ulnar arteries.

Emboli originating from the subclavian and brachiocephalic arteries may also cause vertebrobasilar transient ischemic attacks (TIAs). Occlusions of the proximal subclavian artery may also cause hemodynamic vertebrobasilar symptoms – the subclavian steal syndrome (SSS).

Non-atherosclerotic disorders of the arteries of the arm include Takayasu's and giant cell arteritis and Buerger's disease (*see* vasculitis, p. 312). Irradiation of the chest and/or axilla for malignancy, e.g. breast cancer, may result in long strictures of the subclavian, axillary, and brachial arteries.

Localised arterial lesions distal to the origin of the vertebral artery may be due to compression resulting from thoracic outlet syndrome (TOS). This may result in occlusion of the subclavian artery causing chronic arm ischemia or aneurysm formation causing neurogenic compression and distal embolization. (*See* p. 308.)

Objectives
Identify arterial disease, determine site of arterial lesion, determine cause of arterial lesion, treat effects of arterial lesions, treat arterial lesions, treat cause of arterial lesions.

History
Take a general and vascular history. History of general atherosclerosis affecting the heart and the lower limbs suggests atherosclerosis as the cause of the arm symptoms. A history of cardiac arhythmias or recent MI may suggest a cardiac source of emboli. Patients may present with symptoms related to the arm, but also enquire about vertebrobasilar symptoms.

✧ *Arm symptoms* – forearm fatigue, cold hand, rest pain in the hand, history of embolization (episodes of a pale, cold, painful, weak hand); symptoms may be similar to Raynaud's but are unilateral. Symptoms may be constant with pain, paresthesia, weakness and coldness, or intermittent with claudication, swelling, and color change.

✧ *Vertebrobasilar symptoms (TIAs)* – isolated symptoms are of limited significance. At least three or more of the following symptoms are required for a diagnosis of VBI: unilateral or bilateral simultaneous motor/sensory deficits, ataxia, diplopia, dysarthria, dysphagia, bilateral homonymous hemianopia, vertigo, tinnitus, and transient global amnesia. Drop attacks or loss of consciousness may be the result of embolization or, if they coincide with vigorous use of the arm, represent SSS.

Examination
✧ Perform a general cardiovascular examination. Examine the hands for evidence of ischemia and embolization, e.g. splinter hemorrhages, skin infarcts. Examine for muscle wasting.

✧ Note the rate and rhythm of the pulse. Examine for radial–radial delay. Palpate all the pulses and listen for bruits.

✧ Examine the supraclavicular fossae for the presence of cervical ribs or subclavian aneurysms. Perform a neurologic examination of the arms.

✧ Perform a musculoskeletal examination of the neck and shoulder.
✧ Perform Tinel's and Phalen's test for carpel tunnel syndrome.

Investigations

Routine urinalysis and blood tests. Compare the blood pressure in both arms using the Doppler. Repeat the measurements with the cuff at the upper arm, upper forearm, and lower forearm to detect segmental occlusions of the brachial and forearm arteries. A pressure drop greater than 15 mmHg is significant but may require exercise to produce. Listen with the Doppler over the thenar and hypothenar eminences for arterial signals from the plantar arch.

Take color duplex of the subclavian, axillary, and brachial arteries in different positions to detect stenoses, occlusions, aneurysms, or compression. If vertebrobasilar symptoms are present, this should be combined with insonation of the carotid and vertebral arteries. Visualization of the brachiocephalic and proximal subclavian arteries is difficult with color duplex, but disease in these segments may be associated with damped waveforms more distally. Arch aortogram and selective brachiocephalic/subclavian angiogram is necessary to define the lesions and determine the distal run-off vessels.

Chest X-ray (CXR), cervical spine and thoracic inlet views are required if TOS is suspected and will define bony lesions, e.g. cervical ribs. MRI may detect fibrous bands.

If a cardiac source of emboli is suspected, ECG and cardiac enzymes can be performed. An echocardiogram may be indicated on the advice of a cardiologist.

If an arterial and cardiac lesion is excluded, suspect neurogenic TOS and investigate as appropriate (*see* p. 308).

Treatment

Stenoses of the brachiocephalic and subclavian arteries can be treated with angioplasty alone or combined with stenting. However, stents should not be placed in the thoracic outlet, as compression in this area will lead to failure of the stent. Surgical options include bypass or endarterectomy depending on the location and severity of the disease. Extrathoracic and extra-anatomic procedures tend to be preferred because they do not require thoracotomy, e.g. subclavian-carotid transposition, carotid subclavian bypass, axillo-axillary bypass.

Disease distal to the vertebral origin requires vein bypass. Severe multisegment disease responds poorly to bypass and may respond better to upper thoracic sympathectomy or intermittent prostocyclin infusions.

Subclavian artery stenosis, occlusion, or aneurysm associated with TOS requires resection of the constricting rib or band and repair or bypass of the arterial defect.

Follow-up

If embolization is suspected, admit for inpatient investigation or start anti-embolic therapy and review at short intervals (1–3 weeks) with the results of investigations until the source is identified or serious causes are excluded and the symptoms controlled.

Similarly, severe symptoms of ischemia should be promptly investigated until an arterial lesion has been excluded or confirmed.

Post-operative Follow-up

Review after operation or endovascular treatment to determine the success of the procedure. Detect any residual neurogenic symptoms and treat as appropriate.

Arterial Aneurysms

A true aneurysm is an abnormal dilatation of an artery which affects all three layers of the wall of the artery and where the dilatation exceeds twice its normal diameter. Chronic medial degeneration, particularly of the elastic media, underlies the development of most idiopathic true aneurysms. Aneurysms can be associated with other disease processes including FMD, systemic lupus erythematosus (SLE), Takayasu's arteritis, giant cell arteritis, polyarteris nodosa (PAN), Behet's, Marfan's, and Ehlers–Danlos. Aneurysms can also arise as a result of systemic infection (mycotic aneurysms), dissection of the wall of the artery, or secondary to trauma. These causes typically result in false aneurysms (pseudoaneurysms) where there is a focal disruption of the arterial wall which is contained only by the adventitia or periadventitial tissues.

Many of the examination and study techniques used for the evaluation and diagnosis of arterial insufficiency, described above, are useful for the evaluation of aneurysmal disease. It should be noted that arteriography may be insensitive to the presence of an aneurysm since it only provides luminal definition and the flow lumen of the aneurysm may be relatively small due to the presence of laminated mural thrombus.

Abdominal Aortic Aneurysm (AAA)

The commonest site of arterial aneurysm development is the segment of abdominal aorta below the renal arteries. This is a disease that predominantly affects male smokers. Large AAAs pose a significant risk of rupture, which is nearly universally fatal if not treated promptly; even if surgery is performed, the operative mortality is approximately 50%. Therefore the aim of surgery is to operate before rupture occurs when the peri-procedural mortality is less than 5%. However, not all aneurysms rupture and a number of patients will die of other causes without the aneurysm ever causing any symptoms. Recent large randomized trials have confirmed that surgical exclusion of an AAA does not confer any advantage for aneurysms <5.5 cm in maximal diameter. Surgery should also be performed in the rare instance of a smaller aneurysm which becomes symptomatic.

Objectives

Diagnose AAA, determine size of aorta, determine anatomic suitability of the AAA for various options for exclusion, cardiac, and general surgical risk stratification.

History

The majority of AAA are asymptomatic and are detected on routine clinical examination or imaging of the abdomen performed for other reasons. Patients may present having noticed a pulsatile swelling in the abdomen. The development of symptoms such as backache or abdominal pain, particularly when combined with hypotension and tender abdominal mass, should be presumed to be aneurysm rupture. Assess cardiorespiratory risk factors/symptoms, e.g. angina, exercise tolerance. Enquire regarding family history of aneurismal disease.

Examination

Perform a general and vascular examination with the aim of confirming the diagnosis, detecting aneurysms or stenotic disease affecting other arteries, and determining the general cardiorespiratory fitness of the patient should surgery prove to be necessary.

Investigations

Perform a general atherosclerotic screen of urinalysis and blood tests. B-mode ultrasound is usually adequate to confirm the diagnosis of AAA and gives an accurate estimate of the diameter, but may be insensitive to the presence of aneurysms involving the iliac arteries. CT with intravenous contrast is an excellent modality to evaluate anatomic extent as well as the presence of concomitant occlusive/stenotic vascular disease. Investigations performed prior to surgery include lung function tests, and cardiac risk assessment (e.g. ECG).

Treatment
Correct risk factors and optimise cardiorespiratory function. Asymptomatic AAAs >5.5 cm in diameter should undergo operative repair. Smaller aneurysms are considered for surgery if they are symptomatic. There is some evidence to suggest that women should be treated for AAAs which exceed 5 cm in maximal diameter.

✧ *Open aneurysm repair* is the established operation, performed via a transabdominal approach using a midline laparotomy or via a retroperitoneal approach from a flank incision. The aorta is clamped above and below the aneurysm and the aorta is replaced with an artificial graft. Clamping the aorta puts a major strain on the heart and lungs, which is why a pre-operative assessment is necessary and care in the intensive care unit is necessary post-operatively.

✧ *Endovascular aneurysm repair (EVAR)* involves placing covered stents into the AAA via catheters inserted through the femoral arteries. There are specific anatomic limitations for the use of endografts that are device-specific. As devices evolve and improve, these anatomic limitations are being reduced or eliminated; for example, in some centers juxtarenal aneurysms may be treated with fenestrated or branched endografts.

Follow-up
Small AAAs (3–5.5 cm) typically grow 3–5 cm per year on average, but the growth is discontinuous and unpredictable. Asymptomatic aneurysms less than 5 cm in diameter undergo ultrasound at regular intervals (at least annually) to detect any increase in size. The frequency of evaluation for growth should increase as the AAA approaches 5.5 cm.

All patients are counseled as to the nature of the disease and that any abdominal or back pain should be considered secondary to a leaking AAA requiring urgent repair.

Post-operative Follow-up
Open Repair
At the first visit, confirm wound healing and return to normal activity.

Long-term complications include dilatation of untreated aortic or iliac segments, graft infection or aorto-enteric fistula which may present with hematemesis or rectal bleeding. Other complications may result from adhesions causing intermittent bowel obstruction. Impotence may result from damage to the autonomic nerves on the anterior surface of the aorta/iliac arteries. Stenosis may develop, resulting in ischemic symptoms. Incisional hernia is not uncommon.

Endovascular Repair
Follow-up for all endografts occurs at 1, 6, and 12 months post-procedure with physical examination and CT evaluation of the endograft. The CT scans are used to evaluate for migration of the endograft components and for arterial flow between the endograft and aortic aneurysm wall – termed an "endoleak." Endoleaks are classified as follows:

✧ *Type I* – leak from the upper or lower landing zones; a major defect which needs urgent consideration of correction.

✧ *Type II* – leak from back-bleeding lumbar arteries; usually requires no intervention unless aneurysm continues to expand.

✧ *Type III* – disconnection of graft components or tear in the fabric of the stent; a major problem needing urgent correction.
✧ *Type IV* – due to porosity of the stent material.
✧ *Type V* – unknown source; endotension without identifiable endoleak.

After the first year, annual follow-up CT scans are necessary to detect late complications and endoleaks. With recent concern to reduce radiation exposure to patients, annual duplex ultrasounds supplemented with an abdominal flat plate X-ray is being used instead of CT scans, especially in patients with a stable or shrinking sac; this technique depends on having a qualified ultrasound technician capable of this advanced imaging technique.

Iliac Artery Aneurysm

Iliac artery aneurysm tends to refer to aneurysm of the common and/or internal iliac arteries; the external iliac artery is seldom aneurysmal. Common iliac artery aneurysms often occur in conjunction with AAA and the two are managed simultaneously. Occasionally common iliac aneurysms occur in isolation, or are associated with a small AAA, and merit repair because they have reached a size which presents a substantial risk of rupture or are associated with distal embolization. Internal iliac aneurysms are less common but may also rupture or embolize.

Objectives
Diagnose iliac artery aneurysm, determine size and rupture risk, treat iliac artery aneurysm.

History
Take a general and vascular history. Like AAA, the majority of iliac aneurysms are asymptomatic and are detected on routine clinical examination or on abdominal/pelvic imaging performed for some other indication. The patient may have noticed a pulsatile swelling in the abdomen. Symptoms such as backache or abdominal pain may indicate a rapidly enlarging aneurysm which requires urgent repair.

Iliac artery aneurysms may give rise to embolization and the patient presents with distal limb ischemia. Internal iliac aneurysms may compress structures in the pelvis such as nerves, producing symptoms of sciatica or obturator neuralgia.

Examination
Perform a general and vascular examination with the aim of confirming the diagnosis, detecting aneurysms or stenotic disease affecting other arteries, and determining the general cardiorespiratory fitness of the patient. The aorta bifurcates at the level of the umbilicus so an iliac aneurysm may be palpable below the umbilicus.

Investigations
Perform a general atherosclerotic screen of urinalysis and blood tests. CT with contrast defines the extent of the aneurysm and its relationship to surrounding structures, which is useful in planning surgery. Appropriate surgical/anesthetic risk stratification should also be performed.

Treatment
The normal diameter of the common iliac artery is 1.0–1.5 cm. Data for rupture risk of isolated iliac aneurysms is not as well developed as that for AAA, but the standard

threshold for repair is typically set at 3 cm.

✧ *Isolated common iliac aneurysm* (normal diameter 1–1.5 cm) – endovascular stenting or open repair with Dacron graft.

✧ *Common iliac aneurysm and coexisting AAA* – bifurcated aortic aneurysm repair via open or endovascular technique. Endovascular repair nearly always requires sacrifice of the ipsilateral hypogastric artery – usually with embolization. Unilateral hypogastric exclusion, particularly on the right, is usually well tolerated. Bilateral exclusion of the hypogastrics should not be undertaken lightly. Future devices may allow for maintaining patency of the hypogastric artery when excluding an aneurysmal common iliac.

✧ *Internal iliac aneurysm* (normal diameter 0.75–1.0 cm) – if the contralateral internal iliac artery is patent, treatment can consist of embolization or ligation of the aneurysmal internal iliac. If both internal iliac arteries are aneurysmal, ligate one and use PTFE or vein to revascularize the other.

✧ *External iliac aneurysm* (normal diameter 0.5–1.0 cm) – seldom aneurysmal.

Follow-up
Review with investigations and decide on need and fitness for surgery.

Post-operative Follow-up
Follow-up and complications are the same as for AAA. There is a risk of pelvic ischemia with hypogastric occlusions, including ischemia of the colon.

Thoraic and Thoraco-abdominal Aneurysm (TAA)
Thoraco-abdominal aneurysms are classified based on the Crawford classification system, as types I–IV.

✧ *Type I* affects the descending thoracic aorta and abdominal aorta to just above the renal arteries.

✧ *Type II* affects all the descending thoracic and abdominal aorta and can include the ascending thoracic aorta.

✧ *Type III* affects most of the descending thoracic aorta and all the abdominal aorta.

✧ *Type IV* affects all the abdominal aorta from the diaphragm.

Like AAA, large TAAs pose a significant risk of rupture with high associated mortality. These aneurysms can also present with complications associated with compression or erosion of neighboring structures such as nerves or viscera in the chest or abdomen. Isolated ascending or arch aortic aneurysms are typically managed by cardiac surgeons.

Objectives
Diagnose TAA, determine fitness for surgery, treat those fit for surgery.

History
Take a general and vascular history. Symptoms may include pain in the chest of abdomen secondary to expansion or compression. Compression of the trachea or bronchus can cause cough, wheeze, or evidence of chest infection. Compression of the esophagus can cause dysphagia. Compression of liver or bile ducts may cause jaundice. Vagus nerve traction may present as a hoarse voice.

Assess for symptoms of increased surgical risk, e.g. exercise tolerance, angina, shortness of breath, etc.

Examination

Perform a general and vascular examination. Examine for evidence of atherosclerosis and aneurysmal disease. Assess cardiorespiratory risk profile.

Investigation

Perform a general atherosclerotic screen. Generally, a CT scan or MRI with intravenous contrast is required to determine the extent of aneurysm. LFTs and cardiac assessment (e.g. ECG) are obtained as indicated.

Treatment

The decision to intervene depends on a number of factors to balance the risks of the procedure with the symptoms and risk of natural history of the disease. The risk of rupture is determined by the maximum diameter of the aorta and possibly other features on imaging. Pre-operative preparation includes addressing correctable risk factors and improvement of cardiorespiratory function. Open repair of a TAA involves an extensive thoracic and retroperitoneal exposure. For aneurysms which involve the visceral vessels, many experienced surgeons employ femoral-femoral or atrio-femoral bypass. This procedure carries a high risk of a variety of morbidities as well as mortality.

Endovascular devices have now been adapted for use in excluding thoracic aneurysms with appropriate anatomy. Endovascular repair has mainly been used to treat aneurysms of the descending thoracic aorta, but hybrid techniques, combining open bypass of visceral vessels and endovascular surgery, have been used to treat more extensive lesions.

Follow-up

Serial imaging as with AAA for small thoracic and thoracoabdominal aneurysms.

Post-operative Follow-up

Major complications include paraplegia, limb loss, and death. Endovascular repairs require imaging follow-up as with endoluminal AAA repair. Complications include endoleaks and device occlusion.

Other Peripheral Artery Aneurysms

A peripheral artery is aneurysmal when it is twice the normal diameter. Medial degeneration similar to that affecting the AAA can result in true aneurysms of peripheral vessels as well. Other causes include trauma, congenital, FMD, arteritis, and infection (mycotic). When infection is the cause, the aneurysm often arises suddenly and may be related to a systemic infective episode, e.g. *Salmonella* infection.

The natural history of peripheral aneurysms is not typically to rupture (although this can occur), but these aneurysms tend toward thrombosis or embolization resulting in ischemia.

Objectives

Diagnose aneurysm, differentiate true from false aneurysm, determine whether symptomatic or asymptomatic, determine need for conservative or interventional therapy, treat aneurysm.

History

Try to identify an underlying cause according to those listed above. Determine whether it is aneurysm or pseudoaneurysm. Pseudoaneurysms will usually have been preceded by some trauma or puncture of the artery, most commonly performance of an angiogram.

Symptoms may consist of pain due to expansion or pressure on adjacent structures, distal embolization, or ischemia.

Examination
Palpate all peripheral arteries and pulses to detect coexisting aneurysm or evidence of arterial occlusion and distal ischemia. Palpate for coexisting iliac aneurysm or AAA.

Investigations
Duplex ultrasound is the primary investigation which will confirm the diagnosis, differentiate between true and false aneurysms and provide an accurate estimate of the size and extent of the aneurysm. For true aneurysms of femoral or popliteal segment, evaluation of the aorta should be performed to rule out concomitant AAA. Blood cultures are indicated if mycotic aneurysm is suspected.

Treatment
Pseudoaneurysms due to trauma are typically repaired primarily or with a short interposition graft if the damage to the vessel is severe. Reconstruction of mycotic aneurysms requires extra-anatomic bypass, particularly if the infection is severe or Gram-negative. An in-line reconstruction with native vessel may be considered if the infection is not severe.

✧ *Common femoral aneurysm* (normal diameter 0.5–1.0 cm) – open repair with Dacron or PTFE graft.

✧ *Superficial femoral artery aneurysm* (normal diameter 0.4–0.8cm) – a focal aneurysm affecting one segment of artery, or fusiform aneurysmal disease affecting the whole length of the artery. For focal disease, carry out open repair with PTFE or Dacron graft. For fusiform disease, bypass the whole length of the artery using vein or PTFE with ligation of the superficial femoral artery (SFA) proximally and distally.

✧ *Popliteal artery aneurysm* (normal diameter 0.5–1.0 cm) – can be saccular or fusiform extending into the SFA. Perform saccular or fusiform bypass using vein or PTFE with proximal and distal ligation of the aneurysm.

✧ *Subclavian/axillary artery aneurysm* – open repair and PTFE graft; often associated with a cervical rib or band which will also need treatment.

Post-operative Follow-up
Post-operative follow-up is similar to that for aortic aneurysms. If vein is used for reconstruction, the vein grafts are entered into the vein-graft surveillance program with regular duplex scans to detect developing stenoses.

Visceral Artery Aneurysm
Visceral artery aneurysms are very rare but are associated with a high mortality rate if they rupture, therefore large or symptomatic aneurysms should be repaired. Causes include infection (mycotic), fibromuscular dysplasia, or idiopathic medial degeneration. Any splenic artery aneurysm in a pre-menopausal woman should be repaired as the rupture risk (and associated mortality) is high with pregnancy.

Disorders of the Venous System
By far the most common venous disorder presenting to the vascular clinic is varicose veins. However, careful assessment of all varicose veins is important to detect the underlying cause of venous abnormalities. The evaluation for venous disease is similar in many ways to the evaluation for arterial disease, but additional imaging techniques are listed below.

It should be recognized that certain vascular malformations may present with dilated veins in the leg, e.g. arteriovenous fistulas or venous malformations. The Klippel–Trenaunay syndrome presents with a dilated varicose vein running down the outside of the leg but is associated with hypoplasia of the deep veins. Surgery to remove this unsightly vein may seriously impair the venous drainage of the leg.

Chronic superficial and/or deep venous incompetence may present as varicose veins, leg swelling, or venous ulceration.

Imaging Techniques
Ascending Venography
✧ *Technique* – a vein in the foot is canulated and low osmolar contrast is injected with a tourniquet inflated at the ankle at sufficient pressure to prevent filling of the superficial veins and direct the contrast into the deep veins.
✧ *Advantages* – good for outlining the deep venous system and identifying deep venous thrombosis, post-thrombotic scarred irregular veins, and perforators.
✧ *Disadvantages* – an invasive technique, and cannot reliably identify reflux. Much of the information can be obtained by color duplex.

Descending Venography
✧ *Technique* – the common femoral vein is canulated and contrast is injected. Reflux is induced by generating a standardized Valsalva maneuver by the patient blowing into a manometer device for 10 seconds with a 60-degree head-up tilt on the X-ray table.
✧ *Advantages* – mainly used to demonstrate the extent of deep and superficial venous incompetence.
✧ *Disadvantages* – an invasive technique. Much of the information can be obtained by color duplex. Segmental reflux in the femoral vein can occur in normal subjects.

Varicography
✧ *Technique* – contrast is injected directly into a varicose vein to demonstrate the distribution and connections with the deep venous system.
✧ *Advantages* – a reliable technique which is mainly used to identify the origin of recurrent varicose veins. Provides the surgeon with a "road map."
✧ *Disadvantages* – an invasive technique. Similar information (though not as detailed) may be obtained with color duplex.

Chronic Venous Insufficiency
Chronic venous insufficiency occurs when venous return is impaired by reflux, obstruction and calf muscle pump failure. Sustained venous hypertension leads to edema, varicose veins and leg swelling, eczema (especially around the medial malleolus), lipdermatosclerosis, and eventually ulceration. Swelling initially consists of edema fluid but eventually results in subcutaneous fibrosis and induration.

Objectives
Diagnose venous hypertension, detect underlying cause, correct underlying cause, prevent or treat venous ulceration.

History
Take a general and vascular history. Previous history of deep vein thrombosis, leg swelling, prolonged immobilization or long-bone fractures may suggest deep venous incompetence,

while the presence of varicose veins, past or present, may suggest a superficial venous cause. Symptoms associated with chronic venous hypertension include pruritis, aching pain, limb swelling. Occasionally the patient may complain of venous claudication which consists of a bursting calf pain on walking a certain distance which is not relieved purely by rest and requires elevation of the limb.

Examination
Perform a general and vascular examination. Examine for the presence of varicose veins, limb swelling, lipodermatosclerosis, ulceration, and coexistent arterial disease.

Investigations
Color duplex scanning is useful to identify both superficial and deep venous reflux and may identify scarred, thickened, or obstructed deep veins. Ascending venography is useful to identify scarred, thickened, or obstructed deep veins while descending venography is useful to identify deep and superficial reflux, although these techniques are rarely required. The resting and post-exercise venous pressure and refilling time at the ankle can be measured directly by ambulatory venous pressure measurements.

ABI or arterial duplex scans are performed to exclude coexisting arterial disease, especially if compression therapy is considered. Compression in the presence of arterial disease can result in critical ischemia, gangrene, and limb loss.

CEAP Classification System
After a complete evaluation of patients with lower extremity venous insufficiency, the findings should be condensed into the CEAP (Clinical-Etiology-Anatomy-Pathophysiology) nomenclature. This is a classification system which allows for common communication of all of the components of venous failure, and provides a framework to select appropriate therapeutic measures.

The classification system was revised in 2004. The various levels of each class are given below.

Clinical
- C0 – no visible or palpable signs of venous disease.
- C1 – telangiectasies or reticular veins.
- C2 – varicose veins; distinguished from reticular veins by a diameter of 3 mm or more.
- C3 – edema.
- C4 – changes in skin and subcutaneous:
    - ∝ C4a – pigmentation or eczema
    - ∝ C4b – lipodermatosclerosis or atrophie blanche
- C5 – healed venous ulcer.
- C6 – active venous ulcer.
- S – symptomatic, including ache, pain, tightness, skin irritation, heaviness, and muscle cramps, and other complaints attributable to venous dysfunction.
- A – asymptomatic.

Etiology
- Ec – congenital.
- Ep – primary.
- Es – secondary (post-thrombotic).
- En – no venous cause identified.

Anatomy
- ✧ As – superficial veins.
- ✧ Ap – perforator veins.
- ✧ Ad – deep veins.
- ✧ An – no venous location identified.

Pathophysiology
- ✧ Pr – reflux.
- ✧ Po – obstruction.
- ✧ Pr,o – reflux and obstruction.
- ✧ Pn – no venous pathophysiology identifiable

Treatment
Treatment of all presentations should focus on graduated compression which generates higher compression at the ankle and lower levels of compression at the knee. Compression stockings are used to prevent ulceration in non-ulcerated or healed legs with deep venous incompetence.
- ✧ Class I stockings generate 14–17 mmHg pressure at the ankle.
- ✧ Class II stockings generate 18–24 mmHg.
- ✧ Class III stockings generate 25–35 mmHg.
- ✧ Class IV stockings generate 36–50 mmHg.

Below-knee stockings Class II are adequate for most patients, but compliance can be a problem due to difficulties putting the stockings on or discomfort in hot weather. Non-compliance is greater for classes III–IV and full-leg stockings. Leg elevation reduces the venous pressure at the ankle to 12–15 mmHg, and is useful to reduce leg swelling in grossly swollen legs prior to compression therapy.

Surgical treatment may be indicated for patients with a C2S or greater clinical score.
- ✧ *Coexisting venous and occlusive arterial disease* – any concomitant arterial insufficiency should be addressed first in most cases.
- ✧ *Venous reflux* – patients with As or Ap should be considered for surgical ablation of the incompetent veins as described below.
- ✧ *Radiofrequency ablation (RFA) or endovenous laser ablation (EVLA)* – the refluxing greater/lesser saphenous vein is punctured with a 19G needle under ultrasound control at the knee. A guidewire is passed through the needle up to the saphenofemoral/popliteal junction, and over this is passed a catheter which delivers laser or radiofrequency energy to locally heat the saphenous vein or perforator vein to cause involution. Dilute local anesthetic is infiltrated around the full length of the vein to protect surrounding tissues.
- ✧ *Perforator ligation or subfascial endoscopic perforator surgery (SEPS)* – perforator vein incompetence can be managed by direct ligation of the refluxing vein. When the skin overlying the vein is severely diseased, however, it may be less morbid to perform perforator ligation via a remote incision – the SEPS procedure.
- ✧ *Venous outflow obstruction* – typically this is due to DVT. Treatment with anticoagulation has been the mainstay of therapy, but the risk of post-thrombotic venous insufficiency is high with this management routine. Ongoing studies are evaluating the value of early thrombolytic recanalization of thrombosed iliofemoral venous segments. Surgical venous reconstruction may be useful in select cases, but long-term results can be poor.

Follow-up

Review with results of investigations and decide on appropriate treatment. Venous ulcers undergoing compression are followed at 1- to 3-month intervals, and progress to compression stockings once the ulcer is completely healed.

Post-operative Follow-up

Patients are usually reviewed 4–6 weeks after operation. Common complications are usually related to the wound. After saphenous vein ablation, early duplex evaluation for DVT is necessary to determine whether there has been extension of the superficial thrombus into the deep system. Residual veins not associated with reflux can be treated by avulsions under local anesthetic or sclerotherapy.

Complications

- ✧ Complications of saphenous ablation procedures include bruising in the groin or along the track of the treated long saphenous vein. A cord of thrombus may be palpable along the line of the treated vein. Both will usually resolve.
- ✧ There may be small areas of skin paresthesia in relation to any wound or avulsion site due to damage to cutaneous nerves – once again, this should resolve if mild.
- ✧ Saphenous neuritis is caused by damage to the great saphenous nerve below the knee. This can cause distressing pain, tingling, and paresthesia in the distribution of the great saphenous nerve and referral to the pain clinic may be required in some cases.
- ✧ Tattooing of the skin can occur if incisions are made through (avoid this) ink marks placed pre-operatively to mark the vein. Plastic surgical referral may be necessary for severe tattooing.
- ✧ Avulsions at certain sites should be avoided to remove the risk of damage to other structures, e.g. around the neck of fibula to avoid the common peroneal nerve, the posterior tibial vessels behind the medial malleolus and the sural nerve in the medial line of the posterior calf.

Varicose Veins

Varicose veins are dilated superficial veins in the leg caused by venous outflow obstruction or incompetent valves allowing high-pressure blood to reflux into the superficial veins. Some patients may present with dilated superficial veins which are not varicose or having become worried by the cosmetic appearance of thread veins with or without associated varicose veins. Occasionally, visible veins are either normal or caused by some congenital abnormality or underlying pathology for which varicose vein surgery would be inappropriate.

Objectives

Diagnose varicose veins, exclude other pathology, determine the most appropriate treatment (operative versus non-operative).

History

Most patients will describe the presence of these veins for several years. In females their appearance may coincide with pregnancy. Exclude previous DVT or conditions which may have led to this, e.g. long-bone fractures, prolonged bed-rest, etc.

Determine the symptoms caused by the veins. Patients may complain of local tenderness in the region of a prominent vein or general symptoms of discomfort, aching, or throbbing. There may be a history of acute hemorrhage from a prominent vein or episodes of superficial thrombophlebitis. Alternatively, there may be no symptoms and the main concern is cosmetic.

Examination

Examine the patient standing and determine whether the varicose veins affect the long saphenous system (medial side of thigh and calf) or short saphenous system (mainly lateral calf and originating from the popliteal fossa – but not all). Determine the site of incompetence using a tourniquet. Occasionally there is a communicating vein between the two systems.

Examine for signs of venous stasis – edema or lipodermato-sclerosis spreading from the medial malleolus. The presence of venous stasis should prompt investigations to exclude deep venous incompetence.

Examine for the presence and extent of thread veins. Thrombophlebitis may result in firm, tender cord-like veins caused by thrombosis and fibrosis surrounded by erythema.

Investigations

Color duplex ultrasonography is preferable for confirming the site of incompetence, identifying short saphenous reflux and excluding deep venous reflux. Varicography is the more invasive alternative but is often not required.

Treatment

All patients should be evaluated as above for chronic venous insufficiency, and treatments instituted to resolve underlying significant causes. In many cases, appropriate management of underlying venous insufficiency will resolve varicosities. For varicosities or other prominent veins not associated with venous insufficiency, local therapies may be employed.

✧ *Spider veins* – most patients can be treated by sclerotherapy. Sclerotherapy is a means of chemically causing vein sclerosis. Complications include local and systemic reactions to the sclerosant.

✧ *Superficial veins* not associated with reflux can be treated by sclerotherapy or avulsions.

Follow-up

Most of these problems are routine and there is no urgency for investigations unless DVT is suspected. For those patients who have undergone sclerotherapy, late complications include local skin ulceration due to extravasation of sclerosant (slow to heal but no specific treatment). Superficial thrombophlebitis is caused by a clot in the vein due to inadequate compression; the clot can be aspirated under local anesthetic. If the bandages cause an allergic skin rash, advise patient to wear a cotton stocking under the bandage. Nerve damage may occur but is usually transitory. There may be skin staining; most fades with time.

Post-operative Follow-up

See follow-up recommendations for chronic venous insufficiency (p. 299).

Superficial Thrombophlebitis

Thrombophlebitis is inflammation of a vein due to thrombosis which can occur in normal or varicose veins. When thrombophlebitis occurs in varicose veins this is usually as the result of stasis, but all patients with thrombophlebitis are at increased risk of DVT (25% association) and this should be excluded. Patients who have thrombophlebitis extending to the saphenofemoral junction (SFJ) may have a tongue of thrombus protruding into the femoral vein and are at risk of pulmonary embolus.

Objectives
Diagnose thrombophlebitis, exclude the underlying cause, exclude DVT, treat thrombophlebitis.

History
Take a general and vascular history. Patients complain of tender inflammation over the superficial limb veins. There may be a history of varicose veins and/or DVT. Enquire regarding symptoms of systemic disease, and about a family history of thromboses.

Examination
Perform a general and vascular examination. Examine for the presence of varicose veins and limb swelling. The skin overlying the affected vein is red, inflamed, and tender and may appear infected. Supportive thrombophlebitis may need to be ruled out, but this is unusual in the absence of local trauma. The vein may be palpable as a firm, thrombosed cord underneath the skin. Determine the extent of the thrombophlebitis.

Investigations
The diagnosis is essentially clinical. Duplex will define the extent of the thrombus and exclude protrusion of thrombus through the SFJ and a DVT. CBC, erythrocyte sedimentation rate (ESR) and thrombophilia screen are performed to investigate underlying causes. Depending on the results of the history and examination, appropriate investigations are performed to exclude underlying malignancy.

Treatment
Uncomplicated thrombophlebitis is treated with analgesia, NSAIDs, and compression. DVT is treated with anticoagulation. Varicose veins are treated appropriately once inflammation has subsided.

Extensive thrombophlebitis extending to the SFJ is treated by immediate ligation of the SFJ and anticoagulation, e.g. low-molecular-weight heparin or warfarin, is considered. Underlying causes are treated as appropriate.

Females with thrombophlebitis should stop the contraceptive pill and be counseled regarding their increased risk of DVT.

Follow-up
If extensive thrombophlebitis or DVT is suspected, admit for further investigation and anticoagulation as an inpatient. Otherwise, follow up early (1–4 weeks) with results of investigations. Refer to relevant specialty if an underlying cause is found. Advise regarding increased risk of DVT.

Post-operative Follow-up
Post-operative follow-up is as for venous insufficiency.

Disorders of the Lymphatic System
The primary causes of lymphedema may be familial or non-familial and present at different ages. Lymphedema congenita occurs at <1 year of age (Milroy's), praecox occurs at <35 years, and tarda occurs at >35 years.

Secondary lymphedema occurs due to a blockage of primarily normal lymphatics by malignant disease, surgery, radiotherapy, and infection (parasitic; pyogenic – beta-hemolytic *Streptococcus*, *Staphylococcus aureus*; or TB).

Imaging Techniques
Contrast Lymphangiography
✧ *Technique* – a mixture of local anesthetic and vital blue dye is injected subcutaneously into the first web space. The dye is taken up by the lymphatics and outlines the main channels in the foot. One of these channels is canulated and contrast is infused over a period of 1 hour. Serial X-rays of the leg, groin, pelvis, abdomen, and chest are taken over the first few hours, at 24 hours or even several days later.
✧ *Advantages* – provides anatomic detail of the lymphatics. Useful for imaging the thoracic duct, lymph leaks in the pelvis, abdomen, and chest, and distinguishing reactive from malignant lymph nodes.
✧ *Disadvantages* – an invasive technique largely superseded by isotope lymphangiography.

Radio-isotope Methods
Isotope Lymphangiography
✧ *Technique* – radiolabeled technetium colloid is injected into the second to third web space of the toes. Gamma cameras track the progress of the marker.
✧ *Advantages* – a very specific method which can demonstrate such abnormalities as delayed transit, presence of collaterals, dermal backflow, and reduced uptake in one or more groups of nodes.
✧ *Disadvantages* – an invasive method, involving use of radioactivity.

Classification
Lymphedema can also be classified according to the mechanism of lymphedema:
✧ *Obliterative* – the lymphatics are progressively obliterated from distal to proximal. Represents 80% of lymphedema cases, predominantly affects females.
✧ *Proximal obstructive* – lymphatic obstruction is caused by disease in the abdominal, pelvic or inguinal lymph nodes. Usually unilateral.
✧ *Lymphatic valvular incompetence* and hyperplasia – the lymphatic equivalent of varicose veins.

Objectives
Diagnose lymphedema, identify the underlying cause, treat lymphedema.

History
Take a general and vascular history. The history is one of slow, progressive swelling of the limb or limbs starting at the toes and spreading proximally. Enquire about possible secondary causes. Enquire about recurrent episodes of cellulitis.

Examination
Perform a general and vascular examination. Lymphedema swelling tends to be uniform and non-inflamed, non-pigmented, and pits on pressure in the early stages. The toes are affected early and become square. Later there may be hyperkeratosis of the toes and skin fissuring secondary to fungal infection. Later, chylous vesicles may appear on the pretibial area but ulceration in pure lymphedema is rare. Examine for evidence of secondary causes and chest, abdominal, and pelvic pathology.

Investigation
The diagnosis of lymphedema is mainly clinical. Color duplex is often performed to exclude DVT. The diagnosis can be confirmed and the type of lymphedema classified using isotope or contrast lymphangiography. CT/MRI can be used to exclude pelvic and

abdominal disease and can also demonstrate the typical honeycomb appearance of the lymphatic tissue in the tissues of the affected limb.

Treatment
The aims of treatment are to decrease limb swelling and weight, decrease the risk of infection, and improve function. Pitting edema can be reduced by bed rest. Later, when fibrosclerosis occurs, regular massage therapy is necessary. Diuretics are useful as a short-term treatment only. Compression bandaging can also be used to reduce the swelling and the effect continued by compression stockings; usually class II–IV stockings are necessary. The legs are washed daily and the feet protected with well-fitting, comfortable shoes.

Surgical management is indicated only rarely and only for the most severe cases.

Follow-up
Follow-up is at regular intervals to review the results of investigations, monitor the effectiveness of treatment and detect complications. Once a long-term management plan has been instituted and is controlling symptoms, the patient can be discharged with advice to return if deterioration occurs.

Post-operative Follow-up
Review to determine the success of the procedure and to detect complications.

Other Vascular-associated and Non-vascular Conditions Managed by the Vascular Surgeon
Vasospastic Disorders of the Arteries
Raynaud's Phenomenon
Most commonly, Raynaud's describes an abnormal arterial vasospasm in response to cold usually affecting the fingers. Classically the fingers turn white and numb on exposure to cold, and the static blood becomes de-oxygenated producing a blue color; then the vasospasm is released and a reactive hyperemia occurs and the fingers turn bright red. Two forms are recognized:
- ✧ Raynaud's disease (primary) is the most common form and has no underlying disease. The symptoms are usually mild and seldom produce tissue loss.
- ✧ Raynaud's syndrome (secondary) has an underlying disease, although Raynaud's symptoms may precede the systemic illness. The symptoms may be more severe and associated with ulceration and tissue loss.

There are numerous variations to the classic description. Triphasic color change is not necessary for diagnosis; blanching and reactive hyperemia are sufficient. Vasospasm can be provoked not just by cold but also by emotion, hormones, trauma, chemicals, vibration, and tobacco exposure. Vasospasm does not just affect the fingers; toes are also commonly affected, but the vasospasm can also be systemic affecting the nose, ear lobes, cerebral and coronary arteries, lung vessels producing pulmonary fibrosis, and esophagus producing dysphagia.

Venous spasm produces intense venous congestion and a purple color change, and has the same primary and secondary forms as Raynaud's. Acrocyanosis is the term for venous vasospasm, and venous infarcts are commonly known as chilblains.

Underlying Disorders
- ✧ Immunologic – systemic sclerosis (90%), SLE, mixed connective tissue disease, dermatomyositis/polymyositis, rheumatoid arthritis, cryoglobulinemia, Sjögren's.

✧ *Occupational* – vinylchloride workers, vibration white-finger, ammunition workers, outside workers, frozen-food packers.
✧ *Obstructive* – TOS, Buerger's.
✧ *Drugs* – ergotamines, beta-blockers, cytotoxics, cyclosporin.
✧ *Others* – malignancy, endocrine (hypothyroidism), uremia, hepatitis B, reflex sympathetic dystrophy, arteriovenous fistula.

Objectives
Diagnose Raynaud's, exclude secondary causes, treat Raynaud's, treat any underlying disease.

History
Take a general and vascular history. A history of blanching is usually adequate for diagnosis. Recent onset, especially in children or in middle age, is suggestive of secondary Raynaud's. Determine the provoking factors. Enquire about underlying disorders according to the list above.

Raynaud's is usually bilateral. Raynaud's affecting just one hand is suspicious of a local traumatic or obstructive cause e.g. cervical rib. Confusion can also be caused by Buerger's disease predominantly affecting the upper limbs.

Examination
Perform a general and vascular examination. In primary Raynaud's, the fingers are usually normal to inspection and all pulses are present and normal. In severe and secondary Raynaud's, there may be scars on the finger pulps from previous ulcers or ulcers may be present.

Look for evidence of secondary infection. Examine for any underlying causes. Absent pulses may suggest an atherosclerotic cause, Buerger's disease, or a mechanical cause such as TOS.

Use an ophthalmoscope on high power to examine the skin proximal to the nailfold. Normally, capillary vessels underneath the skin are not visible. If they are this is evidence of significant ischemia usually associated with secondary Raynaud's.

Investigations
The diagnosis of Raynaud's is mainly clinical. Some centers define Raynaud's as a drop in systolic finger pressure on cooling the hand under controlled laboratory conditions, but the results are not totally sensitive and specific. The most important investigations are to exclude a secondary cause.

Carry out CBC, thyroid function tests (hypothyroidism), ESR, and urinalysis for renal disease, CTD, or diabetes. Take a CXR to detect lung fibrosis or malignancy, and thoracic inlet views to detect a cervical rib. Upper limb duplex is useful to exclude major arterial disease. Immunologic tests include autoantibody screen for rheumatoid factor, antinuclear antibody (ANA) for SLE, anticentromere for localized systemic sclerosis (SSc), and antitopoisomerase for diffuse SSc. These investigations may need to be repeated every few years if the symptoms persist or deteriorate.

Treatment
General measures are to stop smoking, change occupation, change medications, stop the contraceptive pill if there is a clear link. Heated gloves and socks or chemical hand-warmers are also beneficial. Mild to moderate primary Raynaud's will often respond to a combination of these general measures to control the symptoms.

If the symptoms are still affecting lifestyle or employment, or secondary Raynaud's is present, drug therapy may be necessary. Dihydropyridine calcium-channel blockers are excellent first-line agents. Other agents which may be effective include inositol nicotinate and naftidrofuryl oxalate (Praxilene). Inpatient treatment is used for infusion of iloprost, as a stable prostocyclin analogue given intra-arterially may terminate a prolonged, severe attack.

Treat any infection or ulcers aggressively with antibiotics (note that the usual signs of infection are often absent). Severe ulceration or gangrene may require surgical debridement or amputation. Treat any underlying connective tissue disorder.

Carotid Body Tumor (CBT)

The carotid body is derived from neural crest cells of the third branchial arch and is located behind and between the internal and external carotid arteries. The correct term for a tumor of this gland is a paraganglioma, and when these occur 5% are bilateral and 10% are malignant. Although not strictly a vascular condition, these lesions are often referred to vascular surgeons because their treatment sometimes requires reconstruction of the carotid arteries. Some cases may rarely be associated with pheochromocytoma.

Differential diagnosis includes carotid artery aneurysm, lymph node mass, branchial cyst, and cystic hygroma.

History

Patients commonly present because they have noticed a pulsatile swelling in the neck. Other symptoms include headache, neck pain, dizziness, hoarse voice, and dysphagia caused by local invasion or cranial nerve compression. CBT seldom causes cerebral ischemia but occasional symptoms of flushing, dizziness, arrhythmias, and hypertension are caused by neuroendocrine secretion by the tumor.

Examination

A mass in the neck may be palpable, which is pulsatile because of its close proximity to the carotid arteries but not expansile. Classically these tumors can be moved from side to side but not up or down. Perform a neurologic exam and examine for cranial nerve lesions (IX, X, XI, XII) – indirect laryngoscopy may be required. Occasionally there may be a Horner's syndrome. Examine for neuroendocrine effects.

Investigation

Growth of the tumor tends to splay the carotid bifurcation which can be detected by color duplex or angiography. The blood supply from the external carotid artery and the very vascular nature of these tumors may also be demonstrated. CT/MRI may be useful to define the relation of the tumor to other structures, to define its extent and to exclude bilateral disease. The Shamblin classification grades these tumors from I to III based on size, site, and degree of difficulty for resection. Grade III may require resection of the external carotid artery or the internal carotid artery and vein graft repair.

Treatment

Tumors require surgical excision and sometimes carotid artery reconstruction. Some centers recommend pre-operative embolization of the blood supply of the tumor to reduce vascularity.

Follow-up

Patients should be reviewed quickly (1–4 weeks) with results to confirm or exclude the diagnosis. The majority of pulsatile lumps turn out to be a prominent or tortuous but otherwise normal carotid artery, and the patient can be reassured and discharged. Confirmed CBTs require prompt treatment. Other causes are managed appropriately. Exclude pheochromocytoma in hypertensive patients.

Post-operative Follow-up
Review histology to confirm complete excision and exclude malignancy. Malignant lesions require oncology referral and long-term follow-up. The complications of the operation are the same as for carotid endarterectomy. Patients can be discharged if unilateral benign disease is confirmed, wounds have healed, and the patient is symptom-free.

Arterial Fibrodysplasia
Fibrodysplasia describes a group of disorders of unknown etiology but which are neither inflammatory nor atherosclerotic and result in stenosis, occlusions, and aneurysms. Variations of the disorder include intimal fibroplasia, medial hyperplasia, medial fibroplasia and perimedial dysplasia. The most important of these conditions is renal artery fibrodysplasia, which affects 0.5% of the population and is the second most common surgically correctable cause of hypertension.

The pathogenesis is unclear, but the underlying cause may represent mural ischemia from inadequate vaso-vasorum blood flow.

✧ *Intimal fibrodysplasia* – primary intimal fibrodyplasia presents in children and young adults as a focal smooth stenosis or web in otherwise normal arteries and may represent residual or persistent neonatal intimal cushions.

✧ *Medial hyperplasia* – hyperplasia of the media causing a stenosis but without accompanying fibrosis. This is rare, affects mainly females, age range 40s to 50s, and presents as a focal stenosis in the main renal artery.

✧ *Medial fibroplasia* – this represents 85% of dysplastic renovascular disease. Two forms are recognized: (i) peripheral – confined to the outer media; and (ii) diffuse – affects the whole media. It tends to progress from the periphery. Compact fibrous tissue replaces smooth muscle and ground substance. Adventitial tissues are not involved but the internal elastic lamina fragments.

✧ *Perimedial dysplasia* – represents 10% of renal artery dysplasias and may coexist with medial fibrodysplasia. Produces focal or multiple stenoses of the main artery but without aneurysmal formation. Microscopically there are collections of amorphous tissue in the adventitia.

The Diabetic Foot
The feet of diabetic patients are prone to the development of infection, ulceration, and gangrene due to a combination of neuropathy, peripheral arterial disease, and arthropathy. Sensory neuropathy reduces the sensation of the feet and makes them more prone to minor injury, which leads to the development of ulcers. Motor neuropathy leads to muscle imbalance and increased shear stresses on the skin which can also cause ulceration. This also leads to joint and gait abnormalities which increase shear stress on the skin and decrease the efficiency of the ankle joint and the calf muscle pump, decreasing the efficiency of the venous circulation of the leg which also predisposes the limb to ulceration. Peripheral arterial disease renders the tissues more prone to ulceration, and once ulceration has occurred healing is delayed or prevented until the blood supply to the area can be improved.

Assessment and management of diabetic foot problems often requires a multi-disciplinary approach involving an endocrinologist, vascular surgeon, and podiatrist.

Objectives
Classify ulcers as *neuropathic, vascular,* or *mixed.* Then as *simple* (superficial infection, minimal necrosis) or *complicated* (infection and extensive tissue necrosis). Assess diabetic control, assess vascular, neuropathic, and orthopedic systems, treat ulcer, treat underlying conditions.

History
✧ Take a general and vascular history. Assess the diabetic control.
✧ Assess the neurologic system – symptoms of central neuropathy include fainting spells, dizziness, nausea, vomiting of retained foods, impotence. Symptoms of peripheral neuropathy include motor weakness, dry feet, numbness or loss of sensation in the feet, hyperesthesia (burning feet) or pain in the legs.
✧ Vascular symptoms include claudication, although rest pain or ulceration may be the first symptom in diabetics. Ask about previous ulcers and healing. Ask about other vascular causes of ulceration, e.g. venous incompetence.

Examination
Perform a general examination. Assess the characteristics of the ulcer. Assess the neurologic, vascular and orthopedic systems.
✧ *The ulcer* – site, size, character: neuropathic, vascular or mixed; simple or complicated.
✧ *Neuropathy* – there is usually a glove and stocking pattern. Examine the lower limb for decreased sensation to light touch (cotton wool), sharp and blunt, vibration (tuning fork on the big toe or malleolli), temperature (coldness of tuning fork on the skin).
✧ *Vascular* – perform a general vascular examination.
✧ *Orthopedic* – observe the patient walking for abnormalities of gait. Examine the foot for evidence of muscle imbalance, e.g. pes cavus, hallux valgus. Examine the joints of the lower limb for swelling, tenderness, range of movement, crepitus, etc.

Investigations
More quantitative tests for neuropathy such as nerve conduction studies are recommended. Arterial ABI is performed. If the arteries are incompressible ABI is unreliable, although arterial stenoses may be suspected from the detection of abnormal waveforms. Toe pressures and/or the toe–pole test are alternative tests.

Arterial color duplex scans are required, and/or angiography with magnified foot views. Take X-rays of joints and bones underlying ulcers for evidence of osteomyelitis.

Carry out tests of diabetic control and perform venous duplex if indicated. Take swabs of ulcers for microbiology. Biopsy ulcers if long-standing, to exclude Marjolin's or vasculitis.

Treatment
✧ *Ulcers:*
 ∝ *Complicated* – antibiotics, clean ulcer, bed-rest and limb elevation. Debridement may be required.
 ∝ *Simple* – predominantly neuropathic – bed rest, remove callus around ulcer, refer to podiatry for appropriate footwear.
✧ *Diabetic arthropathy* – treatment is similar to Charcot's – footwear and surgery to stabilize the foot.
✧ *Neuropathy* – improve diabetic control. Bed rest, remove callus around ulcer, refer to podiatry for appropriate footwear.
✧ *Vascular ulcers* – angioplasty or bypass including popliteal-pedal bypass. Amputations may be required for ongoing infections without possibility of adequate revascularization.

Follow-up
Refer to a multidisciplinary diabetic foot clinic to assess results of investigations and monitor the effect of treatment.

Post-operative Follow-up
Standard vascular follow-up, depending on procedure performed.

Vascular Lesions of the Upper Limb
The same arterial, venous, and lymphatic pathologies can occur in the upper limb as in the lower limb; however, the frequency and pattern of disease tends to be different. Also, the anatomy of how blood vessels leave the chest and nerves leave the neck to pass over the first rib and under the clavicle to enter the arm play an important role in the development of pathology in this region – the thoracic outlet syndrome (TOS).

Vascular lesions of the upper limb are less common than those of the lower limb because atherosclerosis is less common in the vessels of the arm. When atherosclerosis does occur, it tends to affect the proximal segments of arm vessels within the chest rather than the vessels in the arm itself. For the majority of cases, atherosclerosis affects the aortic arch, brachiocephalic and subclavian arteries proximal to the origin of the vertebral artery. Because of the origin of the vertebral artery, stenotic or embolic disease of the brachiocephalic and subclavian arteries may present with symptoms of vertebrobasilar ischemia (VBI) rather than arm ischemia.

Lesions of the subclavian artery occurring distal to the origin of the vertebral artery are most commonly due to TOS and less commonly due to atherosclerosis. However, 95% of the symptoms of TOS are neurogenic in origin rather than arterial. Neurogenic and arterial symptoms are very similar, and it can be difficult to differentiate between the two on initial assessment. In such cases it seems reasonable to investigate the arterial tree first, as arterial lesions are more likely to be limb-threatening than neurogenic lesions. If an arterial lesion is detected, the site of the lesion in relation to the origin of the vertebral artery will suggest the pathology. A lesion of the subclavian artery distal to the origin of the vertebral artery is likely to be due to TOS and to coexist with neurogenic compression. Investigations are then performed to define the anatomy of the thoracic outlet and plan appropriate treatment.

If an arterial lesion is excluded, the arm symptoms are most probably due to neurogenic TOS. Investigations are then organized to exclude other neurologic causes and to define the anatomic abnormality at the thoracic outlet in order to plan the appropriate treatment.

Venous thrombosis and obstruction can occur as a result of thoracic outlet obstruction and present with a swollen cyanotic arm, but this is uncommon. Iatrogenic causes are much more common, such as subclavian vein canulation. Lymphedema and other causes of a swollen arm can occur and the underlying pathologies are similar to the lower limb.

Thoracic Outlet Syndrome (TOS)
The arteries, veins, and nerves of the upper limb pass through a narrow space over the first rib, between the sternomastoid and scalene muscles, and under the clavicle to supply the arm. In some patients, especially young athletes, this space is very narrow and these structures can be compressed resulting in the symptoms and signs of TOS. In the majority of patients (95%), symptoms are caused by compression of the nerves of the upper or lower brachial plexus. In 5% of patients, the subclavian artery and/or vein is compressed.

The causes of TOS include cervical ribs, abnormal scaleneus anterior or medius muscles, fibromuscular bands, abnormal first rib, callus or exostoses from the clavicle or first rib, and neoplasms near the thoracic outlet.

Conditions which may cause similar symptoms in the arm and need to be excluded include cervical spondylosis, cervical disc herniation, cervical spinal cord and plexus lesions, shoulder joint and capsule abnormalities, ulnar nerve compression at the elbow, median nerve compression (carpal tunnel syndrome), multiple sclerosis and motor neurone disease, and cardiac angina.

History

Take a general and vascular history. Most patients describe symptoms of pain, paresthesia, weakness, coldness, numbness, claudication, swelling, or color change. Symptoms may have occurred spontaneously or have been precipitated by trauma or physical overactivity, e.g. painting the ceiling. Symptoms may be worse during physical activity of the arm, e.g. carrying shopping, or occur when the arm is elevated. Symptoms may become constant in long-standing cases.

✧ *Upper plexus symptoms* (C5, 6, 7) are suggested by pain in the neck, shoulder tip, upper chest, supra-scapular area, the outside of the upper arm, and the volar surface of thumb and index finger.

✧ *Lower plexus symptoms* (C8, T1) are suggested by pain in the back of the neck and adjacent scapular area, axilla, medial side of arm, ring, and little fingers.

Color change, numbness, and paresthesia can simulate Raynaud's but represent chronic microembolization from an arterial lesion. Other arterial symptoms include arm claudication, arm fatigue, and weakness with exercise.

Venous symptoms include limb swelling and cyanotic color change, and heaviness accentuated by exercise and relieved by rest. Elevation of the arm may aggravate the symptoms by increasing the compression of the subclavian vein at the thoracic outlet.

Ulnar nerve compression at the elbow produces symptoms in the ulnar nerve distribution distal to this point. Median nerve compression at the wrist – carpal tunnel syndrome – affects the median nerve in the hand only.

Lateral cervical disc prolapse tends to press on one nerve root, causing burning pain in the relevant dermatome and muscle weakness and decreased reflexes in the relevant myotome. Simultaneous pressure on half the spinal cord may cause Brown–Séquard syndrome. Intra-foraminal osteophytes occurring with cervical spondylosis can affect and cause symptoms in several nerve roots without an associated Brown–Séquard syndrome.

Examination

Perform a general and vascular examination. Examine the hands for evidence of ischemia and embolization, e.g. splinter hemorrhages or skin infarcts. Note the rate and rhythm of the pulse. Examine for radial-radial delay. Palpate all the pulses and listen for bruits. Examine the supraclavicular fossae for the presence of cervical ribs or subclavian aneurysms. Examine for arterial lesions as described above.

Examine for muscle wasting of the arm and hand and perform a neurologic examination. Examine for muscle tone and motor weakness, reflexes and loss of sensation to pin-prick and light touch. Perform Tinel's and Phalen's test for carpel tunnel syndrome.

Perform Roos' test – the arms are raised to the level of the shoulders, 90 degrees abducted and externally rotated, like a soldier surrendering. The hands are then repeatedly clenched and unclenched for 1–2 minutes. Patients with TOS can seldom complete more than 30–40 seconds of this before pain forces them to stop. The hand may also go pale and become hyperemic when the position is released.

Perform a musculoskeletal examination of the neck and shoulder. Palpate for tenderness and restricted movement which may indicate cervical spondylosis, disc prolapse, or shoulder joint lesions, e.g. rotator cuff injuries.

A cyanotic, swollen arm with prominent venous collaterals suggests venous TOS.

Investigations

Investigate arterial lesions as described above. Because arterial lesions are potentially limb-threatening, it is reasonable to exclude these lesions initially. Usually color duplex scan is sufficient to investigate both arterial and venous TOS, however arteriograms and venograms may be necessary.

CXR, cervical spine, and thoracic inlet views are required if TOS is suspected and will define bony lesions, e.g. cervical ribs. MRI may detect fibrous bands.

Nerve conduction studies, electromyography and other neurophysiologic tests are often normal in TOS but are useful to exclude other neurologic causes, e.g. spinal cord lesions, ulnar and median nerve lesions.

Ultimately, the diagnosis of neurogenic TOS is clinical after exclusion of other pathologies by the investigations described.

Treatment

In the absence of arterial and venous lesions, the initial management of neurogenic TOS is conservative with analgesia, NSAIDs, and physiotherapy to strengthen the neck and shoulder girdle. Embolic symptoms are treated with aspirin or anticoagulation initially, or treatment of the embolic source.

Surgery is reserved for cases where conservative measures have failed to relieve symptoms, there is impaired function of the limb, or there are associated arterial or venous lesions.

✧ The transaxillary approach may be used if lower brachial plexus symptoms predominate, for resection of the first rib, and if there is no cervical rib or arterial or venous compression.

✧ The supraclavicular approach is used for excision of a cervical rib, if upper brachial plexus symptoms predominate, there are lesions of the subclavian artery or vein which need correction, or fibrous bands or scalene muscle requires division. If the first rib requires resection, then a second infraclavicular incision is required to access the anterior part of the rib.

Post-operative Follow-up

Patients are reviewed to assess the success of the procedure and to detect complications. Initial complications include traction injuries to the brachial plexus, phrenic, and long thoracic nerves, and will usually resolve within 6 months. Injuries may also occur to the subclavian vessels and the thoracic duct.

Vascular Malformations

In contrast to common terminology, vascular malformations refer to arterial and venous abnormalities which have normal endothelial turnover and are present from birth, but may not cause symptoms until later in life. Hemangiomas occur in infants, develop after birth, demonstrate endothelial hyperplasia, and tend to resolve spontaneously, although this may not be complete.

Vascular malformations may be classified as high-flow lesions or low-flow lesions. High-flow lesions consist of arteriovenous malformations. Low-flow lesions may be capillary, venous, lymphatic, or mixed malformations, but there is no arteriovenous shunting.

Acquired arterial and venous abnormalities may result from trauma or iatrogenic procedures. Certain malignant tumors may mimic the features of a vascular malformation and must be excluded; these tumors include angiosarcomas and renal and thyroid metastases.

Objectives
Differentiate vascular malformation from hemangioma, exclude malignant tumor, classify vascular malformation into high flow and low flow, treat lesions conservatively or with intervention.

History
Take a general and vascular history. Patients may describe a lesion which has been present from birth but may have become symptomatic or increased in size at puberty, pregnancy, or after an episode of trauma.

Patients with high-flow lesions may complain of pain, excessive sweating over the lesion, and even ulceration and bleeding. Extremities may be painful due to ischemia caused by arteriovenous shunting proximal to their blood supply.

Patients with low-flow lesions also complain of pain. For capillary lesions, pain may be the predominant symptom with little skin-staining or swelling evident, though local hyperhidrosis is common. Large venous lesions may cause pain due to engorgement and episodes of spontaneous thrombosis. Pain may be worse after exercise and last for days. Limb soft tissue and skeletal overgrowth is common, as is overlying eczema and ulceration.

Lymphatic lesions are associated with deformity, exudation of fluid and are prone to cellulitis. For acquired vascular malformations, there may be a history of trauma or iatrogenic injury.

Examination
Perform a general and vascular examination. Assess the cardiac status. Note that examination may be normal despite the presence of a significant lesion. A small cutaneous discoloration may indicate a large underlying malformation.

If a mass is present, examine it for size, consistency, tenderness, pulsation bruits. Venous lesions tend to be soft, easily compressible with rapid refilling, and engorge with dependency. Calcified phleboliths may be palpable with the lesions. Lymphatic lesions may transilluminate. High-flow lesions tend to be firm, pulsatile, and poorly compressible.

Examine for limb length, and soft-tissue and skeletal hypertrophy, e.g. the Parkes–Weber limb. Tissue in such a limb does not pit on pressure, tends to be warmer than the contralateral limb, and may be associated with a machinery-type murmur. Such a limb may demonstrate Branham's sign – inflation of a tourniquet above arterial pressure proximal to the high-flow lesions is associated with slowing of the pulse, indicating a significant arteriovenous shunt.

Traumatic lesions may be associated with scars.

Investigation
Perform routine hematology and biochemistry. Cardiac assessment may be indicated for large lesions. Duplex is a useful first-line investigation to differentiate high-flow from low-flow lesions. MRI scan or spiral CT is then used to define the extent of the lesion and identify any suspicious characteristics. X-rays may be useful to define bony lesions, and biopsy for histology may be required to exclude malignancy.

For those lesions where intervention is considered appropriate, angiography for high-flow lesions or venography for low-flow lesions are useful to delineate the lesions and plan appropriate treatment.

Treatment

Treatment is multidisciplinary, involving a vascular surgeon, vascular radiologist, cardiologist, plastic surgeon, orthopedic surgeon, and sometimes a maxillofacial surgeon. Half of all lesions can be managed satisfactorily with compression hosiery and analgesia as required. In addition, small superficial arteriovenous malformations may be cured by surgical excision. For larger lesions not appropriate for conservative treatment because of site or size, or for symptoms not controlled by conservative measures, further intervention consists of embolization or surgical treatment.

✧ *High-flow lesions* – tend to be treated by repeated bouts of arterial or direct puncture embolization to control symptoms over many years. Those lesions thought to be suitable for surgical excision can be pre-treated with embolization to decrease intra-operative vascularity and blood loss.

✧ *Low-flow lesions* are treated by direct puncture sclerotherapy under imaging control and either local or general anesthetic. This tends to control the lesions rather than cure them, and may need to be reviewed at regular intervals. Bony and tissue overgrowth abnormalities are treated by plastic and orthopedic surgeons.

Follow-up

Patients are followed up at short intervals (1–4 weeks) with the results of investigations until malignant tumors are excluded and the extent of the lesions is defined. Patients considered suitable for conservative therapy are reviewed at regular intervals (1–6 months) until the symptoms and condition are stable, and are then discharged or given an open appointment.

Post-operative Follow-up

Complications of embolization include inadvertent embolization of other arteries, passage of emboli into the venous circulation, and the post-embolization syndrome of pyrexia, leukocytosis, and malaise. Most of these complications occur while an inpatient, but post-embolization syndrome may last for weeks. Infarction of overlying skin is not uncommon but usually resolves.

Lesions are seldom cured by therapeutic procedures, e.g. embolization, and these need to be repeated if and when the symptoms return as the lesion enlarges again. Therefore, long-term follow-up with repeated duplex ultrasound to monitor the size of the lesions is advised.

Vasculitis

Vasculitis is the term used to describe a group of conditions characterized by inflammation of the blood vessel wall. Vasculitis tends to present to the vascular surgeon as skin ischemia of the lower limbs which mimic large-vessel disease or embolic phenomena. Suspicion is raised by finding a raised ESR or CRP, and screening for autoantibodies is performed. However, arterial biopsy is required for a diagnosis in most cases and should be considered in all suspicious cases unless tissues are too ischemic to support wound healing.

Buerger's Disease (Thromboangiitis Obliterans)

This uncommon disorder can affect all races but is more common in the Middle and Far East. It occurs in smokers and predominantly affects men, although women are increasingly becoming affected. Buerger's is an inflammatory occlusive disease involving muscular, medium-sized arteries of the extremity which produces a granulomatous reaction with giant cells within thrombus. Later, the occluded artery becomes contracted with the artery and vein bound tightly together by fibrous tissue. The disease affects the very distal arteries first and progresses proximally.

History
Smoking history is positive. Foot claudication is the characteristic symptom caused by involvement of the foot arteries. Calf claudication can occur with infrapopliteal disease. The majority of patients are male and most have at least 3–4 limbs affected. It is very rare to have a single limb affected, although upper limb symptoms may predominate and resemble Raynaud's. Initial symptoms include coldness, paresthesia, skin color changes, skin lesions, rest pain, and intermittent claudication. *Note* that gangrene and ulceration may precede claudication.

Examination
Affected digits are purplish red, cold, and damp. Venous filling in the foot is very slow. Gangrene and ulceration may be present. Proximal pulses are normal. In the acute phase there may be redness and tenderness of the skin over the affected vein/artery. There may be phlebitis migrans. There may be evidence of an underlying CTD in women.

Investigations
Perform a general atherosclerotic screen and ESR and autoantibody screen. If tobacco is denied, measure cotinine levels in the urine (a level >50 ng/mL indicates smoking). Carry out ABI – ankle pressures may be normal in the presence of disease affecting foot arteries only; compare ankle and toe pressures. Arteriography tends to be diagnostic, showing multiple segmental occlusions of distal extremity arteries. Occlusions may be tapered or abrupt with extensive reticular collaterals around each occlusion – corkscrew collaterals. The arterial walls are smooth, not irregular as in atherosclerosis. Biopsy of the artery provides a histologic diagnosis.

Treatment
Correct positive risk factors, stop smoking, and introduce walking training for foot claudication to develop collaterals. To heal ulcers, intra-arterial prostaglandin E1 (PGE1) or prostacyclin (PGI2) infusions may be effective, as may sympathectomy. Hyperbaric oxygen therapy has also been proposed. Epidural analgesia for short periods (1–2 weeks) may be useful to allow pain-free time for healing to occur. Transcutaneous electric nerve stimulation (TENS) is an alternative for long-term analgesia. Surgical debridement and amputations are performed as appropriate.

Follow-up
Follow-up depends on severity and on patient behavior. If the patient stops smoking and the condition is mild, it tends to stabilize. Review at regular intervals (1–3 months) and discharge once stable. More severe cases need to be reviewed at shorter intervals to detect the need for inpatient therapy.

Post-operative Follow-up
Use standard post-operative follow-up to determine the success of procedures. This usually consists of ensuring the healing of amputation sites.

Takayasu's Disease (Non-specific Aorto-arteritis)

Takayasu's arteritis mainly affects the aorta and its branches, causing segmental stenosis, occlusion, dilatation, and aneurysm formation. It occurs all over the world but is most common in females from the Far East, usually under the age of 40 years although it can affect any age. Lesions are characterized by intimal proliferation and fibrosis of the medial and adventitial layers. Active lesions have a lymphoplastic infiltrate, Langhans and foreign body giant cells.

✧ *Acute phase* – patients complain of fever, myalgia, arthralgia, weight loss, and pain over the arteries. Pulses are present, blood pressure is elevated, bruits are present, and there are early signs of ischemia.

✧ *Late phase* – inflammation is chronic, pulses are absent, and symptoms of vascular insufficiency predominate.

Takayasu's is divided into 4 types:
✧ *Type I* – affects the aortic arch.
✧ *Type II* – affects the descending and abdominal aorta.
✧ *Type III* – combines types I and II.
✧ *Type IV* – is type II plus pulmonary artery disease.

The most commonly affected vessels are the subclavian, descending aorta, renal, carotid, mesenteric, ascending aorta, and abdominal aorta.

Objectives

Diagnose Takayasu's, differentiate from other arteritis, connective tissue disorder (CTD) or atheromatous disorders, treat Takayasu's.

History

General symptoms include dizziness, syncope, claudication, angina, stroke, MI, and upper or lower limb ischemia depending on which arteries are affected.

Examination

Perform a general examination. Pulses may be absent, especially the carotid and in the upper limbs. Hypertension may be present secondary to RAS or coarctation of the aorta. This may result in congestive cardiac failure due to hypertension, aortic insufficiency or coronary ischemia. Erythema nodosum and pyoderma gangrenosum may be present and associated with juvenile rheumatoid arthritis, sarcoid and inflammatory bowel disease.

Investigations

In the acute phase, CBC may show anemia and a leukocytosis, and the ESR is elevated. An autoantibody screen should be performed to exclude CTD.

Angiography is diagnostic and may show either variable lengths of narrowing of the aorta and other arteries progressing to segmental occlusion, or arterial dilatation and fusiform and saccular aneurysm formation – or a combination of the two (seen in the majority of cases).

Treatment

Long-term steroids, cyclophosphamide, or methotrexate. Angioplasty is useful in the chronic stage, especially for RAS. Surgery is avoided in the acute phase if possible. A bypass of affected areas is performed. Endarterectomy is seldom possible. Therefore, carotid and vertebral disease is treated by bypass procedures taken from the ascending aorta. Aneurysms are resected in younger patients.

Follow-up

Follow up with joint care with relevant physicians. All patients require long-term follow-up. The condition is monitored using serial duplex scanning, angiography, or MRI angiography.

Post-operative Follow-up

Routine post-arterial surgery follow-up, depending on procedure performed.

Polyarteritis Nodosa (PAN)

A systemic necrotizing vasculitis affecting small and medium-sized muscular arteries. It is associated with hepatitis B and most frequently diagnosed in men between ages of 40 and 60 years, although any age can be affected. Damage to the blood vessel wall can result in aneurysm formation.

History

Take a general and vascular history. Symptoms depend on the artery affected. General symptoms include malaise, abdominal pain, weight loss, fever, and myalgia. GI involvement is common and manifests as abdominal pain, nausea, and vomiting. This can proceed to bowel perforation and hemorrhage.

Examination

Hypertension is a frequent finding due to renal artery involvement. Skin manifestations include nailfold infarcts, palpable purpura, and livedo reticularis. Aneurysms may be palpable. Mononeuritis multiplex commonly occurs. Other important sites to examine are the testes and retina.

Investigations

Urinalysis may reveal proteinuria with renal failure developing in two thirds of patients. A CBC may reveal anemia and the ESR may be elevated. Antineutrophil cytoplasmic antibody (ANCA) may be elevated. Hepatitis B surface antigen and antibody should be checked in all patients.

Angiography shows the characteristic findings of saccular or fusiform aneurysms and arterial narrowing. Arterial biopsy may reveal a vasculitis which is diagnostic when combined with the angiographic appearance.

Treatment

Corticosteroids with cyclophosphamide if control is difficult. Angioplasty may be useful once the acute disease has settled.

Follow-up

Follow-up is at regular intervals by the relevant physician to determine the course of the disease. Long-term follow-up is required to detect late arterial complications.

Giant Cell Arteritis

A systemic granulomatous vasculitis which effects large and medium-sized blood vessels, commonly the cranial branches of the aorta and in particular the ophthalmic artery causing sudden blindness. It occurs mainly in those over 50 years and is 3–5 times more common in women.

History

Fever, weight loss, and fatigue may be the earliest symptoms but these are often missed. Classically the patients present with severe headache. Jaw claudication is described in over half of patients due to facial/maxillary artery involvement. Once blindness is complete it is permanent, but amaurosis fugax is reversible with steroid treatment.

Examination

Perform a general and vascular examination. Tenderness of the scalp over the superficial temporal artery region may be elicited. Examine for disease of the carotid vertebral and subclavian arteries.

Investigations

Diagnosis is usually based on the clinical findings, a raised ESR (positive in 80% of cases), and positive granulomatous histology from a temporal artery biopsy (negative in 50% due to skip pattern). Therefore a negative biopsy in the presence of a strong clinical suspicion should still be treated with steroids. Exclude other causes of amaurosis fugax, e.g. by duplex of carotid arteries.

Treatment

High-dose steroids initially, gradually tailing down to a maintenance dose.

Follow-up

Follow-up is usually by internal medicine physicians, with patients referred to vascular surgeons to perform the temporal artery biopsy.

Post-operative Follow-up

Review with histology and confirm wound healing. Refer to relevant specialty for further management.

Cutaneous Vasculitis

This typically occurs in the post-capillary venules, although capillaries and arterioles are also involved. Most patients have a single episode which is self-limiting and requires no special treatment. Patients with severe or recurrent episodes are investigated by skin biopsy and treated with steroids.

✧ *Idiopathic cutaneous vasculitis* is the most common form; this produces symmetrical palpable purpura typically affecting the lower leg. Lesions occur in crops appearing as a macular erythema progressing to purpura. It is distinguished from urticaria because lesions last longer than 24 hours. Biopsy of lesions shows leukocytoclastic vasculitis with endothelial swelling, often necrosis, hemorrhage, fibrin deposition, and infiltration with polymorphonuclear neutrophils.

✧ *Necrotizing vasculitis associated with infections, drugs, or CTD* – infections are often viruses affecting the upper respiratory tract, e.g. Henoch-Schönlein purpura. The most common associated drugs are penicillin and sulfonamides. Diuretics and NSAIDs can also cause it. Histology shows a leukocytoclastic vasculitis.

✧ *Cutaneous vasculitis as a manifestation of systemic disease* – the most common disease is SLE. Other associated diseases are Churg–Strauss and Behçet's disease.

Questions and Answers

Q1 In a patient presenting with unilateral leg pain exacerbated by ambulation, which of the following symptoms are consistent with intermittent claudication as the source of the pain?

    A Distance of ambulation before symptoms become severe and prevent further ambulation varies between one block and six blocks with unpredictable variation each day of the week.

    B Pain can be associated with prolonged standing or sitting.

    C Relief of symptoms occurs within a few minutes of stopping walking.

    D Pain in legs is described as a sharp, radiating pain extending down along the back of the thigh.

A1 C: Patients with claudication have pain that develops after a predictable distance/effort of ambulation and is relieved promptly with rest. They do not have similar leg pain when sitting or standing, even for prolonged periods. Radiating pain along the posteriolateral thigh is generally consistent with a radiculopathy rather than claudication.

Q2 Which of the following would be an indication for carotid endarterectomy in a patient after a transient ischemic attack (TIA) which caused right-arm weakness?

    A A CT angiogram only significant for a right internal carotid artery stenosis of approximately 60%.

    B A four-vessel neuroangiogram only significant for a focal smooth left internal carotid artery stenosis of approximately 25%.

    C A duplex ultrasound evaluation with B-mode image suggesting an 80% stenosis of the left proximal internal carotid artery and a peak systolic velocity suggesting less than 50% stenosis.

    D A duplex ultrasound evaluation with B-mode image suggesting less than 50% stenosis of the left proximal internal carotid artery and an end-diastolic velocity suggesting a greater than 80% stenosis.

A2 D: Patients with greater than 50% stenosis of a patent internal carotid artery ipsilateral to a symptomatic anterior circulation cerebral event should be considered for treatment with endarterectomy, as the risk of recurrent neurologic events is high. B-mode ultrasound images are an inaccurate way to gauge the degree of stenosis in the internal carotid arteries. Elevation of the peak systolic and end-diastolic velocities by Doppler are a much more reliable and reproducible means to evaluate carotid disease.

Q3 Which of the following is not associated with poor healing of the diabetic foot wound?

    A Impaired motor function of the muscles in the foot.

    B Vascular insufficiency.

    C Increased pain and sensation in the foot.

    D Altered immunologic response to infection.

A3 C: Diabetes can result in neuropathic changes to the foot, including reduced sensation and motor function which can result in Charcot foot and inability to sense minor injuries. Diabetes can also cause accelerated atherosclerotic changes of the limb arterial tree, particularly in the tibial vessels. Hyperglycemia is also associated with impaired immune function and a reduced ability to clear infection.

Q4   Which of the following patients with aneurysms should not be considered for surgical intervention to repair/exclude the aneurysm?

  A   A 68-year-old male patient followed for several years, now with a 5.1 cm abdominal aortic aneurysm seen on routine CT scan today which has increased from 4.7 cm one year ago.

  B   A 70-year-old female patient with a 3.8 cm left common iliac artery aneurysm seen on CT scan for evaluation of benign uterine fibroids.

  C   A 64-year-old female patient with a 5.8 cm abdominal aortic aneurysm seen on CT scan obtained to evaluate a prior umbilical hernia repair.

  D   A 57-year-old male patient with a history of coronary artery disease, gallstones, and a known 4.5 cm abdominal aortic aneurysm who has a two-hour history of epigastric abdominal pain with weakly palpable radial and carotid pulses.

A4   A: The most common aneurysms occur in the infrarenal segment of the aorta (AAA) and pose a significant risk for rupture when they exceed 5.5 cm in maximal diameter. Typical growth rates for these aneurysms averages 3–5 mm per year, although the growth can be episodic. Patients with known AAA, even if less than 5.5 cm, who present with abdominal tenderness and hypotension should undergo emergency aneurysm repair. Asymptomatic common iliac aneurysms with a diameter greater than 3 cm should be considered for exclusion/repair.

Q5   Evaluation of venous insufficiency in a patient should include a summary classification reporting system which consists of all except which component?

  A   Clinical findings.

  B   Pathophysiology of the venous disease.

  C   Ankle–brachial index.

  D   The veins identified to have incompetent valves.

A5   C: The CEAP classification system is a simple means by which to communicate many of the pertinent details of a patient with venous insufficiency. It does not include the evaluation of the arterial supply of the extremity.

Lumps and Bumps

Michael J. Collins and Philip Wai

ELEVEN

Potential Consultations
✧ Skin lumps.
✧ Groin lumps.
✧ Lymph nodes.
✧ Ingrowing toenails.
✧ Scrotal lumps/testicular swellings.

Skin Lesions
The skin consists of epidermis, dermis, and adnexal structures, which include hair follicles, sebaceous glands, eccrine and apocrine sweat glands. Benign and malignant lesions can arise from any of these elements.

Benign Lesions of the Epidermis
Skin Tags (Squamous Papillomas)
History
These are common (found in 25% adults), particularly obese patients. They begin in the second decade, increasing in frequency up to the fifth decade. The axilla, neck, and inguinal region are most affected. Skin tags will catch on clothing or jewelry.

Examination
There is a small, non-inflamed tag of skin which is skin-colored, oval, and mobile with no deep fixation or induration of the base. A short broad-to-narrow stalk lengthens and narrows as it grows. They rarely exceed 1 cm in diameter.

Investigation
None.

Treatment
Excision biopsy.

Post-operative Follow-up
Review with histology and check wound healing.

Common Wart
Caused by papillomavirus. It may occur anywhere on the body, but commonly on the hands and feet.

History
Slow-growing lesions, usually in the second decade of life. They are painful if on the soles of the feet (verrucas), or may catch and bleed.

Examination
Exophytic growth or hard, tender black area on the sole of the foot.

Investigation
None.

Treatment
Cryotherapy, curettage, topical preparations (40% salicylic acid or 5-fluorouracil [5-FU]), laser ablation. May regress spontaneously.

Follow-up
Rarely indicated.

Seborrheic Keratosis
Associated with old age.

History
Painless, pigmented warty plaques which are unsightly and may catch on clothing and bleed.

Examination
Appears as a "stuck-on" brown warty plaque, often with variegated pigment and truncal predominance. They may grow quite large, to 1–2 cm in diameter. They have a greasy texture.

Investigations
None.

Treatment
Curettage or excision. Other modalities include cryotherapy or topical trichloroacetic acid.

Follow-up
Review with histology, and discharge.

Kerato-acanthoma (Molluscum Sebaceum)
This is a benign, rapidly growing, self-healing skin tumor, which clinically resembles squamous cell carcinoma (SCC).

History
Found from the fifth decade onwards, with a male to female ratio of 3 : 1, typically on the face or the dorsum of the hand. It has a rapid 6-week growth phase, then involutes over the next 6 months. Usually painless, but may catch and bleed.

Examination
It appears as a globular tumor, with keratin plug/horn and radial symmetry.

Investigation
Excision biopsy to exclude SCC.

Treatment
Excision. May require reconstruction depending on size and position.

Follow-up
Review with histology

Pre-malignant Lesions of the Epidermis
Actinic and Solar Keratosis
These pre-malignant lesions usually occur on skin which is chronically exposed to sunlight (face and hands). Approximately 5% become SCCs.

History
Occur from middle-age onwards. The patient presents with erythematous macules and papules with coarse, adherent whitish scales. These are slow-growing lesions, not usually associated with pain or bleeding.

Examination
The patient has erythematous, rough or scaly macule or papules, which may be ulcerated. Examine lymph node fields.

Investigation
Excision biopsy is often indicated, especially in immunosuppressed (e.g. renal transplant) patients as there is a higher rate of conversion to SCC.

Treatment
Cryotherapy, topical 5-FU, excision. Less commonly, topical immune modulator (imiquimod) or photodynamic therapy (PDT) may be used.

Follow-up
Follow-up is long-term to detect recurrence or new lesions in the same or other areas.

Bowen's Disease (Intra-epidermal SCC in situ)
The principal etiology is sun damage. Bowen's disease of the glans penis is termed erythroplasia of Queyrat. Bowen's disease of the nipple is associated with underlying ductal carcinoma.

History
There is a slow-growing, red scaly plaque, which may irritate and occasionally bleed.

Examination
A well-defined red hyperkeratotic plaque is seen. There is clear potential for invasive transformation; ulceration suggests invasion.

Investigation
Skin biopsy under local anesthetic. It is critical to exclude an underlying malignancy (e.g. in the breast).

Treatment
5-FU, photodynamic therapy, cryotherapy, excision.

Follow-up
There is no long-term follow-up once the patient is adequately treated.

Malignant Lesions of the Epidermis
Basal Cell Carcinoma (BCC)
This is the most common skin cancer in white races. It is locally invasive; metastasis is extremely rare.

History
A slow-growing skin lesion which gradually ulcerates and may bleed. It is not painful unless advanced.

Examination
Usually found on skin chronically exposed to sunlight and in areas rich in pilosebaceous follicles, hence more than 90% occur on the face. Lesions are characterized by a pinkish color, pearly edges, and telangiectasia. There are many subtypes, which may be broadly grouped as: *localized* (e.g. nodular/nodulocystic), *superficial*, or *infiltrative* (e.g. morphoeic).

Superficial BCCs are less easy to diagnose clinically, as they may simply present as a persistent erythematous macule. Infiltrative (morphoeic) lesions tend to "ghost" under the skin.

Investigation
✧ Carry out incision/excision biopsy if diagnosis is uncertain.
✧ Uncommonly, in advanced lesions, morbidity arises from invasion into underlying structures – nares, sinuses, external auditory meatus, orbit, or brain; therefore MRI/CT may be required.
✧ Gorlin's syndrome (autosomal dominant inheritance) comprises multiple BCCs (lifelong), palmar pits, and jaw cysts.

Treatment
✧ Surgical excision with a 2–3 mm margin, but a wider margin (5 mm) if the border is indistinct or with larger lesions.
✧ For superficial BCCs, consider dermatology referral for topical 5-FU, topical immiquimod, or photodynamic therapy.
✧ Recurrent or infiltrative BCCs in anatomically sensitive areas may require micrographic surgery.
✧ Also consider radiotherapy, particularly in elderly patients.

Follow-up
Review histology, and discharge if excision is complete. Incomplete excision generally requires further excision.

Follow up long-term for multiple recurrences or in lesions narrowly excised in anatomic areas at high risk of deeper invasion.

Squamous Cell Carcinoma
This is the second most common skin cancer in white races, yet the incidence is still only one quarter that of BCC. Associated factors include exposure to sunlight, Bowen's disease, chronic ulcers and burns (Marjolin). It is prone to local recurrence (well differentiated 7% risk; poorly differentiated 28% risk) and metastases (lymph node metastases at presentation in 2–3% of cases). Increased metastatic potential is determined by location (sun exposeure, e.g. lip and ear), diameter (>2 cm), depth of invasion (>4 mm thick), poor differentiation and perineural invasion, host immunosuppression.

Differential diagnosis includes keratoacanthoma, BCC, Bowen's disease, actinic keratosis, malignant melanoma, pyogenic granuloma, and traumatized seborrheic keratosis.

History
Patients describe a quickly growing lump which ulcerates and bleeds.

Examination
The edge of the ulcer is often raised and everted. Examine for regional lymphadenopathy.

Investigations
Diagnosis is confirmed by biopsy.

Treatment
Wide local excision (5–10 mm margin). Therapeutic lymph node dissection is performed if indicated. Treatment is coordinated through the local skin cancer multidisciplinary team (MDT). Radiotherapy may be considered by the MDT if there is a close margin or the cancer is recurrent or inoperable.

Follow-up
Discuss within the forum of the local MDT. Review histology to confirm diagnosis and complete excision. Incomplete excision generally requires further surgery.

Long-term follow-up is by the plastic surgeon/dermatologist for high-risk lesions – histologically thick lesions, poorly differentiated or in a difficult anatomic site.

Benign Lesions of the Dermis
Dermatofibroma (Fibrous Histiocytoma)
History
This is a usually slow-growing, irritating, brownish nodular lesion. Approximately 20% are preceded by trauma or insect bite.

Examination
Presents as a well-circumscribed reddish brown nodule which is firm to palpation due to abundant fibrous stroma. It usually occurs on the legs, and typically is <1 cm in diameter.

Treatment
Excision biopsy.

Post-operative Follow-up
Review histology.

Hypertrophic Scar
This is an abnormal scar limited by the initial boundary of the incision or wound. Proposed etiologies include increased wound tension, infection, and delayed healing. There is a higher risk with certain anatomic sites (sternum, shoulders, deltoid). The scars often regress spontaneously as they mature.

History
Hypertrophic scars develop within weeks of wound healing, and there is some degree of improvement with time. There is little in the way of a familial history.

Examination
A raised, thickened, pinky-red, often irritating scar confined to the injury site.

Investigation
None.

Treatment
Expectant management initially. Otherwise, topical silicone gels/silicone sheets or pressure garments (for at least 6 months). Finally, re-excision should only be considered if etiology is clear, as otherwise there is a high risk of recurrence; consult with plastic surgery.

Keloid Scar
An abnormal scar which develops months after injury, shows no regression and may get worse between 6 and 12 months. It is more common in black African races, and has a familial tendency. Common sites include the face and earlobes (piercings). The original wounds are often trivial and not under tension.

History
Exuberant scar formation progressing beyond 6 months. It is itchy, hard, and often painful. There is a similar reaction in previous wound scars.

Examination
Examination shows a heaped-up, exuberant, overgrown scar, defined by firm scar tissue that extends beyond the boundaries of the incision or wound. By contrast, a hypertrophic scar does not extend beyond these boundaries.

Investigation
None.

Treatment
Generally, refer to a plastic surgeon for management. Intralesional steroid, pressure garments, or topical silicone may be indicated. Excision surgery is a last resort and should be performed only in conjunction with other modalities – steroid injection, pressure splints, or radiotherapy.

Follow-up
Response rates for all treatments are variable, and follow-up depends on treatment modality. There is a high chance of recurrence whichever modality is chosen.

Malignant Lesions of the Dermis
Metastatic Carcinoma
These occur most commonly from primary sites of tumor in the breast, lung, and bowel.

History
There are small, hard, painless nodules in the skin, which may or may not be related to the site of a previous tumor or irradiation.

Examination
Small hard nodules are found in an area adjacent to a previous surgical scar or radio-therapy field. If arising in independent areas, exclude undiagnosed underlying primary malignancy.

Investigation
Incision/excision biopsy.

Treatment
Excision if possible; defects from larger lesions may require plastic surgical reconstruction. Otherwise, consider adjuvant therapies as appropriate. Ensure adequate ongoing management of primary cancer.

Follow-up
Confirm diagnosis with histology, and arrange appropriate therapy as indicated for primary tumor.

Pigmented Skin Lesions
Most suspicious pigmented lesions are referred to a dermatology or plastic surgery clinic for excision if malignancy is suspected. However, knowledge of these lesions is necessary for the general surgeon, as they may be referred as simple skin lesions for day-case excision without appreciating that they may be malignant, especially if not pigmented.

Melanocytes are specialized cells located at the basal layer of the epidermis. They synthesize melanin and store it in vesicles called melanosomes. Melanosomes are distributed to surrounding cells. Melanin production is stimulated by sunlight and a pituitary hormone, melanocyte-stimulating hormone (MSH). All races have approximately the same number of melanocytes, but the baseline activity of these cells varies.

Nevus cells are melanocytes which have entered the dermis; they have a distinct phenotype – more spherical, fewer dendritic processes, and aggregation in nests.

Benign Pigmented Lesions
Benign pigmented lesions may be subdivided into those containing *melanocytes* (melanocytic nevi) and those containing *nevus cells* (nevocellular nevi).

Melanocytic Nevi
✧ *Simple lentigo* – benign melanocytic nevus of the *epidermis* characterized by a tan or brown macule with slightly irregular borders.
✧ *Blue nevus* – benign melanocytic nevus of the *dermis*. Appears as a round area of blue-black discoloration deeper in the skin.

Nevocellular Nevi
Benign nevocellular nevi which include *congenital* (giant hairy nevus or non-giant hairy nevus), *acquired* (junctional, compound, intradermal) or *special* (spitz, dysplastic, halo).
✧ *Congenital nevus* – histologically similar to a compound nevus, containing junctional and intradermal components. It may be disfiguring, causing great parental anxiety and concern. There are dark brown papules of variable size; these can be very large and often hairy (giant hairy nevus). One to two percent undergo malignant transformation, mainly within the first 5 years of life. Sacral lesions are associated with spina bifida or meningocele. Treatment is by serial excision; also dermabrasion, curettage, laser.

✧ *Junctional nevus* – nests of nevus cells clustered at the epidermal–dermal junction. These are deeply pigmented macules, with a well-defined border, and often occur on the trunk. They typically occur in the first and second decades of life and progress to compound or intradermal nevus with age.

✧ *Intradermal nevus* – nests of nevus cells clustered within the dermis. They are flesh-colored or light tan dome-shaped papules, often occurring on the face or neck and typically in the second and third decades of life.

✧ *Compound nevus* – contains junctional and intradermal components. Appears as a dark brown papule with well-defined, regular borders. Often occurs on the trunk and typically arises up to early adulthood.

✧ *Dysplastic (atypical) nevi* – irregular outline, variegated pigmentation, and a diameter >5 mm. They are often multiple (dysplastic nevus syndrome). There is a 5–10% risk of malignant change to superficial spreading melanoma.

Treatment
Excision biopsy if recent changes are suspicious of melanoma (see below).

Follow-up
Review histology. For dysplastic nevi, re-excision with wider margins (up to 5 mm) may be indicated.

Malignant Pigmented Lesions
There are a number of pigmented malignant skin lesions (e.g. pigmented BCC). However, by far the most important to exclude is malignant melanoma, due to its high metastatic potential and unpredictability. Absence of pigment does not exclude melanoma – a diagnosis of amelanotic malignant melanoma should always be considered.

Malignant Melanoma
This is a malignant tumor of epidermal melanocytes. There are four main subtypes:

✧ *Superficial spreading melanoma* – the most common type of melanoma (60%). Has a flat, irregular border, heavy and irregular pigmentation, and a raised surface. Ulceration indicates invasion. There is equal incidence in males and females, on sun-exposed areas – backs in men, lower legs in women. Radial growth occurs prior to vertical growth.

✧ *Nodular melanoma* – the second most common melanoma (20%). There is early vertical growth, and therefore a poorer prognosis. It is typically uniformly black, but may be amelanotic.

✧ *Melanoma arising in lentigo maligna* – comprises 5–10% of all melanomas. The precursor lesion is lentigo maligna (Hutchinson's freckle), which equates to melanoma in situ (radial growth only), 40% of which will become invasive.

✧ *Acral lentiginous melanoma* – comprises 2–8% of all melanomas in Caucasians, and 40–60% in dark-skinned races. They arise on the palms, soles, mucocutaneous junctions, and subungually. Subungual melanoma are most common in the big toe, then the thumb. Biopsy is needed to distinguish from pigmented nevus of the nail matrix. It is treated by amputation of the affected digit.

Secondary Melanoma (Primary not Identified)
Lymph node disease is the main presentation (primary lesion regressed). Non-lymph node metastatic sites include the skin, brain, lung, bone, spinal cord, and adrenals. Abdominal obstruction or intussusception is a possible presentation of metastasis.

Objectives
Exclude melanoma, stage and treat melanoma in context of a regional melanoma MDT meeting.

History
Most patients present because they have noticed a new mole or a change in an existing mole. The UK National Institute for Health and Clincial Excellence (NICE) suspected cancer referral guidelines (2005) detail three "major" suspicious features of a mole – *change in size, irregular shape*, and *irregular color*. There are four "minor" features – *largest diameter >6 mm, inflammation, oozing*, and *change in sensation*. Major features score 2 points, and minor features 1 point; a total of 3 points should trigger referral to the local melanoma service for excision biopsy.

Examination
Examine lesion for suspicious features (as above). Check for satellite nodules, in-transit metastases, palpable regional nodes, lymphedema, and hepatomegaly.

Investigation
◇ All suspicious pigmented lesions which are not obviously benign on clinical examination require full-thickness excision biopsy for histological confirmation. At this stage ensure a minimal (2 mm) margin until histological diagnosis is certain. A cuff of subdermal fat should be included in the biopsy to allow accurate histologic analysis of depth of invasion. Orientate the excision biopsy ellipse on the limbs in the longitudinal axis to facilitate future wide local excision.
◇ Histologic analysis of the depth of invasion provides useful prognostic information. The Breslow thickness (BT) classification measures the depth of invasion from the stratum granulosum of the epidermis to the deepest part of the tumor.
◇ Melanoma staging is based on the TNM system with modifications from the American Joint Committee on Cancer (2001). Invasion of less than 1.0 mm carries a good prognosis. Invasion greater than 2.0 mm carries a high risk of metastases.
◇ Other histologic features associated with poor prognoses include ulceration, mitotic activity, neurovascular invasion, and microscopic satellites.

Treatment
Treatment is in accordance with the NICE cancer service guidelines 2006 (Improving Outcome for People with Skin Tumors including Melanoma). Early referral to a local melanoma service is mandatory, with referral prior to excision biopsy if there is a high clinical index of suspicion. There should be immediate referral to a regional melanoma MDT following excision biopsy diagnosis. Subsequent management will include wide local excision down to fascia, with margins determined by BT (1 cm if BT <1 mm; 2 cm if BT >1 mm). Therapeutic regional lymphadenectomy is undertaken for nodal metastases and local control. Sentinel node biopsy remains controversial, and is only undertaken in selected centers in the context of clinical trials. Chemotherapy, radiotherapy, and immunotherapy should be guided by the oncologist in the context of clinical trials.

Follow-up
Undertaken by plastic surgery, dermatology, and oncology.

Vascular Skin Lesions

✧ *Campbell de Morgan spots (cherry angiomata)* – small (1–3 mm) bright red spots are found on sun-exposed skin in older patients. These lesions are an arteriovenous fistula of a dermal capillary. They are benign and require no treatment.

✧ *Pyogenic granuloma* – a rapid-growing benign vascular nodule, consisting of proliferating capillaries in a loose stroma of connective tissue. The differential diagnosis includes amelanotic melanoma, glomus tumor, and Kaposi's sarcoma.

History

There is usually a history of trauma at the site, followed by a rapidly growing lesion, which may bleed.

Examination

This presents as a dark red nodule of exuberant granulation tissue which may have ulcerated. Common sites are fingers, upper chest, lip, and toes.

Investigation

Excision biopsy to exclude malignancy.

Treatment

Lesions often recur after cautery, as proliferating vessels extend deep into the dermis. Hence, they generally require excision biopsy.

Post-operative Follow-up

Review with histology, and discharge.

Port Wine Stain

This is usually present at birth (0.3% of live births). It is classified as a capillary vascular malformation. There is deep reddish-blue discoloration of the skin, mostly on the face (cranial nerve V distribution), and rarely the trunk and extremities. It grows in proportion to the child and persists lifelong. Two thirds of patients develop hyperplastic skin changes (cobblestoning) by adulthood.

The most well-known associated syndrome is Sturge–Weber syndrome (ophthalmic cranial nerve V1 distribution) characterized by intracranial lesions causing intractable epilepsy. Others include Klippel–Trenauney–Weber syndrome (extremity distribution) and Cobb syndrome (truncal distribution). Treatment is by cosmetic camouflage or argon/pulsed-dye laser therapy. However, laser therapy shows no benefit in 20% of cases, and 50% may recur after 4 years.

Strawberry Nevus

These are red, soft, compressible, fleshy lesions arising within or just after the first 2 weeks of life on the head and neck. They are classified as a capillary hemangioma and are relatively common. Multiple hemangiomas may be associated with internal hemangiomas of major organs. There is a cycle of proliferation (strawberry phase) and involution. Lesions tend to grow for 6–8 months and then the majority regress with time; typically 50% of lesions will have regressed by the age of 5 years. Therefore, treatment is generally non-operative; observation only.

However, urgent treatment is required for peri-orbital hemangiomas if they are obstructing visual fields (there is a risk of deprivation amblyopia). If symptomatic (bleeding) or in an anatomically difficult site, then refer to plastic surgery. Excision, pulsed dye laser or intralesional steroid injection may all be considered. Regressed lesions may leave a redundant skin-fold requiring excision.

Spider Nevus (Acquired Telangiectasia)

This is a small red lesion (angioma) consisting of a central feeding arteriole with radiating capillaries, which blanches on pressure. The presence of up to five is normal. They are common in pregnancy but disappear postpartum. Large numbers are associated with cirrhosis of the liver. They also occur in hyperthyroidism, carcinoid, post-irradiation, after topical steroid use, in systemic lupus erythematosus (SLE) scleroderma, and dermatomyositis. They may be treated with pulsed dye laser.

Glomus Tumor (Angioneuromyoma)

Glomus bodies are small arteriovenous anastomoses involved in thermoregulation. Tumors are associated with nerve and muscle and classically occur in the fingers and toes, particularly in the nailbed where they cause nail ridging. They are dark bluish-red, cold intolerant, and exquisitely tender due to association with nerves. Treatment is by surgical excision.

Kaposi's Sarcoma

This is a malignant tumor of endothelial cells and perivascular connective tissue cells. It may occur in immunosuppressed patients and is commonly seen in AIDS patients (50%).

History

Patients complain of a slightly tender, raised nodule. There may be a history of immunosuppression.

Examination

Examination shows a raised purplish nodule, which may be single or multiple.

Investigation

Excision biopsy.

Treatment

Excision biopsy. Local radiotherapy or cytotoxic therapy for multiple lesions. Ensure that etiological factors are investigated and managed (e.g. immunosuppression).

Follow-up

Refer to the appropriate specialty: dermatology, plastics, infectious diseases.

Lesions of Skin Appendages
Epidermoid Cyst (Sebaceous Cyst)

These arise due to blockage of the duct of a sebaceous gland. Sebaceous glands are common on the scalp, face, neck, and back.

History

Appears as a slow-growing lump which occasionally discharges or becomes infected and inflamed.

Examination
There is a soft/firm, spherical lump with a central punctum on the skin surface. It arises within the dermis and often extends deeper, but is tethered to the epidermis. There may be discharge through the punctum.

Investigation
None.

Treatment
Surgical excision. If acutely infected, allow to settle first with antibiotics. An abscess may require incision and drainage. At excision, failure to remove the cyst wall completely may result in recurrence.

Post-operative Follow-up
Review histology and confirm wound healing. Wound infection is common, especially if the cyst ruptures during excision; this usually responds to antibiotics. Failure to remove the entire cyst wall will result in recurrence.

Dermoid Cyst
Dermoid cysts may be *congenital* or *acquired*.
✧ *Congenital cysts* are usually present in young children. They are most common at the embryologic fusion lines of the head and neck (inclusion cysts), usually at the outer angle of the eyebrow (external angular dermoid).
✧ *Acquired cysts* are a complication of trauma, where a piece of epidermis is translocated into deeper tissue (implantation cyst). They are commonly seen following hand injuries.

History
There is a firm subcutaneous lump arising at a site of trauma or previous surgery. Alternatively, there is a soft, slow-growing lump, typically at the eyebrow, noticed in early childhood with no history of trauma.

Examination
Examination finds a firm, discrete lump under the skin, located at embryologic fusion lines (congenital) or associated with a previous scar (acquired).

Investigation
Excision biopsy. Congenital cysts are referred to pediatric surgery or plastics for work-up (CT/MRI for deep extension).

Treatment
Excision biopsy.

Follow-up
None.

Pilonidal Sinus
This is a chronic infection of the skin caused by penetration of hairs into the skin and subcutaneous tissues. A sinus is formed which leads to a cavity filled with hair and granulation tissue. Common sites include the natal cleft, between the fingers (hairdressers), or

occasionally the umbilicus or axilla. The differential diagnosis includes perianal fistula, hidradenitis suppurativa, and simple boils.

History
There is a chronically discharging skin infection which fails to clear despite courses of antibiotics. Repeated episodes of inflammation and discharge may occur.

Examination
Perform a general examination. Depending on the site, there will usually be evidence of one or more sinuses and hairs may be visible within these. There is usually evidence of chronic inflammation or discharging sinus.

Investigation
Microbiology, blood sugar, urine dipstick.

Treatment
Treatment is conservative – careful wound toilet and shaving of surrounding hair. Use antibiotics in acute phases; incision and drainage for acute abscesses. Surgical excision is performed in chronic disease; there may be a requirement for plastic surgical reconstruction.

Post-operative Follow-up
Review histology and confirm healing.

Hidradenitis Suppurativa
A chronic, indolent disease of the skin and subcutaneous tissue in apocrine-gland-bearing areas; characterized by recurrent deep abscesses in the axillae, groins, perineum, and perianal areas. *Staphylococcus aureus* is the usual organism, but occasionally coliforms are cultured.

Differential diagnosis includes folliculitis, carbuncle, cellulitis, or, in the perianal area, pilonidal sinus or perianal fistula.

History
Recurrent inflammation and infection which fails to respond to repeat courses of antibiotics. It is most common in young adult females.

Examination
There is an involved area of skin which is indurated and fibrotic with evidence of chronic inflammation. Chronic discharging sinuses may be present.

Investigations
Microbiology.

Treatment
Non-surgical treatment should include advice on weight loss and stopping smoking (both are strong risk factors). Encourage careful personal hygiene and antiseptic washes (chlorhexidine). Consider dermatology referral for advice on long-term antibiotics (clindamycin) and anti-androgens (cyproterone acetate) in females. Abscesses require incision and drainage.

In severe disease, excision of the affected hair/gland-bearing skin may be indicated. Healing is by secondary intention or primary closure for small defects. Alternatively, larger defects are reconstructed with split skin grafts or a local flap (plastic surgery).

Follow-up

Review at regular intervals (1–3 months) to monitor the effect of conservative therapy and to decide if surgical intervention is indicated.

Subcutaneous Lesions

Lipoma

A soft, benign tumor of adipose tissue, usually occurring singly but may be multiple. It is commonly subcutaneous, but can be intramuscular. Lipoma are normally painless. If tender, then it is more likely to be an angiolipoma. Rarely, liposarcomatous change can occur in a benign lipoma. There should be a higher index of suspicion for malignant change if the lesion is large, rapidly growing, or painful.

History

There is a slow-growing lump under the skin; usually asymptomatic.

Examination

Examination reveals a lump in the subcutaneous tissue not attached to the dermis. It is often lobulated. Absence of punctum helps differentiate this from an epidermoid cyst. Contraction of underlying muscle helps distinguish between subcutaneous and intramuscular location.

Investigation

Usually none. If diagnosis is uncertain or unusual features are present, ultrasound or CT/MRI is indicated. Consider fine-needle aspiration (FNA) cytology if the lesion is suspicious.

Treatment

Most lesions can be excised (shelled out) under local anesthetic. Large or intramuscular lipomas require excision under general anesthetic. Liposuction may be considered with larger lesions to minimize scarring, but is associated with a higher recurrence rate.

Follow-up

None unless reviewing with the results of investigations or to assess wound healing following large lipoma removal.

Neurofibroma

This is a benign tumor arising from neural tissue and supporting stromal cells. It is a soft, fleshy tumor which is either sessile or pedunculated. Neurofibromatosis (von Recklinghausen's disease) patients have multiple tumors, arising throughout life. It is a disfiguring condition which causes great distress to sufferers.

Commonly, it is caused through autosomal dominant inheritance following sporadic mutation. Type 1 neurofibromatosis is associated with mainly cutaneous features, and type 2 neurofibromatosis is associated with central nervous system (CNS) tumors (neurofibromas). Occasionally, malignant change to neurofibrosarcoma occurs (with increase in size and pain).

History

Single or, more commonly, multiple soft cutaneous lumps over the body. Otherwise asymptomatic, although it may become traumatized leading to inflammation or infection. There may be a positive family history.

Examination
There are usually several fleshy lesions which may be tender to palpation. Neurofibromataosis is associated with café-au-lait patches and axillary freckles.

Investigation
Excision biopsy to confirm the diagnosis.

Treatment
Excision if symptomatic or there is suspicion of neurofibrosarcomatous change. Delayed healing is common.

Post-operative Follow-up
Review with histology and confirm wound healing. Discharge with advice or refer to clinical genetics.

Disorders of the Nails
Ingrowing Toenail (Onychocryptosis)
This is a common condition mainly in young people, and usually affects the lateral edge of the big toenail. A sharp edge of the nail traumatizes the nailbed causing pain, ulceration, infection, and a granulation tissue response which exacerbates the condition.

History
There is pain, recurrent inflammation and infection at the side of the nail.

Examination
Most commonly the lateral side of the big toe is affected, but it can affect both sides or other toes. The affected skin at the side of the nail is inflamed, boggy, swollen, and with onycholysis and creeping overgranulation.

Investigation
None. Microbiology, including fungal scrapings, is carried out if diagnosis is unclear.

Treatment
⬦ Mild cases may respond to antibiotics and chiropody.
⬦ Other cases require surgical treatment. Surgical procedures include simple nail avulsion, wedge excision and phenolization, and Zadek's procedure (total excision of germinal matrix).

Follow-up
Follow-up is at regular intervals (1–3 months) for conservative management. Proceed to surgery if this fails.

Post-operative Follow-up
Review to determine wound healing. Complications include infection, prolonged wound healing and recurrence.

Onychogryphosis
This is a "ram's horn" deformity of the toenail, usually affecting the big toes of elderly people.

History
Patients complain of increasing thickening and deformity of the nail, which is difficult to cut and interferes with footwear.

Examination
The nail is thickened, yellow, and hooked. Etiology includes trauma and fungal infections.

Investigation
Microbiology – fungal scrapings.

Treatment
Initially, chiropody. Otherwise, removal of the nail or Zadek's procedure.

Follow-up
None.

Post-operative Follow-up
Review to confirm healing. Complications are the same as for ingrowing toenail.

Subungual Exostosis
A bony lump arising from the distal phalanx, that grows underneath the nail. It usually affects the big toe.

History
A young patient complains of pain and deformity of the toenail. It may have failed to respond to treatment for ingrowing toenail.

Examination
The toenail appears to be pushed up by a lesion arising underneath the nailbed.

Investigation
X-ray of the toe reveals the bony exostosis.

Treatment
Consider plastic or orthopedic surgery referral for removal of the nail, and excision of the bony nodule with careful nailbed preservation.

Post-operative Follow-up
Review with histology before discharge.

Groin Lumps
One of the most commonest presentations in general surgery is with a lump in the groin. The differential diagnosis is large, but in practical terms the *main* distinction is between *hernias* and *other causes*.

Differential diagnosis of a lump in the groin:
- *Skin and soft tissues:*
  - ∝ Sebaceous cyst
  - ∝ Lipoma.
- *Hernias:*
  - ∝ Inguinal

∝ Femoral.
✧ *Vascular*:
   ∝ Femoral artery aneurysm
   ∝ Sapheno varix.
✧ *Lymphadenopathy*:
   ∝ Generalized versus localized.
✧ *Renal/urogenital system*:
   ∝ Ectopic or maldescended testis
   ∝ Transplanted kidney.

Inguinal Hernias
History
There may be a sudden onset related to abdominal straining. There is a reducible lump, which may be increasing in size.

Examination
Examination reveals a reducible lump in the groin arising from above the inguinal ligament (usually above and medial to the pubic tubercle). There is an expansile cough impulse. Direct hernias appear medial to the deep ring.

Investigation
None or ultrasound.

Treatment
Can be observed if the lump is not incarcerated and the patient is unfit for surgery, but most are repaired surgically by either open mesh techniques or laparoscopically using either a transabdominal (TAP repair) or an extraperitoneal (TEPP repair) approach.

Follow-up
None or review with the results of investigations.

Post-operative Follow-up
Review to confirm successful repair and wound healing at around 2–4 weeks.

Femoral Hernias
History
There may be a sudden onset related to abdominal straining, typically in the female. There is a reducible lump, which may be increasing in size.

Examination
Examination reveals a reducible lump in the groin arising below the medial end of the inguinal ligament (below and lateral to the pubic tubercle).

Investigation
None or ultrasound.

Treatment
Surgical repair.

Follow-up
None or review with the results of investigations.

Post-operative Follow-up
Review to confirm successful repair and wound healing at 2–4 weeks.

Lymph Node Mass
Enlarged lymph nodes in the groin can be a great source of diagnostic confusion.

The femoral canal normally contains a lymph node, which if enlarged can be mistaken for a femoral hernia. Lymph nodes overlying the femoral artery may transmit the pulsation and resemble a femoral artery aneurysm.

If enlarged lymph nodes are recognized, then their management is the same as for lymph nodes elsewhere in the body.

Objectives
Determine whether the enlargement is *localized* or part of a *generalized* lymphadenopathy. If localized, examine the *whole drainage area* for a cause, i.e. infective, neoplastic.

History
✧ Ask about local symptoms for the drainage area of that group of lymph nodes, e.g. leg, perineum, anus, scrotum, lower abdomen, and back.
✧ Ask about other lumps elsewhere on the body.
✧ General symptoms include weight loss and night sweats.

Examination
✧ Examine the lump, noting size, consistency, etc. Determine whether the lump is isolated or part of a general enlargement.
✧ Perform a general examination of all lymph node sites, including liver and spleen.
✧ Perform a thorough examination of the drainage area of the lymph for a possible infective or neoplastic cause for lymph node enlargement.
✧ Include a rectal examination for possible anal tumor.

Investigation
Excision biopsy of the enlarged lymph node is not the first investigation. Laboratory tests include CBC and peripheral smear, ESR, and monospot/Paul Bunnell (for glandular fever). FNA of non-pulsatile lumps is carried out for cytology and microbiology, including Ziehl–Neelsen (ZN) stain and tuberculosis (TB) culture. Use ultrasound to exclude other causes. Perform an excision biopsy for lymphoma.

Treatment
Treatment depends on the results of investigations.

In children and young people, *once lymphoma is excluded* the cause is usually infective and will settle. Similarly, the management of TB lymphadenopathy is the relevant chemotherapy.

In cases related to generalized lymphadenopathy, e.g. lymphoma/leukemia or glandular fever, management is of the underlying condition. Local causes may include SCC, melanoma, genital infection/neoplasm, an infective lesion on the leg, etc.

Follow-up
Follow up at short intervals until cancer is excluded. Determine whether excision biopsy is necessary.

Post-operative Follow-up
Review histology and confirm wound healing. Treat any underlying condition appropriately.

Possible complications include damage to surrounding structures, lymphocele, infected lymphocele, and non-healing. Non-healing wounds are particularly associated with TB or neoplastic causes, and respond to treatment of the underlying condition.

Lipoma
See above.

Sebaceous Cyst
See above.

Hydrocele of the Cord
Usually, hydroceles are confined to the scrotum. Isolated hydroceles can occur in the spermatic cord and present with lumps in the inguinal canal.

History
There is a slow-growing, non-reducible lump in the groin.

Examination
Examination reveals a non-reducible lump in the groin which does not arise from the deep inguinal ring. The lump is usually mobile but has no expansile cough impulse, and may be made to transilluminate. The lump moves down with traction on the ipsilateral testis.

Investigation
None, or ultrasound and/or FNA.

Treatment
Aspiration or surgical excision.

Follow-up
None or review with the results of investigations.

Post-operative Follow-up
Review histology and confirm wound healing at 2–4 weeks. Complications are similar to those for inguinal hernia.

Undescended/Maldescended Testis
Undescended testes are seldom palpable in the groin except in the thinnest of individuals, but maldescended testes may lie in an abnormal position after emerging through the external inguinal ring.

History
There is a tender lump in the groin, upper thigh or lower abdomen. A testicle is absent on one side of the scrotum. Ask whether the testicle has always been absent or has been noticed in the scrotum at some time.

Maldescended testes are usually asymptomatic. If symptoms occur, it may be that the testicle is now diseased.

Examination
Examination reveals the absence of a testis in the scrotum. There is a testicle-like lump in one of the above sites.

Investigation
None, or ultrasound to identify testicular internal architecture.

Treatment
If the patient is pre-pubertal, replace the testis in the scrotum if it is normal to inspection at operation. After puberty, orchidectomy is performed as the testis is unlikely to function and carries an increased risk of tumor formation. Consultation with urology is recommended.

Follow-up
Review with the results of investigations.

Post-operative Follow-up
Review histology (if orchidectomy performed) and confirm wound healing. Complications are similar to those for inguinal hernia or hydrocele repair.

Sapheno Varix
A sapheno varix may best be described as a venous aneurysm of the long saphenous vein just before its junction with the femoral vein in the groin.

History
There is a soft lump in the groin which disappears on lying down. Usually there is a history of varicose veins.

Examination
Examination reveals a soft, reducible lump in the groin, arising below the middle of the inguinal ligament. The lump disappears on lying down. Varicose veins are usually visible in the affected leg.

Investigation
None or venous duplex scan.

Treatment
Varicose vein operation.

Follow-up
Review with the results of investigations.

Post-operative Follow-up
Review to determine success of the operation and confirm wound healing. Complications are those described for varicose vein operation.

Femoral Artery Aneurysm

✧ *True femoral aneurysms* involve all three layers of the artery wall and often occur in conjunction with abdominal aortic or popliteal aneurysms, which may also require treatment.

✧ *False femoral aneurysms* usually occur after arterial injury or cannulation of the femoral artery. Blood escapes from the lumen of the artery but is "contained" by the adventitia of the artery to produce a swelling which transmits a pulsation.

History
True femoral aneurysms usually present with a history of a gradually increasing firm pulsatile lump in the groin. Femoral aneurysms may embolize and block off distal arteries, so ask about claudication, rest pain, or blue toes. If there is a history of recent injury or cannulation, e.g. cardiac angiography, then consider false femoral aneurysm as the cause.

Examination
✧ Examination reveals a pulsatile lump in the groin which does not reduce or disappear when lying down. A true aneurysm is expansile in three directions at once (medial, lateral, anterior). A false aneurysm has only transmitted pulsation.

✧ Examine all other arteries for aneurysmal disease. Examine for evidence of distal embolization and peripheral ischemia.

Investigation
Duplex ultrasound of aorta, iliac, femoral, and popliteal arteries.

Treatment
Surgical repair of both forms of aneurysm.

Follow-up
Review with the results of investigations.

Post-operative Follow-up
Review to confirm graft function and wound healing.

Scrotal Lumps/Testicular Swellings
Although disorders of the testes and scrotum are increasingly being referred to urologists, these are still a common problem in general surgery clinics.

By definition, scrotal lumps originate in the scrotum and on examination it is nearly always possible to get above the lump. If the lump is confirmed as scrotal, the next questions are: Does the swelling involve the whole scrotum or is it localized to one side or one part of the scrotum? Does the swelling arise from the skin and connective tissue of the scrotum, the coverings of the testicle (i.e. tunica vaginalis), the appendages of the testicle (e.g. epididymis), or the body of the testicle itself? Is the lump cystic or solid? *The most important objective in all scrotal lumps is to exclude testicular cancer.*

✧ *Skin* – sebaceous cysts, warts, chancre, and skin cancer, e.g. epithelioma (chimney sweeps, tar workers).

✧ *Connective tissue* – lymphedema; idiopathic lymphedema occurs spontaneously or in response to friction, etc.; secondary lymphedema may result from generalized edema, e.g. congestive heart failure, renal failure. Infections may cause lymphatic obstruction, e.g. *Wuchereria bancrofti* produces the well-known elephantiasis of the scrotum. Pelvic cellulitis, ascites, and skin infection are other causes.

✧ *Tunica vaginalis* – this describes a double-walled covering of the testis. In health this contains a small amount of fluid which acts as a lubricant for movement of the testis. A large amount of fluid can accumulate to produce a hydrocele. Hydroceles may occur spontaneously or secondary to underlying disease of the testis, e.g. infection, tumor. Blood may also accumulate in the same way and is known as a hematocele. In cases of gross infection, pus may accumulate to produce a pyocele.

✧ *Testicular appendages* – cysts and swellings occur in the epididymis and spermatic cord, producing lumps which are palpable and separate from the testis, e.g. epididymal cyst, varicocele.

✧ *Testis* – lumps arising from the body of the testis are tumor until proven otherwise.

Hydrocele

Hydroceles are a collection of fluid in the tunica surrounding the testes. Hydroceles may be *primary* or *secondary*. Primary hydroceles occur spontaneously and there is no underlying cause; they usually occur in men over the age of 40 years. In secondary hydroceles, fluid accumulates because of underlying inflammation, infection, trauma, or tumor of the testis; it occurs in younger men.

Primary hydroceles may be classified as:

1. *Vaginal hydrocele* – occurs within the tunic vaginalis and surrounds the testis, and does not communicate with the peritoneal cavity.
2. *Congenital hydrocele* – is associated with a hernial sac and communicates with the peritoneal cavity.
3. *Infantile hydrocele* – extends from the testis to the deep inguinal ring but does not communicate with the peritoneal cavity.
4. *Hydrocele of the cord* – occurs anywhere along the spermatic cord; can occur in women – hydrocele of the canal of Nuck.

Objectives

Diagnose hydrocele, differentiate primary from secondary, treat hydrocele, and treat underlying cause.

History

Patients complain of a gradually increasing swelling of the scrotum. In primary hydroceles this is usually painless, although patients may report a dragging sensation. In secondary hydroceles there may be a history of tenderness, inflammation and systemic illness. Ask about genitourinary infections. In children with congenital hydroceles, these may fill up during the day when upright and empty at night when supine.

Examination

✧ Examine the scrotum, inguinal region, and the testes. Confirm the presence of a scrotal lump and assess the swelling according to the criteria in the introduction to scrotal lumps.

✧ If the testis is not palpable separately from the lump, then a hydrocele is likely.

✧ Does the lump transilluminate? All primary hydroceles transilluminate because they contain clear watery fluid. Secondary hydroceles may not transilluminate to the same extent because they may contain turbid fluid, pus, or blood.

✧ A hydrocele of the cord moves down when traction is applied to the testis.

✧ Aspiration of a tense hydrocele may be necessary to allow palpation of the testis.

Investigation

✧ *Primary hydroceles* – ultrasound may used to confirm difficult cases. A sample of fluid may be aspirated and sent for cytology and microbiology. The testis is then palpated to confirm a normal shape, contour, and smooth surface.

✧ *Secondary hydroceles* – ultrasound is usually performed to confirm the presence of a hydrocele and to examine the underlying testis. A sample of fluid may be aspirated and sent for cytology and microbiology. If tumor is suspected ultrasound is mandatory, and determinations of serum alpha-fetoprotein (AFP) and beta human chorionic gonadotropin (beta-hCG). If urinary tract infection is suspected, a sample of urine is sent for microbiology.

Treatment

✧ *Primary hydrocele* – aspirate to dryness and review in 2–4 weeks. If the hydrocele recurs, a further attempt at aspiration is justified. In the elderly and unfit this can be repeated every 2–3 months, but in most patients surgery is indicated if the hydrocele recurs.

✧ *Congenital hydrocele in children* – an inguinal operation is required to deal with the accompanying hernia sac.

✧ *Secondary hydrocele* – treatment is primarily of the underlying disorder.

Follow-up

Secondary hydroceles should be reviewed at short intervals (1–4 weeks) until cancer is excluded. Thereafter, follow-up is at regular intervals until there is evidence that the underlying condition is responding to treatment.

In primary hydrocele, review every 1–3 months and aspirate or arrange for surgery. Complications of aspiration include infection and hematoma.

Post-operative Follow-up

In primary hydrocele, review after 4–6 weeks to determine the success of the operation and to check wound healing.

Epididymal Cyst

Epididymal cysts are similar collections of fluid to hydroceles but are separate from the testis. Spermatoceles are similar to epididymal cysts but consist of turbid fluid which contains spermatozoa. Both may be multiple or multi-locular.

Objectives

Diagnose cyst, exclude other causes, treat cyst.

History

Patients complain of a gradually increasing lump separate from the testes. There is seldom any secondary history, although patients may report an aching or dragging sensation in the testicle, groin, or lumbar region.

Examination

Perform a general and abdominal examination. Confirm the presence of a scrotal lump – you can get above it. The lump is smooth, oval and separate from, and above and to the lateral side of a normal testis. Epididymal cysts usually transilluminate, and may be multiple and bilateral.

Investigation
None, or ultrasound in difficult cases. Lumps may be aspirated to dryness. Aspiration of clear watery fluid confirms the diagnosis (whitish turbid fluid suggests a spermatocele). Bloodstained fluid should be sent for cytology and microbiology.

Treatment
Aspiration to dryness in the clinic, and review. They tend to recur after aspiration.

Follow-up
Review at 1–3 monthly intervals. If the cyst recurs more than twice, then surgery is indicated. Complications of aspiration include hematoma and infection.

Post-operative Follow-up
Determine the successful removal of the cyst and confirm wound healing. Generally, the scrotum heals very well. Wound infections respond to antibiotics. Successful removal of one cyst does not prevent others from forming in the future.

Hematocele
Hematoceles are similar to hydroceles but contain blood instead of fluid.

Hematoceles may result from aspiration of a hydrocele if the needle causes bleeding within the scrotum. Hematoceles may also complicate surgical procedures of the groin or scrotum, e.g. hydrocele or scrotal hernia repair. Other causes include trauma, torsion, or tumor.

Objectives
Diagnose hematocele, exclude cancer, treat hematocele.

History
Determine the onset of swelling and any precipitating cause, e.g. surgical procedure or trauma. Onset related to trauma or torsion is usually rapid. Tumor causes a more gradual onset, however sudden onset may occur due to rupture of a small vessel involved in the growth. Patients may ascribe this to an episode of trauma which may be mild. Testes involved with tumor are more prone to bleeding after trauma.

Examination
Examine the scrotum, inguinal region, and testes. A hematocele is usually a tense, firm scrotal lump similar on examination to a hydrocele except that it does not transilluminate. In addition, there may be ecchymosis of the scrotal skin.

Investigation
Aspiration of blood confirms the diagnosis but does not establish the underlying cause. If tumor is suspected, then ultrasound should be performed to define testicular architecture and measure serum beta-hCG and AFP.

Treatment
If the patient presents acutely, admit for exploration and evacuation of hematoma once tumor has been excluded. In elderly unfit patients, or if the hematocele is chronic (i.e. organized hematoma), a conservative course can be followed with analgesia and a scrotal support.

Follow-up
If immediate exploration is not indicated, review at short intervals (1–4 weeks) until cancer is excluded. If a conservative course is being followed, review at regular intervals (1–3 months) until there is evidence of resolution. Then discharge or give an open appointment.

Post-operative Follow-up
Review to confirm success of operation and wound healing at 4–6 weeks. Complications are similar to those for hydrocele repair.

Varicocele
Varicocele is a malformation of dilated veins surrounding the testis in the scrotum. Varicoceles may be *primary* or *secondary*.
◇ The vast majority are primary and are congenital. Their importance is that they may inhibit sperm production because they maintain the testis at a higher temperature than is optimal for spermatogenesis.
◇ Secondary varicoceles are rare, but may be caused by obstruction to the testicular vein as it joins the renal vein by thrombus or tumor extending along the renal vein, or by fibrosis caused by excess adrenaline in the blood draining from an adrenal pheochromocytoma.

Objectives
Diagnose varicocele, detect secondary cases, treat varicocele, treat underlying cause.

History
Usually young men (teens and early twenties) complain of a generalized swelling in the scrotum which is worse on standing. They may also complain of heaviness or a dragging sensation. Varicoceles occurring in older age groups or in patients with systemic symptoms suggest kidney tumors or pheochromocytomas. There may be a history of infertility.

Examination
On standing the scrotum feels full – like a bag of worms. The swelling reduces considerably and may disappear on lying down and elevation of the scrotum. The testis is normal to palpation.

Investigation
Ultrasound of the testis and, if indicated, kidney and adrenal gland. If secondary causes are suspected, CT/MRI of kidney and adrenal, urinary free catecholamine levels, CBC.

Treatment
Mild cases do not require treatment, especially if unilateral. The dragging sensation may be helped by a scrotal support.
   More severe cases can be treated by ligation of all but one of the veins in the spermatic cord in the groin, or laparoscopically by clipping the veins inside the peritoneal cavity.

Follow-up
If unilateral and mild, advise and discharge or review once (at 4–6 weeks) after use of a scrotal support to relieve symptoms. If symptoms are persistent or severe, counsel that surgery may be indicated.

Post-operative follow-up
Review after 2–4 weeks to determine success of operation – relief of heavy sensation and resolution of veins – and to check wound healing.

Chronic Epididymo-orchitis
Epididymitis describes inflammation/infection confined to the spermatic cord and epididymis. Orchitis describes inflammation/infection confined to the testis. Epididymo-orchitis describes infection/inflammation affecting both, and can be *acute* or *chronic*.
✧ Acute infections are usually investigated and treated as an inpatient and will not be described again here.
✧ Chronic infections may be referred to the outpatient clinic for repeated episodes of inflammation or investigation of a testicular swelling or hydrocele.

In children and in men over the age of 35 years, acute epididymo-orchitis is usually secondary to bacterial infection of the urinary tract which may have disordered anatomy allowing infection. In younger men, the urinary tract is normal and epididymo-orchitis is usually due to sexually transmitted organisms, e.g. *Neisseria gonorrhoea*, *Chlamydia*, *Herpes simplex* and *Trichomonas vaginalis*.
In all age groups, epididymitis can be secondary to systemic disease, e.g. TB, *Brucella*, sarcoid and *Cryptococcus*. Other rare causes of testicular infection include:
✧ *Pyogenic orchitis* – may occur following an episode of generalized sepsis and will occasionally destroy the testis.
✧ *Viral orchitis* – may occur secondary to influenza and coxsackie virus infection, but is most commonly secondary to mumps. Occurs exclusively in postpubertal patients and starts 4–6 days after the parotitis to give testicular swelling and a hydrocele.
✧ *Granulomatous orchitis* – may occur following trauma, infection, chemicals, or after vasectomy. Testis becomes enlarged and tender.

Objectives
Diagnose epididymitis, exclude tumor or underlying systemic disease, exclude abnormalities of the urinary tract, treat epididymitis, treat underlying condition.

History
Take a general history for symptoms which may suggest a systemic cause. Usually, symptoms are confined to the genito-urinary tract and describe recurrent episodes of pain in the epididymis and testis following episodes of dysuria or urethral discharge. This may settle with a course of antibiotics but not completely resolve, and be a continuing source of symptoms over weeks or months. Ask about sexual encounters to determine the risk of infection and symptoms affecting their sexual partner.
If indicated, ask questions to exclude the rarer causes outlined above.

Examination
Perform a general examination. The scrotum may be erythematous, swollen, and tender. A hydrocele may be present.
Try to determine the point of maximal tenderness, i.e. epididymis or testis or both. The epididymis may feel thickened and hard. The testis may be enlarged, irregular, and firm.

Investigations
Urinalysis or microscopy, culture and sensitivity test (C&S) of urethral discharge. If cultures are not diagnostic, send blood for immunology for immumoglobulin G and M

(IgG and IgM) antibodies to *Chlamydia*. Check urinalysis to exclude evidence of renal impairment. In children and elderly men, further investigation of the urinary tract may be indicated to exclude congenital abnormalities or obstruction.

If tumor cannot be excluded, ultrasound of the testis is indicated, as well as estimations of serum AFP and beta-hCG. If ultrasound suggests disordered testicular architecture, surgical biopsy/orchidectomy of the testis may be indicated; this may also be necessary for the diagnosis of tuberculosis, sarcoid, malakoplakia, etc.

Treatment
Symptomatic treatment includes analgesia, scrotal support, and occasionally drainage of a tense hydrocele. Children and older men are treated for common urinary pathogens. Chronic epididymo-orchitis in young men may require prolonged treatment with doxycycline, erythromycin, etc.

Treatment of secondary conditions is of the underlying condition. Treatment of mumps orchitis is symptomatic.

Follow-up
Follow-up is at short intervals (1–4 weeks) until acute infection settles and tumor or serious causes are excluded. Thereafter, follow up at longer intervals (1–3 months) to allow time for treatment to work and inflammation to settle. Remember to arrange further investigation of the urinary tract in children and elderly men.

Complications of epididymo-orchitis include abscess formation, testicular infarction, and obstruction of sperm. Abscess formation is suspected if infection fails to settle and pain and swelling persist. Ultrasound may demonstrate abscess. Treatment requires incision and drainage or orchidectomy.

Post-operative Follow-up
Review histology and treat underlying cause appropriately. Complications include wound infection, hydrocele, and scarring.

Testicular Tumors
Testicular tumors are the most common tumors affecting young men. The management of such tumors is specialized and the general surgical management consists mainly of diagnosis and referral to a urologist and oncologist. It is important to consider the diagnosis in any patient with scrotal pathology especially since complete cure can be expected if diagnosed sufficiently early.

Tumors may arise from all tissue components in the testis, but 90% of tumors are either teratomas (ages 25–30) or seminomas (ages 35–40). Other tumors account for the remaining 10% and include lymphomas (these tend to develop in elderly men), Sertoli cell and Leydig cell tumors.

Carcinoma in situ has been identified with increasing use of testicular biopsy for investigation of infertility. These patients have a 50% risk of developing testicular cancer within five years.

Objectives
Diagnose testicular cancer, stage cancer, treat cancer.

History
Take a general history. The classic history is of painless enlargement of the testis, but it can present mimicking infection, hydrocele, and trauma. The diagnosis should be considered

in all scrotal swellings. Weight loss, back pain, or shortness of breath may indicate extensive disease. Headaches may indicate brain metastases.

Examination
✧ Perform a general examination.
✧ Examine the scrotum and determine the characteristics of the lump or swelling.
✧ Examine for distant spread, the supraclavicular fossae for lymph nodes, the chest for bronchial lung metastases, pleural effusions, etc.
✧ Examine the abdomen for central lymph node masses, etc.

Investigation
Ultrasound of both testes. Serum estimation of beta-hCG and AFP – raised in 50–90% of non-seminomatous tumors, and may also be raised in seminomas with a teratomatous element.

Definitive diagnosis is by inguinal exploration of testis and testicular biopsy performed by an experienced urologist. Initial staging is by CXR, and thoracic and abdominal CT scan. Bone and brain scans are indicated by clinical findings.

Treatment
Treatment is administered by the urologist and oncologist with a special interest. It consists of radiotherapy and chemotherapy, depending on the stage of the tumor.

Follow-up
Follow-up is by urologist/oncologist.

Questions and Answers
Q1 A 70-year-old man presents to the office with a 1.3 cm firm, pink mass and a palpable cervical lymph node. A biopsy reveals Merkel cell carcinoma. What is the next step in management?
  A Radiation.
  B Chemotherapy.
  C Enucleation.
  D Surgical excision with 1–2 cm margin.
  E Surgical excision with 1–2 cm margin, superficial parotidectomy, and ipsilateral neck dissection.

A1 E: Merkel cell carcinomas are rare cutaneous malignancies that affect patients who are elderly, and can often appear in the face. The mainstay of treatment is aggressive surgical resection; if a clinically palpable lymph node is present, a lymph node dissection should be performed.

Q2 A 45-year-old man presents with a 2 cm pearly white lesion with a rolled border on the center of the forehead. The most appropriate management is:
  A Resection with a 5–10 mm margin.
  B Resection with a 4 cm margin.
  C Sentinel lymph node biopsy.
  D Chemotherapy.
  E Radiation.

A2   A: Basal cell carcinoma is the most common form of non-melanoma skin cancer and it often appears as a pearly white lesion with a rolled border, and is often termed a "rodent" ulcer. Optimal management involves surgical resection with 5 mm margins for low-risk lesions.

Q3   A 43-year-old man working in his shed notices that he has a lesion in the nailbed of his right index finger. This appears to be a melanoma. What is the next most appropriate management step?
A   Isolated limb perfusion with interleukin-2.
B   Sentinel lymph node biopsy in the axilla.
C   Radiation to the index finger and right hand.
D   Resection at the proximal interphalangeal joint, preserving as much function as possible.
E   Radical amputation of the right hand.

A3   D: Subungual melanoma has a poor prognosis and therapy involves amputation, typically one joint space below the affected nail.

Q4   A 56-year-old woman presents with a melanoma on her right calf. The biopsy indicates that it is 2.6 mm deep. What is the appropriate margin of resection?
A   It is appropriate to perform Mohs surgery.
B   A 1 cm margin of resection.
C   A 2 cm margin of resection.
D   A 4 cm margin of resection.
E   You can perform 5 mm resection preserving as much tissue as you can, so long as a sentinel lymph node biopsy is performed.

A4   C: Melanoma with less than 1 mm depth of invasion should require a margin of resection of 2 cm with a sentinel lymph node biopsy. If the depth of invasion is less than 1 mm, sentinel lymph node biopsy is indicated for young age, depth >0.75 mm, evidence of ulceration, or high mitotic rate.

Q5   A 27-year-old woman presents with recurrent hidradentitis suppurativa. She has had multiple resections of her axilla and been treated with antibiotics, and the hidradenitis involves the nipple–areolar complex. What is the most appropriate and definitive management?
A   Intravenous antibiotics without definitive surgical therapy.
B   Chemotherapy.
C   Incision and drainage of the nipple–areolar complex.
D   Topical corticosteroids.
E   Excision of the nipple–areolar complex.

A5   E: Although hidradentitis suppurativa rarely involves the nipple complex, if present then the most definitive management involves excision of the nipple–areolar complex.

Index

Note: entries in **bold** refer to figures and tables.